Study Guide to

CORE CURRICULUM FOR CRITICAL CARE NURSING

Second Edition

Study Guide to

CORE CURRICULUM FOR CRITICAL CARE NURSING

MAURENE A. HARVEY, RN, MPH, CCRN
Consultants in Critical Care, Inc.

Illustrated by Krista Osterberg

W.B. SAUNDERS COMPANY
A Division of Harcourt Brace & Company

Philadelphia / London / Toronto / Montreal / Sydney / Tokyo

W. B. SAUNDERS COMPANY
A Division of Harcourt Brace & Company

The Curtis Center
Independence Square West
Philadelphia, PA 19106

Library of Congress Cataloging-in-Publication Data

Harvey, Maurene A.
Study guide to Core curriculum for critical care nursing / Maurene A. Harvey; illustrated by Krista Osterberg.—2nd ed.
p. cm.
To be used with: Core curriculum for critical care nursing. 4th ed. 1991.
ISBN 0-7216-3500-8
1. Intensive care nursing—Examinations, questions, etc. I. Core curriculum for critical care nursing. II. Title.
RT120.I5C63 1991 Suppl.
610.73′61—dc20 91-30969
CIP

Editor: Thomas Eoyang

Study Guide to Core Curriculum for
Critical Care Nursing .... ISBN 0-7216-3500-8

Printed in the United States of America.

Last digit is the print number: 9 8 7 6 5 4

PREFACE

The majority of my 22-year career in critical care has been devoted to educating practicing nurses. In 1976, I began using the *AACN Core Curriculum for Critical Care Nursing* as the framework for comprehensive courses. Since then I have taught this material approximately 300 times.

In the process, classroom exercises and handout material were developed in an effort to help nurses grasp the key concepts and more difficult content found in the *Core Curriculum*. They were developed based on a review of the literature on adult learning strategies. This became the basis for the first edition of this study guide. The second edition reflects lessons learned over five years using the first. Student feedback has been invaluable in restructuring and improving the material. The end product is presented here with the sincere hope that it adds to your knowledge, enhances your clinical practice, and helps prepare you for CCRN certification.

The input of the following reviewers was tremendously helpful and greatly appreciated:

Tess L. Briones, M.S.N., R.N., C.C.R.N., University of Michigan, Ann Arbor, Michigan;
John L. Carty, R.N., D.N.Sc., Army Nurse Corps, Fort Sam Houston, Texas;
Richard DeAngelis, M.S.N., R.N., San Diego, California;
Sharon Espersen, R.N., M.S., C.C.R.N., Salem Hospital, Salem, Oregon;
Jay L. Falk, M.D., F.A.C.E.P., F.C.C.M., Orlando Regional Medical Center, Orlando, Florida;
Bonnie Mowinski Jennings, R.N., D.N.Sc., L.T.C.(P.), A.N., U.S. Army Nurse Corps, Department of Health and Human Services, Bethesda, Maryland;
Joanne M. Krumberger, R.N., M.S.N., C.C.R.N., Milwaukee, Wisconsin;
Sara R. Neagley, R.N., M.A., Milton S. Hershey Medical Center of the Pennsylvania State University, Hershey, Pennsylvania;
Diana L. Nikas, R.N., M.N., C.C.R.N., C.N.R.N., F.C.C.M., Harbor–U.C.L.A. Medical Center, Torrance, California;
June L. Stark, R.N., M.Ed., New England Medical Center Hospitals, Boston, Massachusetts;
Linda Waite, R.N., M.N., C.C.R.N., Marquette University, Milwaukee, Wisconsin;
Ginger Schafer Wlody, R.N., M.S., C.C.R.N., F.C.C.M., Department of Veterans Affairs Medical Center, Wadsworth Division, Los Angeles, California.

CONTENTS

INTRODUCTION

The *AACN's Core Curriculum for Critical Care Nursing* describes the knowledge base required by nurses caring for the critically ill. It consists of objectives, content outlines, and resources for nine areas: Pulmonary, Cardiovascular, Neurological, Renal, Endocrine, Hematological, Gastrointestinal, Psychosocial, and Legal/Ethical. Each of the first seven covers physiologic anatomy, clinical assessment, the planning, implementation and evaluation of care, and specific pathologic conditions.

This study guide facilitates understanding of the *Core Curriculum*'s content and its application to practice. There are nine sections matching those in the *Core Curriculum,* the length varying with the amount of content and its level of difficulty.

THE CCRN EXAMINATION

Many critical care nurses utilize the *Core Curriculum* in preparation for the CCRN examination. It has been recommended as one of the primary study resources by the AACN Certification Corporation. However, it must be emphasized that the examination is not based on the *Core Curriculum* but on an examination blueprint, the outcome of a Role Delineation/CCRN Validation Study.

In earlier years, the breakdown and content of the examination had been determined by the opinion of experts in the field, a commonly accepted practice in the certification arena. As standards for credentials emerged related to testing of individuals for credentialing purposes, role delineation studies became the most accepted means of collecting data on which to base an examination about one's profession.

AACN's Certification Corporation completed its first Role Delineation Study in 1984. A task force had been commissioned to define the practice of critical care nursing and to develop an examination based on the findings. As a result of this landmark in professional certification research, the task force made recommendations for changes in the CCRN examination to make it a more valid assessment of an individual's knowledge for practice as a critical care nurse caring for adult critically ill patients. The changes were made, field tested, and then incorporated into the bi-annual tests beginning in February 1985. A new test blueprint was constructed and questions were developed based on the cognitive levels of recall/ comprehension, application/analysis, and synthesis/evaluation. Adjustments to the blueprint were made again in July of 1989 to reflect ongoing changes in critical care nursing practice.

Based on the data obtained, the task force assessed which patient care problems or diseases were most commonly encountered and what percent of practice was spent on each of the defined systems. They also identified the specific knowledge required for the care of patients experiencing these problems.

The Distribution of Questions

Here is a comparison of the distribution of questions between content areas before the task force, after the task force, and after the later modifications.

	Pre 2/85	Post 2/85	Post 7/89
Pulmonary	20%	19%	18%
Cardiovascular	20%	19%	21%
Neurological	10%	19%	19.5%
Renal	10%	14%	12.5%
Endocrine	10%	7%	8%
Hematology/Immunology	10%	7%	8%
Gastrointestinal	10%	13%	10%
Psychosocial	10%	*0%	0%
Legal/Ethical	0%	2%	3%

* Psychosocial questions were not eliminated but were included as aspects of care of patients with problems in the other eight areas in a more holistic practice model. All alterations were made as a result of the Role Delineation Study that surveyed critical care nurses to determine how much of their practice was involved with each of the areas.

The Cognitive Level and Number of Questions

Prior to 1985, about 85% of the questions on the CCRN examination were at the recall or comprehension level of learning. The task force study found that the thought processes involved in decision making in critical care required a higher level of understanding. Accordingly, only 36% of the questions test the ability to recall or comprehend (one-step thinking), 39% test the ability to apply and analyze knowledge (two-step thinking), and 25% test the ability to synthesize and evaluate (critical thinking). Mini case scenarios are often used to test the higher cognitive levels. They are similar to the questions in the Comprehensive Examination at the back of this book.

Although the overall level of difficulty of questions is now higher than before, they are written in the context usually encountered in bedside practice. Nurses are used to this type of thought process and may not necessarily find the questions harder to answer. Because there is a time limit of four hours for the examination and it does take longer to think these problems through, the number of questions was cut from 250 to 200 in the tests given from 1985 on.

The Examination Blueprint

The knowledge outlined has become the blueprint for the examination. This means that nurses preparing for the examination can use the blueprint to identify what they need to study. Because of the changing nature of our practice and the need to have the CCRN examination be relevant to current practice, role delineation studies must be repeated.

The AACN commissioned a second task force that completed its work in 1990. The results of this study will form the basis of a new examination blueprint beginning in February 1992. The new breakdown, compared with the one in use since July of 1989, is as follows:

	Post 7/89	**Post 2/92**
Pulmonary	18%	22%
Cardiovascular	21%	39%
Neurological	19.5%	8%
Renal	12.5%	5%
Endocrine	8%	4%
Hematology/Immunology	8%	4%
Gastrointestinal	10%	8%
Legal/Ethical	3%	0%
Multisystem	0%	10%

The decision to eliminate the legal/ethical section was based on the difficulty in testing this area fairly in multiple choice format and the legal differences that occur state to state, not on lack of clinical occurrence. The level of difficulty will still be distributed 36% recall or comprehend, 39% apply or analyze, and 25% evaluate or synthesize. The examination will still consist of 200 multiple choice questions to be answered within a period of four hours.

The blueprint also details what content areas candidates will be held responsible for in each system. It is based on the elements of the nursing process; assessment, planning, intervention, and evaluation. Candidates are typically tested on their knowledge of

A. Anatomy, physiology, and pathophysiology
B. Invasive and noninvasive diagnostic studies
C. Relevant pharmacology
D. Etiology and risk factors
E. Signs and symptoms
F. Nursing and collaborative diagnosis
G. Goals and patient care outcomes
H. Complications
I. Patient care management

Each of these areas is addressed in the relevant chapters of the *Core Curriculum*.

The blueprint then lists Patient Care Problems. The Patient Care Problems for the February 1992 blueprint, along with the pages they are addressed in the *Core Curriculum*, are listed below.

Cardiovascular	**Pages in *Core***
Cardiac trauma	101–105
Dysrhythmias	175–187
Myocardial conduction system defects	184–187
Unstable angina	207–223
Acute myocardial infarction/ischemia	223–242
Acute congestive heart failure/pulmonary edema	242–247

Cardiovascular	**Pages in *Core***
Acute inflammatory disease	247–256
Cardiomyopathies	256–261
Structural heart defects (acquired and congenital)	261–284
Hypertensive crisis	284–289
Acute peripheral vascular insufficiency	289–299
Ruptured or dissecting aortic aneurysm	289–299
Cardiogenic shock	299–309
Hypovolemic shock	299–309

Pulmonary	**Pages in *Core***
Respiratory distress syndrome	84–87
Status asthmaticus	94–97
Acute pulmonary embolus	98–101
Air-leak syndromes	91–94, 101–105
—pneumothorax	
—pulmonary interstitial emphysema	
Thoracic trauma	101–105
—lung contusions	
—fractured ribs	
—hemothorax	
—pulmonary hemorrhage	
Acute respiratory infections	105–109
—acute pneumonia	
Pulmonary aspirations	109–112
—aspiration pneumonia	
Acute respiratory failure (other etiologies)	112–125

Neurological	**Pages in *Core***
Head trauma	386–395
Intracranial hemorrhage/intraventricular hemorrhage	393–395, 407–412, 416–418
Acute spinal cord injury	395–407
Cerebral embolic events	407–412
Aneurysm	412–416
Space-occupying lesions (e.g., brain tumors)	418–423
Neurologic infectious diseases	423–427
Seizure disorders	427–432
Encephalopathy (e.g., hypoxic-ischemic, metabolic, infectious)	
See:	
Shock	299–309
Increased ICP	375–385
Neurologic Infectious Diseases	423–427
Renal Failure	521–543
Hepatic Failure	790–792

Renal	**Pages in *Core***
Acute renal failure (e.g., acute tubular necrosis)	521–543
Life-threatening electrolyte imbalances	573–600
Renal trauma	600–606

Endocrine	**Pages in *Core***
Diabetes insipidus	629–634
SIADH	634–637
Diabetic ketoacidosis	655–662
Hyperglycemic hyperosmolar nonketotic coma (HHNK)	662–667
Acute hypoglycemia	667–672

Hematology/Immunology	**Pages in *Core***
Organ transplantation	Only renal covered
	562–565
Life-threatening coagulopathies	739–741
—disseminating intravascular coagulation (DIC)	
Immunosuppression	(See *Study Guide*, Chapter 6)

Gastrointestinal	Pages in *Core*
Acute pancreatitis	774–781
Hepatic failure/coma	783–792
Bowel infarction/obstruction/perforation	799–803
Acute abdominal trauma	803–809
Acute GI hemorrhage	817–825

Multisystem	Pages in *Core*
Sepsis/septic shock	299–309 (see *Study Guide*, Chapter 6)
Asphyxia	Only under Increased ICP
Toxic ingestion (e.g., drug/alcohol overdose)	447–457
Burns	—

Notice that almost all of the Patient Care Problems are addressed at least in part in the *Core Curriculum*. Organ transplant is only partially addressed. The physiology of rejection is covered in immunology on pages 684 and 688 and renal transplant is covered in the renal chapter. Burns are not addressed at all. If you are using the *Core Curriculum* to prepare to take the CCRN examination, you will need to use a supplemental source for these two areas.

Scoring of the Examination

Currently over 6000 nurses sign up to take each of the bi-annual examinations. Each candidate across the nation, on a given test date, answers the same 200 questions. They are selected from a pool of hundreds of potential questions under the guidance of the Examination Development Committee. Each examination is different from those before. About one-third to one-half of the questions are brand new and the rest may have been used on past tests.

After the test has been administered, the testing company scores the exam and results are statistically evaluated. Raw scores are converted into scaled score units based on this evaluation. You must achieve a predetermined scaled score in order to pass the examination. It usually equates to answering about two-thirds of the questions correctly. Since the AACN has been offering the examination, about two-thirds of the candidates pass each examination.

In addition to your total scaled score, you will also be given the number or percentage of questions answered correctly in each system. This allows you to identify your strengths and weaknesses.

Further Recommendations for CCRN Candidates

It is very important that you obtain an application booklet for the examination you plan to take from the AACN Certification Corporation. It contains the current requirements candidates must meet, the verification of RN licensure and clinical practice forms, the application, the deadlines, the fees, the test date and test sites, as well as a more complete description of the CCRN Certification Corporation's purpose and policies. Many of these change over time.

The examination blueprint is also likely to be modified to reflect the ongoing changes in critical care nursing practice. I cannot overemphasize that to prepare properly for the examination you must obtain the current blueprint for the examination that you apply to take. It is an important means of guiding your study efforts.

Two other very helpful study tools are available through the AACN Certification Corporation: "Evaluating Your Knowledge for CCRN Certification—A

Blueprint for Study'' and ''A Compilation of Sample CCRN Examination Questions.'' There are knowledge statements in the first tool similar to learning objectives that expand on the blueprint and are an excellent guide for study. The sample examination consists of questions retired from previous examinations and is based on the February 1985 blueprint, but it is an excellent way to get a feel for the style and depth of questions. An answer key is provided so that you may also assess your strengths and weaknesses.

There are several more general recommendations for preparing for the examination.

A. The examination focuses on the current standards of care and not on the cutting edge. You will not be held responsible for areas under investigation and not yet common practice.
B. The examination avoids areas of controversy where there is more than one school of thought and lack of consensus.
C. The examination focuses on the knowledge base required for critical care generalists, not that of specialists or those practicing in large teaching centers. Although you are expected to know the indications and limitations for treatment options available in these centers, you do not need experience caring for patients undergoing these interventions to answer the questions. Examples include organ transplant, heart surgery, and intra-aortic balloon counter pulsation.
D. This examination focuses on the care of the critically ill *adult*. The AACN certification is currently developing two additional separate tests, one for pediatrics and one for neonatal intensive care nurses. They are expected to be offered beginning in July 1992.

The AACN can be commended for their efforts to make the certification process a valid method of documenting competence in critical care nursing. They will continue to evaluate the test design and content. Information on continuing changes in the examination can be found in the updated *Candidate Examination Handbook* describing the certification program. This is available from the AACN Certification Corporation, 101 Columbia, Aliso Viejo, California 92565-1458.

INSTRUCTIONS FOR USING THIS STUDY GUIDE

This study guide offers a variety of strategies to facilitate learning the content of the *Core Curriculum* and incorporating the information in the care of the critically ill patients. They are based on concepts found in a review of the literature on adult learning strategies.

Activities include diagrams that illustrate concepts, charts and tables that make comparisons and summarize key points, fill-in-the-blank and multiple choice exercises that test retention, and clinical assignments that encourage application.

Everyone learns differently. You may find some aspects of the study guide more helpful than others and can adjust the way you use it accordingly.

Those preparing to take the CCRN examination should keep in mind that although many of the questions on the certification examination are at the recall or understanding level, some require analysis, application, synthesis, or evaluation. However, *you cannot use knowledge you don't have*. A firm comprehension of the knowledge base must precede thought processes at a higher cognitive level. Some of the examination tests your critical thinking ability and you can perform at this level only if you have understood concepts, not if you have memorized them.

Each section follows the same format. Although concise directions are given at the beginning of each new activity, detailed instructions are provided here to help you get the most from the study guide.

Figures and Tables

A series of figures and tables is provided to help visualize, organize, and compare concepts. The concepts represented by the diagrams are presented in the order in which the concepts occur in the *Core Curriculum* with the page number in parenthesis. While studying the *Core Curriculum,* keep the study guide open and be aware of what the next diagram concerns so you will know when to use it. The tables can also be used to quiz yourself on material by covering the columns one at a time and trying to recall what it says by reading the vertical and horizontal qualifiers.

One of the tables in each system contains "Clinical Applications." It picks out key aspects of anatomy, physiology, or assessment, and describes how and why it is clinically relevant and where you might apply it. It is meant to focus your attention on the physiologic principles and rationale behind patient care phenomena and nursing interventions.

Exercises

Fill-in-the-Blank

This portion restates some of the *Core Curriculum's* key concepts leaving blanks to fill in. Although this requires a significant amount of time, it is based on a key aspect of learning: you remember more of what you write than what you read. When you think you are familiar with the material, use this exercise to help identify areas of strength and weakness. Again, they relate to concepts presented in the same order as they appear in the *Core Curriculum*. They are broken down into major topics within each system with the corresponding pages in the *Core Curriculum* listed. You may answer them one topic at a time or wait until you finish the whole system.

The answers are listed at the end of the exercises along with the appropriate page number in the *Core Curriculum*. Because fill-ins are sometimes general or subjective, there may be a variety of ways to communicate the same idea. Use your common sense to determine whether your response is equivalent to the answer given in the study guide.

Summary of the Pathologies

This exercise asks you to summarize each pathology presented in the section. It requires careful thought in order to synthesize the detailed material presented into concise descriptions of the pathophysiology, etiology and risk factors, signs and symptoms, collaborative diagnosis, complications, management, and goals. It is best to list phrases or words that will help you remember key points. You can then build larger concepts. Another approach is to write down only the things you have difficulty remembering, not the things you already know well. Again, it is well known that you can remember more of what you write than what you read. This section is an important part of the study guide.

Clinical Application

The idea of this exercise is to help make the transition from knowledge to practice. You are asked to care for patients with the diseases you've studied. It is important to make note of where the patients correlate with the typical clinical picture and where they deviate from it. Most nurses remember their experiences in caring for patients longer than they remember what they read. This is a wonderful way to learn as long as each patient's idiosyncracies are identified. Using one patient as an example of what a classic case is like is often misleading.

Although it may seem difficult on a busy day to make time for this commitment to learning, it is the *most helpful thing anyone wanting to master the material can do*. Take the *Core Curriculum* to work and review the descriptions and the suggestions related to your patient while you plan care. At the end of the day you can use it to evaluate care. It may stimulate you to discuss complex or key problems with other team members. Each of these three uses can take as little as 5 to 10 minutes. The knowledge gained is invaluable in developing clinical expertise and in answering questions on the CCRN examination.

Multiple Choice Post Quiz

As a final evaluation of your understanding of the section's content, there is a multiple choice post quiz. The style is reflective of some types of questions on the certification examination and may help you determine whether or not you've studied each system enough.

Whenever taking multiple choice tests, be sure to read each question carefully. Try not to read anything into it but make sure you read what is there. Every word counts.

There is only one right answer. Many questions are purposefully designed to offer more than one possible answer, in which case you must choose the best, the most direct, or the most often true. Others do not provide the most obvious response, and you must find the one that is the next best or indirectly implied.

Another way to use the questions is as a pretest. If you think your knowledge level in a particular system is already adequate, you can take the test to see whether or not you need to study it. You may only have a few weak areas and the answer sheet will refer you to the primary pages of the *Core Curriculum* which cover the questions. If you don't think your knowledge is adequate, you can use the questions as both a pretest and a posttest to evaluate your progress.

Comprehensive Examination

At the end of the study guide is a comprehensive examination requiring knowledge of all systems and utilizing higher cognitive levels. They reflect the more complex kinds of questions on the certification examination. They allow you to practice and get more comfortable with the type of thought processes involved. In answering these, use the same guidelines listed above for the multiple choice tests in each section.

Appendices

There are two appendices. The first is titled "Names to Remember" and simply pulls from all systems a few dozen structures and phenomena with proper names, such as Babinsky's Sign. They are sometimes difficult to remember and may appear in the CCRN examination. They are listed with the page of the *Core Curriculum*. You will find them referenced.

The second is a list of drugs commonly used in critical care. Since this is an important aspect of critical care nursing, there may be several questions involving some of these agents.

STUDYING STRATEGIES

There are many books written on how to take standardized tests. If you have difficulty with tests in general, it may be worth picking one up and reading through it.

Most people do have some degree of test anxiety, but it is worth controlling excessive negative feedback. I frequently hear students muttering such things as:

> "Why did I sign up to take this test—I don't have time to study. Why did I do this to myself? Nobody cares if I'm a CCRN or not."

Such thoughts are not productive and, even if fleetingly felt, should be squelched and replaced with more positive ones such as:

> "Isn't this interesting material? It's nice to have the test as a motivation to fill in all my knowledge weaknesses. I'm glad I'm finally taking the time to do this for me—for my patients."

Remember, lots of benefit always comes from studying for the CCRN examination. It motivates experienced nurses to go back through the whole body and study material they can now relate to a practice base and to continue to incorporate it for the rest of their career. You've embarked on a valuable project of personal growth, so begin and end each study session with a pat on the back.

On the other hand, don't ever expect to get to the point where you will be able to say:

> "There, now I know it all."

The more you learn, the more layers you discover. Take confidence from the fact that while you're studying and especially when you're applying it to patients, you are growing and becoming more knowledgeable. Let the study guide help you solidify what you're accomplishing. Be assured that studying something always results in learning something.

It is especially important to have a constructive attitude as you drive to the examination site and psychologically prepare yourself to approach the four hours of testing. Here is a useful exercise worth repeating. Even if you don't believe each statement, it stimulates the positive and mitigates the negative thoughts.

READ SEVERAL TIMES ALOUD WHILE TAKING S L O W DEEP BREATHS

I AM BRIGHT AND ALERT.

MY MIND IS HUMMING AND CLICKING.

I AM IN A RARE FORM.

I AM THOROUGHLY PREPARED FOR THE EXAM.

NO QUESTION WILL BE TOO DIFFICULT—ONLY STIMULATING.

I AM LOOKING FORWARD TO THE CHALLENGE.

I HAVE STUDIED HARD AND DESERVE TO PASS.

I CAN HARDLY WAIT TO SHOW THEM WHAT I KNOW.

I W I L L DO WELL!!!

TEST-TAKING STRATEGIES

There are some very practical measures that can be helpful on test day. First, make sure you allow plenty of time to find your way to the site, parking, and the room. Anxiety produced by cutting the time close is not helpful.

Read your test admission ticket carefully for time, site, and what to bring (pencils, identification, etc.). Be prepared to be proctored by people the testing company has hired to administer the test. They are following instructions to make sure that each site is run in a secure but fair fashion.

Environments in large rooms are difficult to control and it may be too hot or too cold for your taste. This can interfere with clear thinking so dress in layers to adjust. Also, dress comfortably.

As you wait for everyone to be seated and the test booklets to be handed out, view "butterflies" as a good sign. People think more clearly with a little extra adrenalin pumping. Think about how you're going to take control of the next four hours, to focus your energies on calm concentration, to use your time wisely, to become a CCRN, and to stay one for the rest of your critical care career.

Listen to the instructions read by the proctor carefully. To date, there is no penalty for guessing. That means that you should answer *every* question. Do not leave one blank since you have a good chance of guessing it right.

You are then given four hours to answer all 200 multiple choice questions. They are not arranged by section. Although there is no break, the proctors will usually let you get up to use the restroom or stretch.

Use your time wisely but don't hurry. Most people have plenty of time to get through the whole test. Still, it is a good idea to keep an eye on your watch and make sure you have at least 100 done by the first two hours.

Read each question and each choice carefully. Do not read into the question but do not miss qualifiers. There will be many questions where the answer is not immediately apparent. *Don't panic*. Expect them and have a planned approach. First, cross out choices you know are wrong. Then, start thinking about what you know about the root that may lead to an indirect answer. If you get any vague glimmers pointing to one choice during this mental process, pick that answer. If not, use your gut feeling, pick one quickly, and go on. Don't let it throw you. Everyone in the room is guessing. Guess with skill and then forget about it. You might want to circle those you guess on in case a question later in the test stimulates a glimmer or a thought that would make you want to change your answer. Most authorities recommend *not* changing answers unless you have a good reason. Your first choice is usually the best guess.

This is a three-celebration process. Celebrate first when you decide to take the CCRN certification examination and to enter an accelerated period of career growth and development. Celebrate second when you finish the test and enter the period of confident anticipation. Celebrate third when you get your scores and see how well you do. Good luck!

1

The Pulmonary System

SECTION-RELATED TIPS FOR THOSE STUDYING TO TAKE THE CERTIFICATION EXAMINATION

This section is unique in two ways. First, pulmonary practitioners use many abbreviations. The abbreviations that appear on the certification examination are those used as much by critical care nurses as by respiratory therapists. The rest of the factors are written out rather than abbreviated. However, to study this section and much of the pulmonary literature, it is useful to memorize a few additional abbreviations and their meanings. A list of those commonly encountered follows this introduction and it would be helpful to familiarize yourself with the ones you do not feel comfortable with before continuing.

Second, many calculated variables, such as oxygen content, oxygen transport, and alveolar-arterial oxygen tension gradients, appear in this chapter. Although the certification examination to date does not ask that you calculate variables, it is helpful to practice calculating them to appreciate the impact of the factors involved. Variables may come up in the questions in scenarios, or you may be asked whether they would be high, low, or normal, given certain circumstances. If so, just recall the factors involved and how they impact on that number. For example, suppose you are given a scenario in which the patient has pulmonary edema with a history of chronic obstructive pulmonary disease (COPD) and has recently suffered a myocardial infarction. All of his vital signs, electrolytes, complete blood cell count (CBC), blood gases, and hemodynamic values are given.

The question is: This patient's oxygen transport is

a. high
b. low
c. normal
d. unable to determine

If you know that the only three significant variables that determine oxygen transport are cardiac output, hemoglobin, and arterial hemoglobin saturation, you can then disregard the rest of the information and focus on the right answer. The exercises in this chapter ask you to calculate examples of each of these parameters out of the belief that it will help you appreciate what really affects them.

Please see the Preface for important general suggestions that are relevant to the bulk of the *Core Curriculum* content. They apply to this section as well as to the others that follow.

Abbreviations

A	Alveolar
a	Arterial

A-a gradient (or A-aDO_2 or DA-aO_2)	Alveolar-arterial oxygen tension or pressure difference)
a-$\bar{v}O_2$ difference (or Da-$\bar{v}O_2$ or Ca-$\bar{v}O_2$ difference)	Arterial-venous oxygen content difference
BE	Base excess
CaO_2	Arterial oxygen content
$C\bar{v}O_2$	Venous oxygen content
2,3-DPG	2,3-Diphosphoglycerate
E	Exhaled
F	Fraction or frequency
FEV_1	Forced expiratory volume in one second
FIO_2	Fraction of inspired oxygen
FRC	Functional residual capacity
FVC	Forced vital capacity
H^+	Hydrogen ion
HCO_3^-	Bicarbonate
H_2CO_3	Carbonic acid
I	Inspired
$\overline{m}vO_2$	Mixed-venous oxygen tension or pressure
p	Partial pressure
pAO_2	Alveolar oxygen pressure or tension
paO_2	Arterial oxygen pressure or tension
pB	Barometric pressure
pCO_2	Carbon dioxide pressure or tension
pIO_2	Inspired oxygen pressure or tension
$p\bar{v}O_2$	Venous oxygen pressure or tension
pH	Negative logarithm of the hydrogen ion concentration (is inverse to absolute hydrogen ion concentration)
Q	Quantity of blood flow
$\dot{Q}$	Quantity of blood flow per minute or cardiac output
R	Respiratory or respiratory exchange ratio
REE	Resting energy expenditure
RQ	Respiratory quotient
SaO_2	Percent saturation of hemoglobin in arteries
$S\bar{v}O_2$	Percent saturation of hemoglobin in veins
V	Volume of gas or air
V_A	Effective alveolar gas volume per breath
$\dot{V}_A$	Effective alveolar gas volume per minute
VC	Vital capacity
$\dot{V}CO_2$	Volume of carbon dioxide produced per minute
V_D	Volume of dead space per breath
$\dot{V}_D$	Volume of dead space per minute
V_E	Volume expired
$\dot{V}_E$	Volume expired per minute
$\dot{V}O_2$	Volume of oxygen consumed per minute
V/Q	Ratio of volume of gas to quantity of blood flow
$\dot{V}/\dot{Q}$	Ratio of volume of gas to quantity of blood flow per minute
V_T	Tidal volume

FIGURES AND TABLES

Refer to these figures and tables while reading the Pulmonary Section of the Core Curriculum.

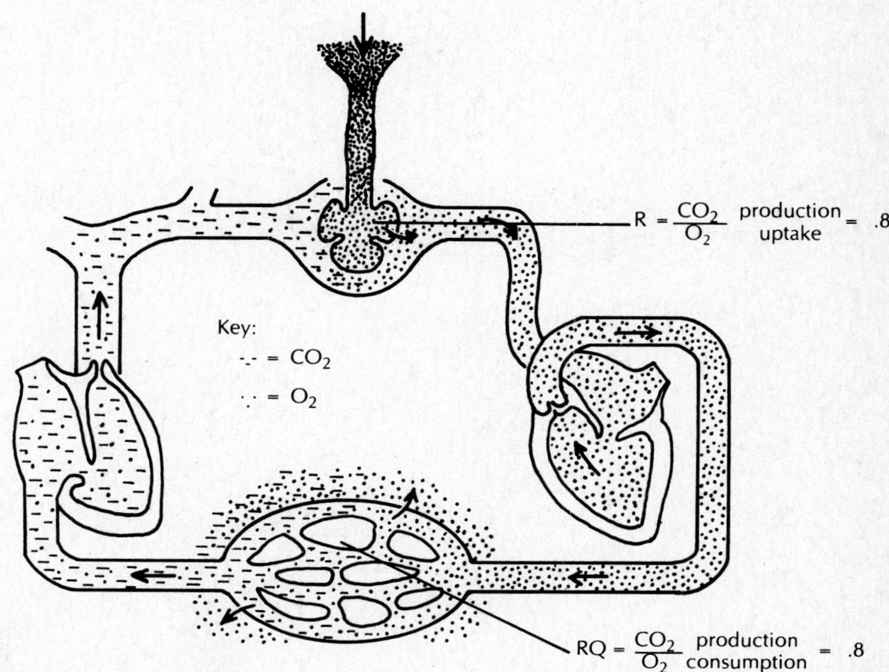

Figure 1–1. Types of respiration. External gas exchange is described as the respiratory exchange ratio (R), internal gas exchange as the respiratory quotient (*page 1*).

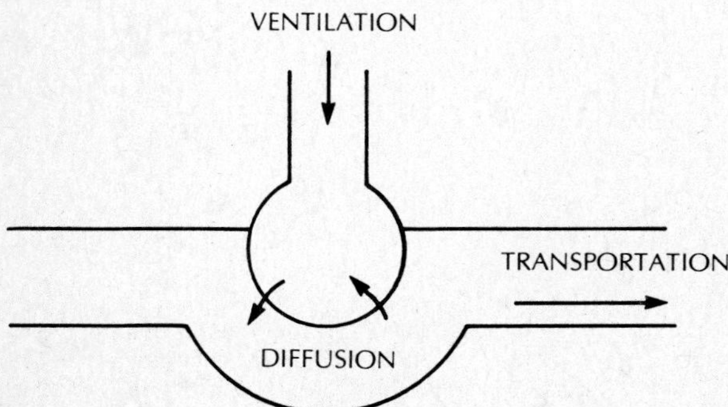

Figure 1–2. Steps in gas exchange. The first three steps involved in respiration are ventilation, diffusion, and transportation. The fourth is cellular diffusion and, although not pictured, is the most important step (*pages 1–19*).

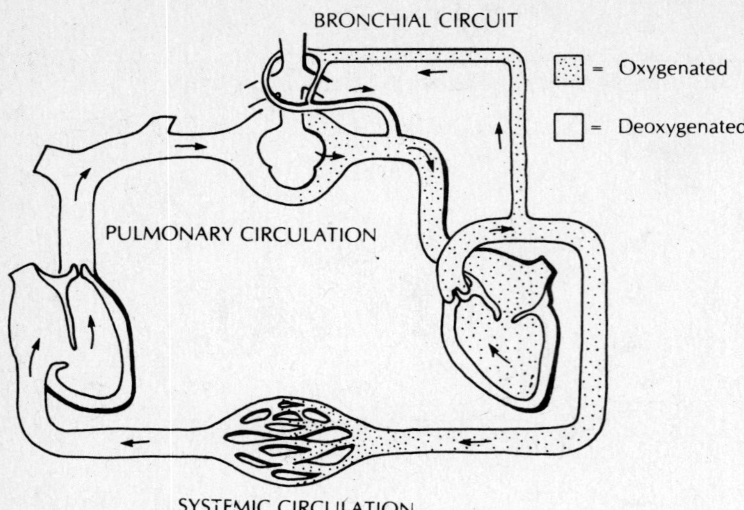

Figure 1–3. Comparison of pulmonary, bronchial, and systemic circuits (*page 2*).

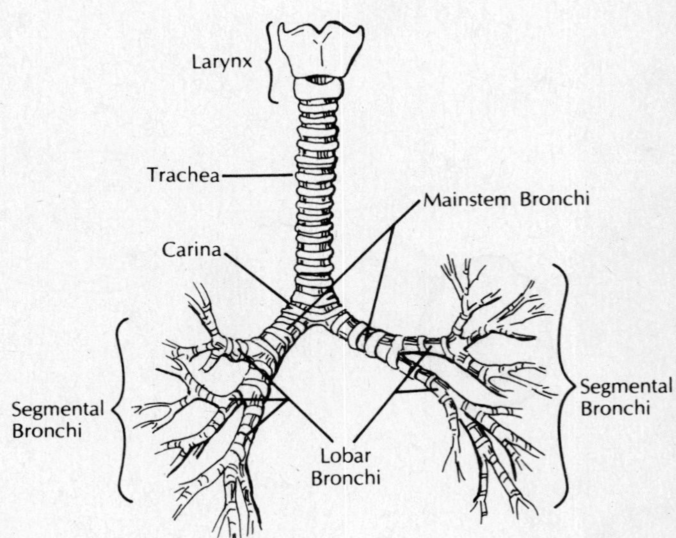

Figure 1–4. Conducting lower airway structures, larynx to lobar bronchi (*page 3*).

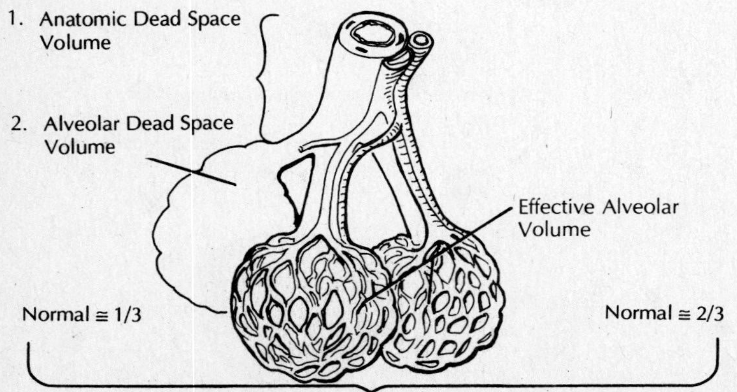

Figure 1–5. Components of minute ventilation include the anatomic and ineffective alveolar dead space volumes and the effective alveolar volume. It is the effective alveolar volume, not the total volume, that determines whether or not ventilation is adequate (*pages 5–7*).

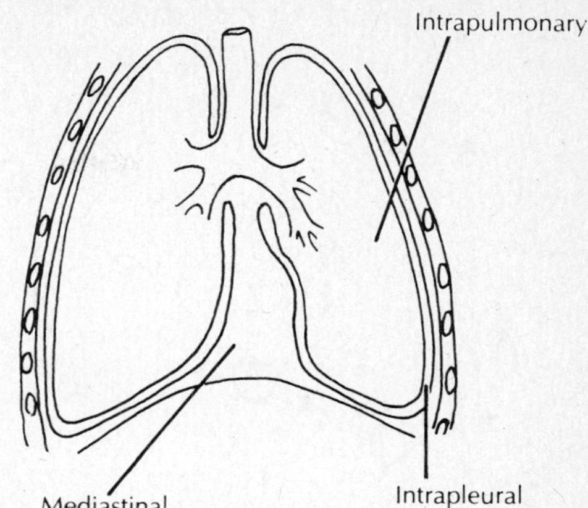

Figure 1–6. Thoracic cage, with the cavities within indicated (*pages 8–9*).

Table 1–1. LUNG MECHANICS (*page 8*)

	Normal Muscle Activity	Accessory Muscles
Inspiration	70% = Diaphragm contraction (innervation via C_3–C_5) 20% = External intercostals (innervation via T_1–T_{11})	Neck muscle contraction
Expiration	Relaxation of inspiratory muscles (passive act)	Contraction of abdominal and internal intercostal muscles

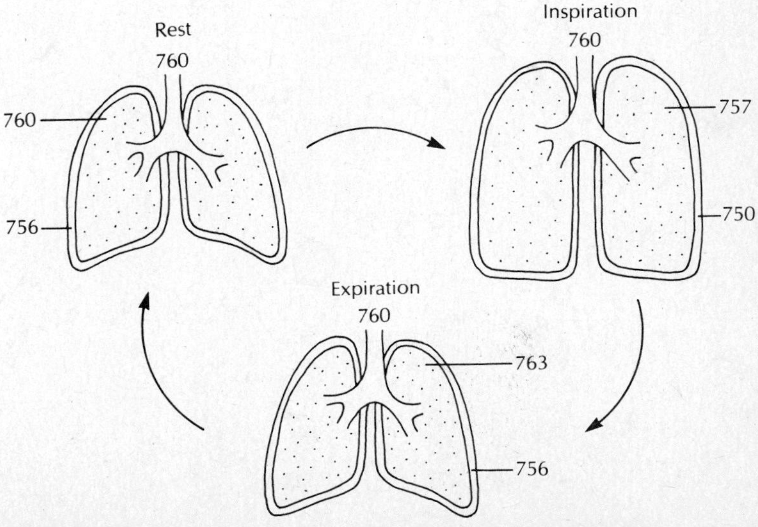

Figure 1–7. Normal changes in intrapulmonary and intrapleural pressures as compared with atmospheric pressures during a ventilatory cycle (*page 9*).

760
760
760
~755 mm Hg in the
INTRAPLEURAL SPACE

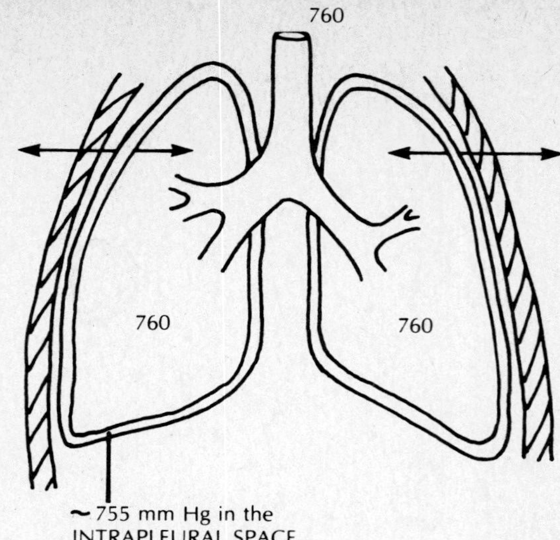

Figure 1–8. Pleural space with subatmospheric pressure created by the tendency of lung tissue to collapse from elastic recoil and of the chest wall to expand (*page 9*).

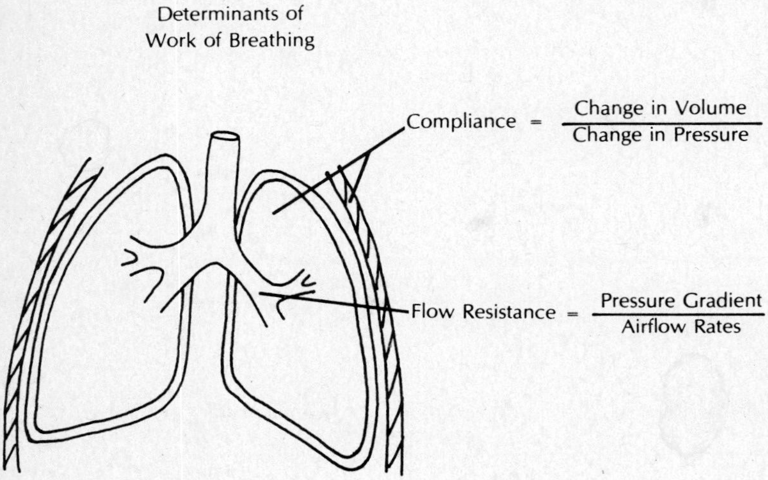

Determinants of
Work of Breathing
Compliance = Change in Volume / Change in Pressure
Flow Resistance = Pressure Gradient / Airflow Rates

Figure 1–9. Types of resistance. Elastic resistance (compliance) and flow resistance can be evaluated by application of basic physics formulas. Together, they determine the work of breathing (*pages 10, 45*).

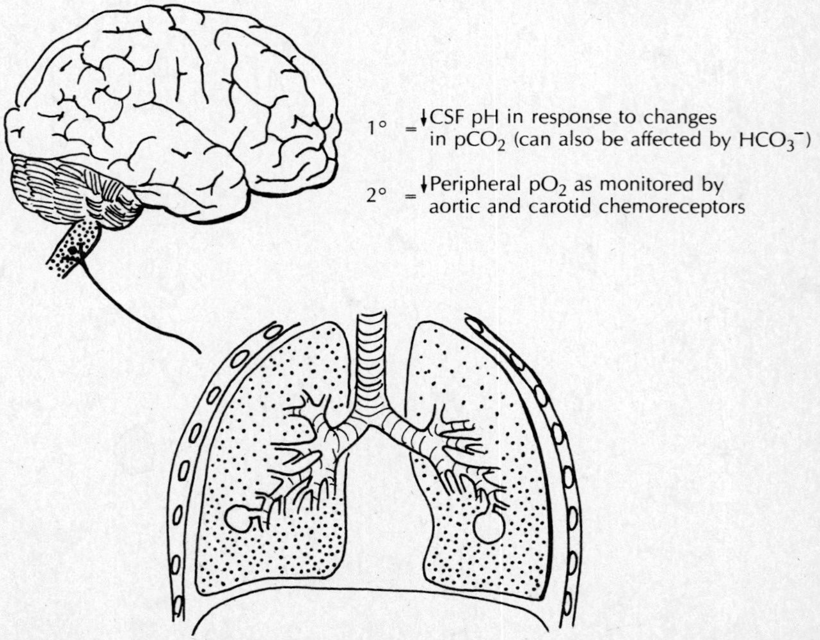

1° = ↓CSF pH in response to changes in pCO2 (can also be affected by HCO3⁻)
2° = ↓Peripheral pO2 as monitored by aortic and carotid chemoreceptors

Figure 1–10. Major components that influence control of ventilation in the medulla (*page 11*).

Table 1–2. COMPARISON OF PULMONARY PARAMETERS (*pages 12–19*)

Measurement	Primary Factors Involved	Comments
$pAO_2 = FIO_2\,(pB - 47) - \frac{paCO_2}{.8}$	Inspired O_2 tension and CO_2 entering alveoli from the bloodstream	Used in A-a gradient and other calculations
A-a Gradient = $pAO_2 - paO_2$	pAO_2 and paO_2	Evaluates ability of O_2 to diffuse across the alveolar capillary membrane. Increased in (1) $\dot{V}/\dot{Q}$ mismatch (2) Shunting (3) Diffusion block Normal = ↓ 10–20 mg on room air (also directly related to FIO_2 and cardiac output).
CaO_2 = $(Hgb \times 1.34 \times SaO_2) + (.0031 \times paO_2)$	Hgb and SaO_2 normally determine 97% of the CaO_2; the paO_2 only 3%	Reveals the actual volume of O_2 in each 100 cc of blood. Normal = 20 cc vol %
O_2 Transport = $(CaO_2 \times 10) \times CO$	CaO_2 and CO are both important in ensuring adequate O_2 delivery	Reveals the volume of O_2 delivery to the tissues per minute. Normal = 1000–1200 cc/min
a-$\bar{v}O_2$ Content Difference = $CaO_2 - C\bar{v}O_2$	Hgb, SaO_2, and $S\bar{v}O_2$ normally determine most of the difference in contents	Reveals volume of oxygen taken up by tissues. Increased when: (1) Tissue supply decreases (decreased SaO_2, Hgb, or CO) (2) Tissue demand increases (fever shivering, convulsing, struggling) Normal = 4.5–6 vol %
$S\bar{v}O_2$	Inversely related to the a-$\bar{v}O_2$ content difference	Trends the interaction between tissue's oxygen supply and demand. Increases when: (1) Tissue supply increases (increased SaO_2, Hgb, or CO) (2) Tissue demand decreases (hypothermia, decreased metabolic rate)

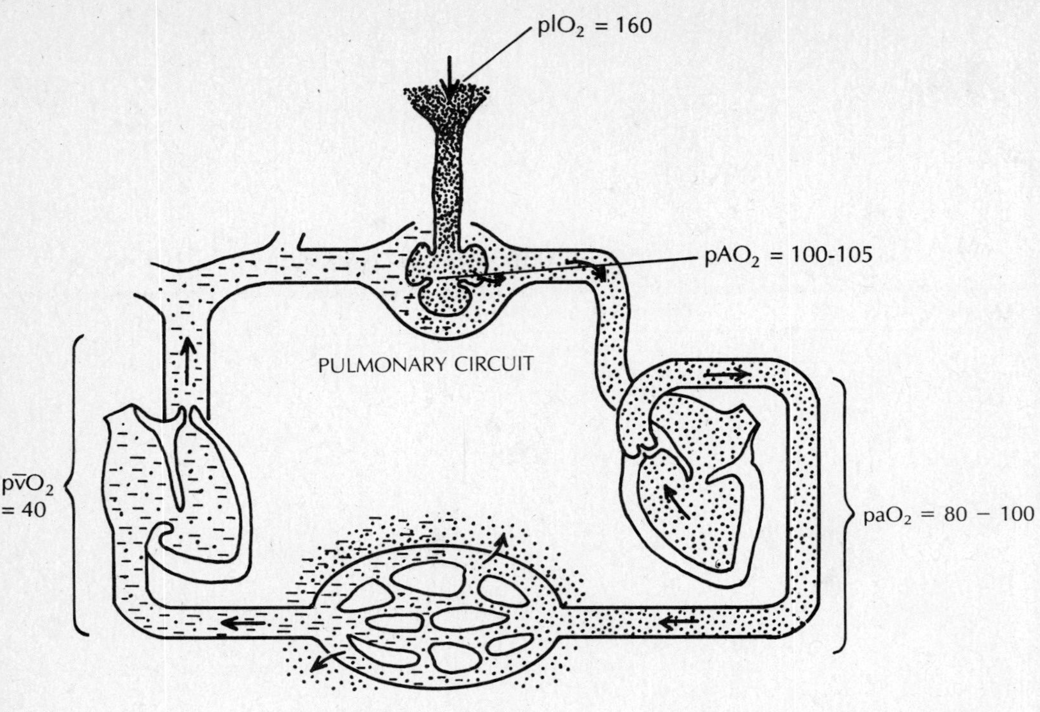

Figure 1–11. Comparison of partial pressures of oxygen in inspired (pIO_2), alveolar (pAO_2), arterial (paO_2), and venous ($p\bar{v}O_2$) gases. Values are those for patients on room air and are in mm Hg (*pages 12–19*).

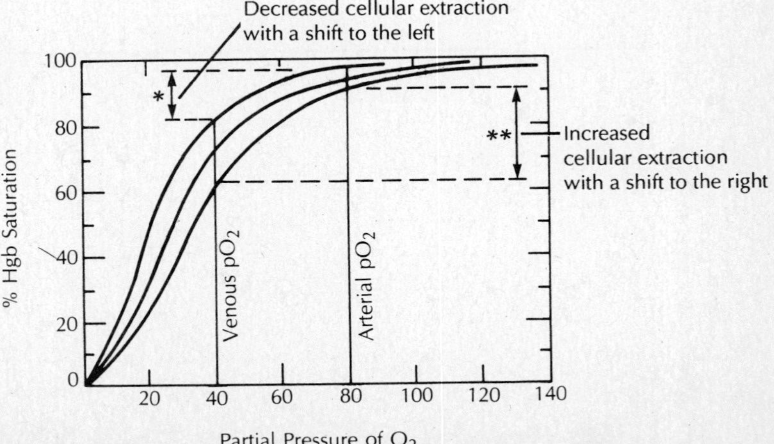

Figure 1–12. Comparison of shifts to the right and left. Cellular extraction is demonstrated as the difference between standard arterial and venous values (*pages 14–15*).

O$_2$ Extraction

Arterial

Venous

CaO_2 – $C\bar{v}O_2$

↑ Supply or ↓ demand will ↓ extraction
↓ Supply or ↑ demand will ↑ extraction
$S\bar{v}O_2$ is inversely related to O_2 extraction

Figure 1–13. Evaluation of cellular oxygen extraction by arterial-venous content differences (*page 15*).

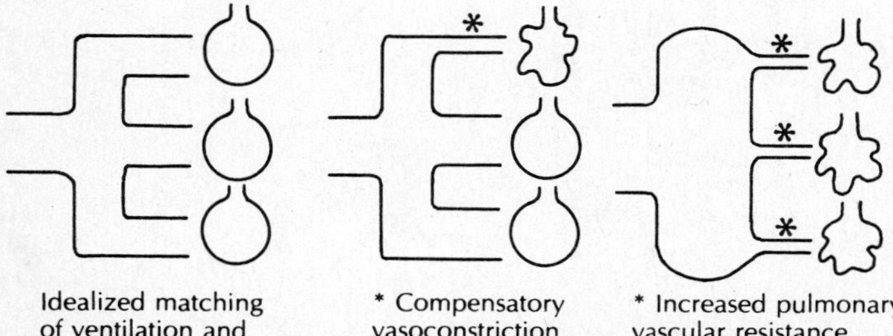

Figure 1–14. Comparison of effects of local and diffuse hypoxic vasoconstriction (*page 18*).

Table 1–3. COMPARISON OF MECHANISMS OF HYPOXEMIA (*pages 19–22*)

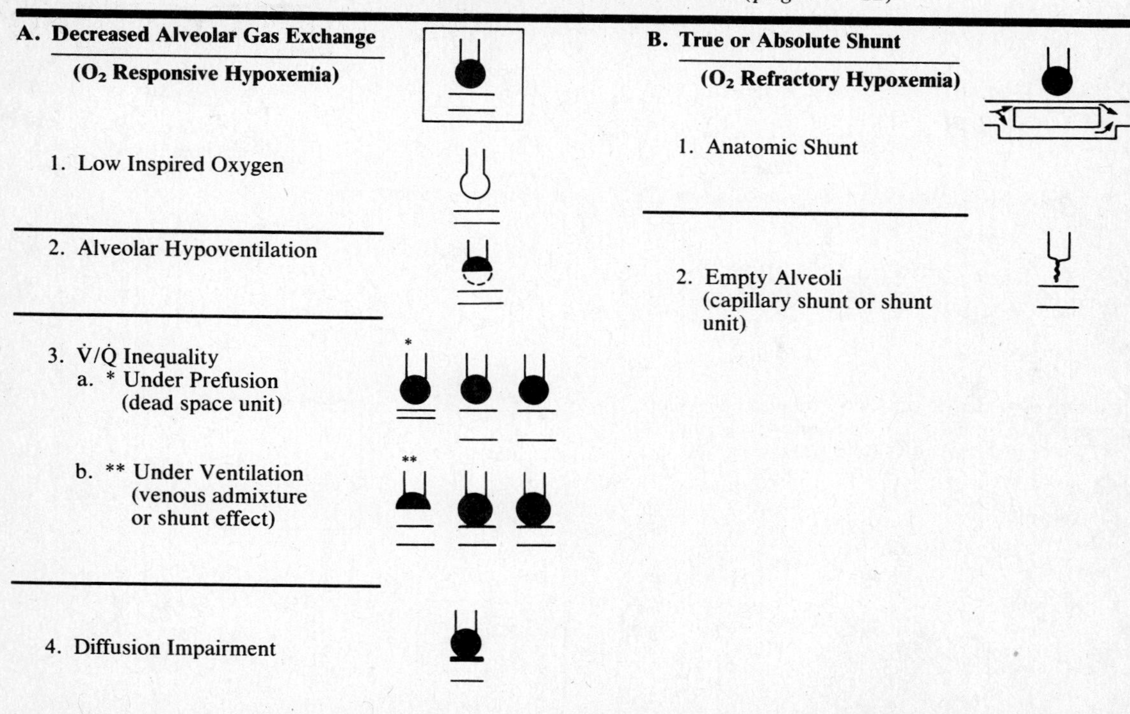

A. Decreased Alveolar Gas Exchange (O_2 Responsive Hypoxemia)	B. True or Absolute Shunt (O_2 Refractory Hypoxemia)
1. Low Inspired Oxygen	1. Anatomic Shunt
2. Alveolar Hypoventilation	2. Empty Alveoli (capillary shunt or shunt unit)
3. $\dot{V}/\dot{Q}$ Inequality a. * Under Prefusion (dead space unit) b. ** Under Ventilation (venous admixture or shunt effect)	
4. Diffusion Impairment	

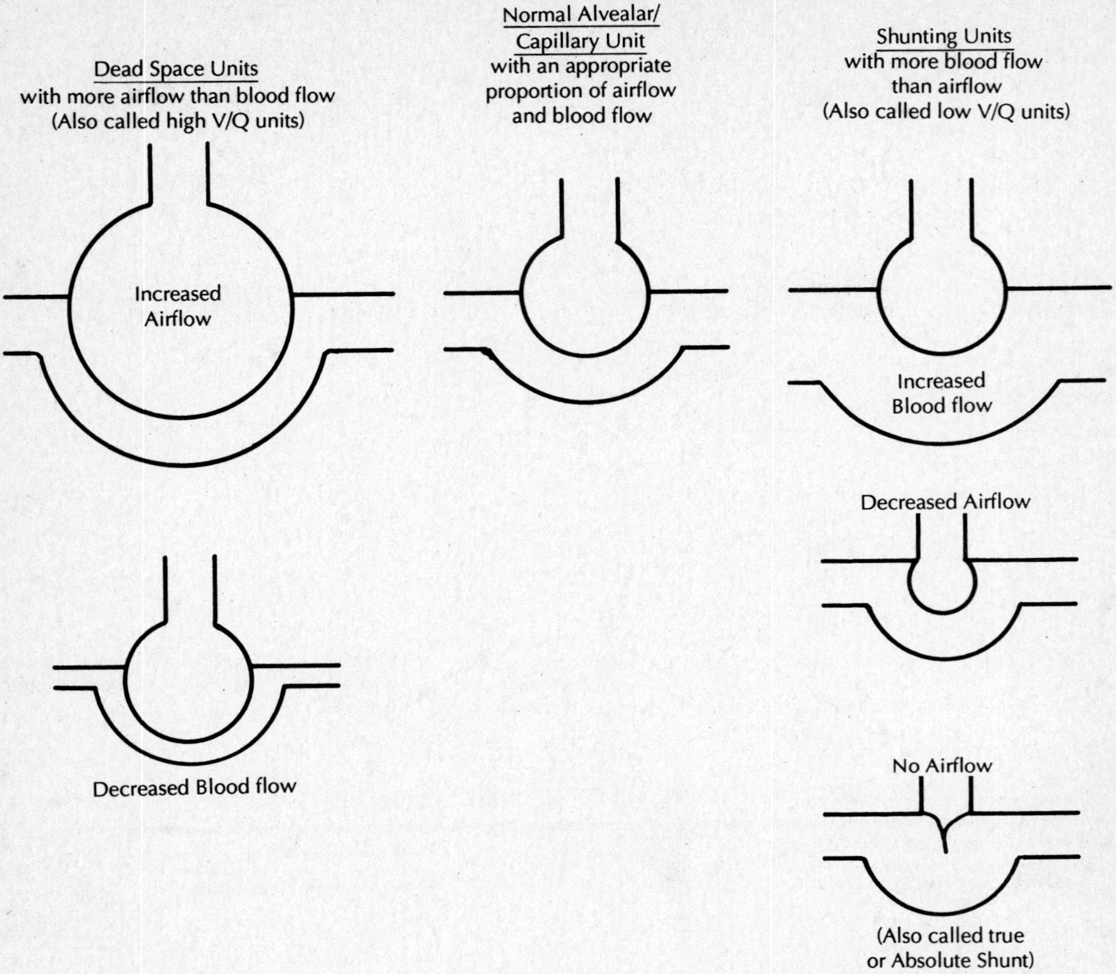

Dead Space Units
with more airflow than blood flow
(Also called high V/Q units)

Increased
Airflow

Decreased Blood flow

Normal Alvealar/
Capillary Unit
with an appropriate
proportion of airflow
and blood flow

Shunting Units
with more blood flow
than airflow
(Also called low V/Q units)

Increased
Blood flow

Decreased Airflow

No Airflow

(Also called true
or Absolute Shunt)

Figure 1–15. Comparison of alveolar dead space and alveolar shunting. Various types of each are depicted (*pages 6, 19–22*).

Figure 1–16. Example of changes in hydrogen ion (H^+) concentration caused by addition of carbonic acid (H_2CO_3) or by bicarbonate (HCO_3^-) (*page 22*).

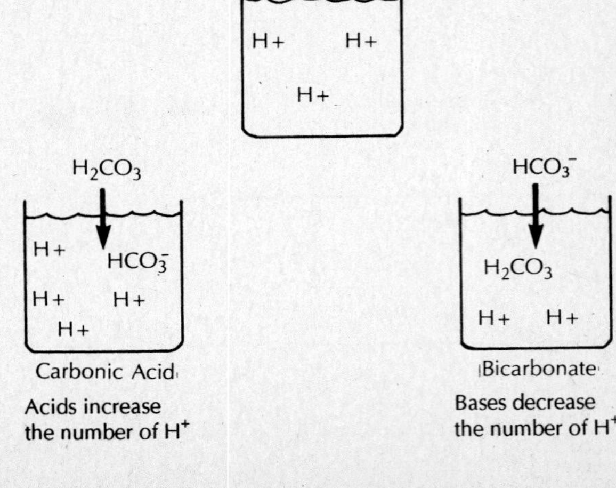

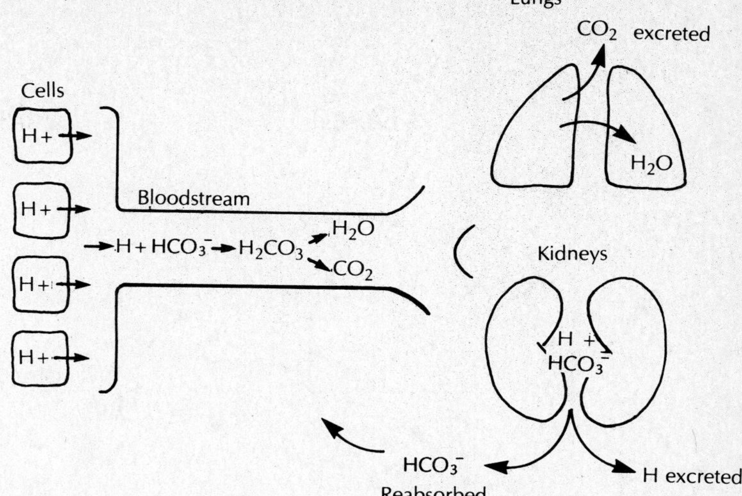

Figure 1–17. Representation of the production of hydrogen ions by cells, the primary buffer system in the bloodstream, and the elimination of hydrogen ions in the lungs and kidneys (*page 22*).

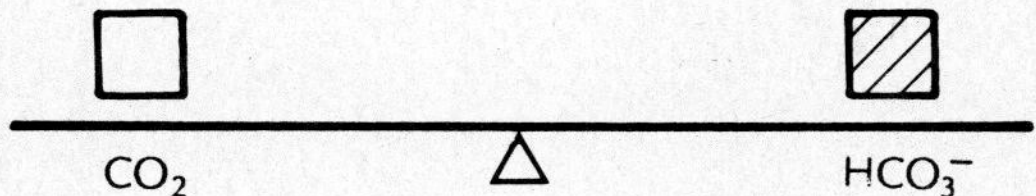

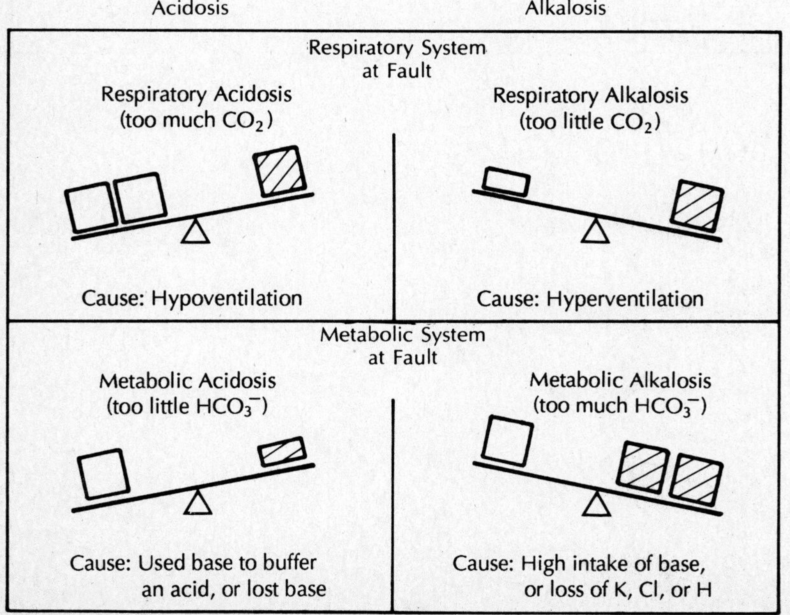

Figure 1–18. Comparison of the four primary acid-base imbalances in terms of changes in carbon dioxide (CO_2) and bicarbonate (HCO_3^-) (*pages 22–25*).

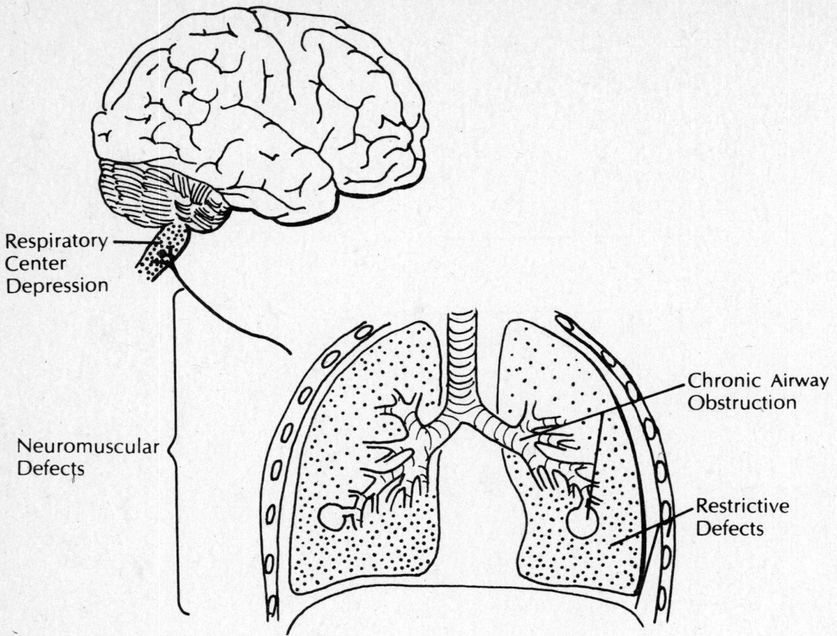

Figure 1–19. Etiologic factors that cause alveolar hypoventilation or respiratory acidosis (*page 23*).

Figure 1–20. Changes in anions (−column) that occur in metabolic acid-base imbalances. In the left-hand diagram "x" represents anions created by certain diseases and poisonings. This particular type of metabolic acidosis is recognized by the presence of a higher than normal anion gap. The anion gap is calculated as: $(Na^+ + K^+) - (Cl^- + HCO_3^-)$. The normal difference is less than 16 (*page 24*).

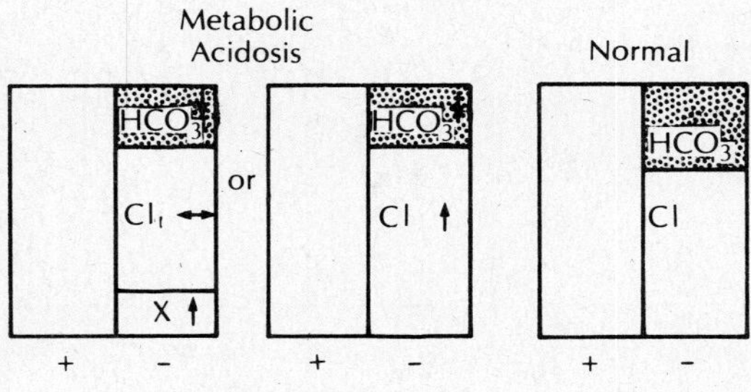

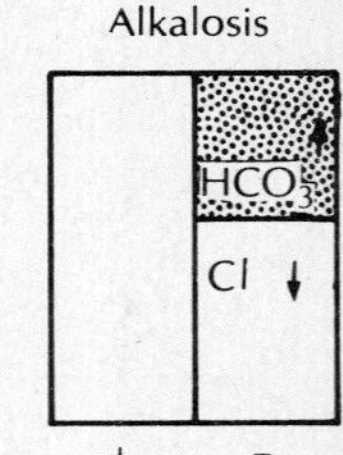

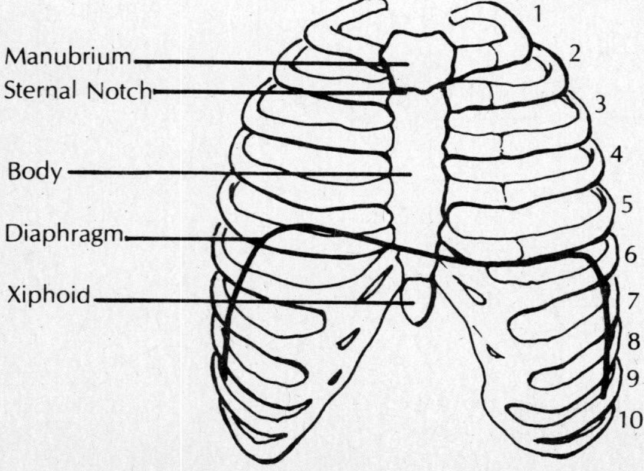

Figure 1–21. Key landmarks of the thoracic cage, with the first ten ribs numbered (*page 31*).

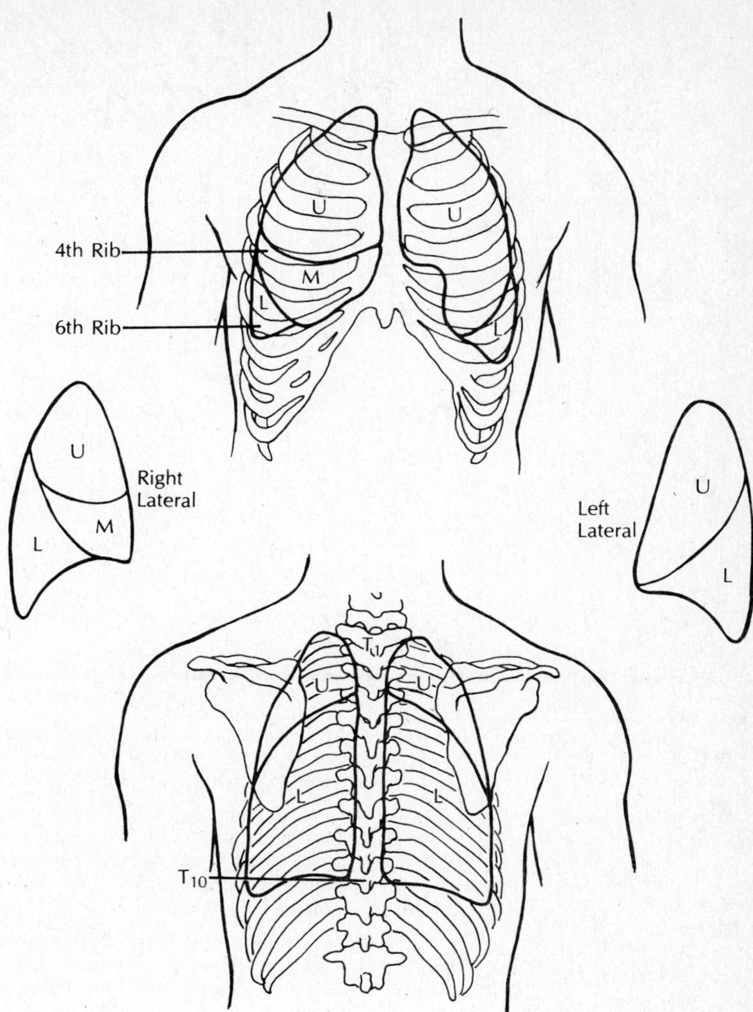

Figure 1–22. Borders of the upper (U), middle (M), and lower (L) lobes of the lungs from anterior (top), lateral (labeled), and posterior (bottom) views (*page 31*).

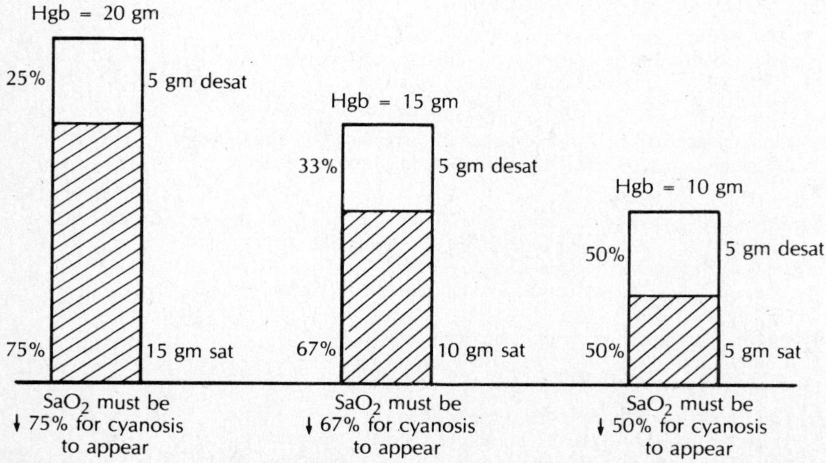

Figure 1–23. Comparison of the SaO_2 required to cause cyanosis in patients with high, normal, and low hemoglobin levels (*page 34*).

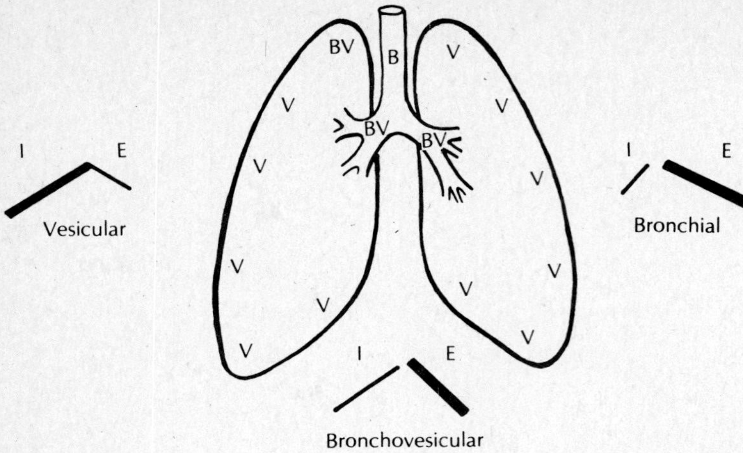

Figure 1–24. Normal sites in thoracic area for vesicular (V), bronchial (B), and bronchovesicular (BV) breath sounds. Breath sounds are compared using standard diagrams, with upslope indicating the length and intensity of inspiration (I) and downslope that of expiration (E) (*pages 38–39*).

Table 1–4. CLINICAL APPLICATIONS OF PULMONARY PHYSIOLOGIC ANATOMY (*pages 1–27*)*

Factor	Clinical Application	Page No.
Respiratory Quotient	Diets in which extra calories are given in the form of glucose produce much higher quantities of CO_2 than those in which extra calories are given in the form of lipids.	1
Bronchial Artery	Since the lungs have a dual blood flow, pulmonary emboli may not lead to pulmonary infarction. Since both arteries drain into the pulmonary veins, the full saturation of hemoglobin achieved by normal pulmonary capillaries is not appreciated in the arterial blood gas samples monitored.	2
Endotracheal and Tracheal Intubations	Bypass the nose and its ability to warm, filter, and humidify air. Open the glottis and interfere with its ability to protect the airway from aspiration or to participate in gag, cough, swallow, or Valsalva maneuver. May stimulate the cough reflex centers in the larynx or carina if not positioned carefully. Mechanically irritate the airway, which increases mucus production and inhibits ciliary activity. Distort vocal cords into a strained position.	2, 7, 8, 51–54
Tracheal Innervation	Parasympathetic nerves cause bronchoconstriction and increased mucus production, whereas the sympathetic nerves cause bronchodilation and decreased mucus production.	3
Terminal Bronchioles	Since alveolar CO_2 is directly related to pulmonary blood flow, the terminal bronchioles dilate in response to increasing alveolar CO_2, making it an important mechanism in matching airflow to blood flow.	3
Alveolar Type II Cells	Since these cells are primarily insulted in patients with ARDS, the decreased ability of the cells to produce substrates like surfactant leads to the following potential consequences: (1) Alveolar collapse (atelectasis and decreased functional residual capacity) (2) Increased work of breathing and decreased pulmonary compliance (3) Loss of detoxification functions of type II cells	4, 5, 87–90
Alveolar Ventilation	The functional portion of the total volume of gas inhaled, i.e., the part that participates in gas exchange. It is not synonymous with minute ventilation. It is monitored indirectly by subtracting estimated dead space from the total minute ventilation or by monitoring the pCO_2 and pH for the adequacy of ventilation.	5–7

Table 1–4. CLINICAL APPLICATIONS OF PULMONARY PHYSIOLOGIC ANATOMY (*pages 1–27*)* *Continued*

Factor	Clinical Application	Page No.
Dead Space Ventilation	The measurable portion of the minute ventilation that does not participate in gas exchange. It is also estimated by assessing the three types (alveolar, anatomic, and mechanical).	5, 6, 50, 64
Muscles of Respiration	May be assessed by inspection and palpation. Excessively developed respiratory muscles indicate chronically increased work of breathing. Use of accessory muscles at rest indicates current increased work of breathing. Resting the diaphragm, on alternating breaths, indicates diaphragm fatigue and is easily recognized by lack of abdominal rise during inspiration.	9, 32, 33
Pressure Changes During Spontaneous Ventilation	In normal spontaneous breathing, air flows into the lungs as the passive end result of lung expansion decreasing intrapulmonary pressures ("negative pressure ventilation"). In almost all mechanical ventilators used today, air is pushed into the lungs actively ("positive pressure ventilation").	9, 56
Control of Ventilation	Normally, the CSF pH responding to changes in pCO_2 affects ventilation instantaneously. However, HCO_3^- can also cross the blood-brain barrier and alter ventilation by altering the CSF pH.	11, 25
Shifts in the Oxygen-Hemoglobin Dissociation Curve	Conditions that cause shifts to the right (acidemia, hypercapnea, and fever) result in lower saturation of hemoglobin but also potentially in increased tissue oxygenation. Conditions that cause shifts to the left (alkalemia, hypocapnea, and hypothermia) result in better saturation of hemoglobin and potentially in decreased tissue oxygenation.	15
Pulmonary Hypoxic Vasoconstriction	Helps mitigate hypoxia in patients with localized pulmonary disorders. In such patients drugs that cause pulmonary vasodilation may increase the degree of hypoxemia. In patients with widespread diffuse disease, it may lead to pulmonary hypertension, and pulmonary vasodilators may be used to treat resulting right heart failure.	18
Shunting	The definition of shunting is not well standardized in the literature. Many sources use the term to refer to any state where blood flows from the right side of the heart to the left side without getting perfectly resaturated with oxygen. Causes of shunting include: (1) Diffusion block (2) Low V/Q units (3) Anatomic right-to-left shunts (4) Blood flowing through airless alveoli Neither (3) nor (4) are treatable with oxygen therapy.	19–21
Refractory Hypoxemia	When the patient's paO_2 does not respond to high-dose oxygen, the cause is usually absolute or true shunting where there is no gas exchange between airflow and blood flow [see (3) and (4) above].	21
Anion Gap	When only the basic four serum electrolytes are compared (sodium plus potassium compared to chloride plus bicarbonate), the anions normally are no more than 16 mEq below the cations. When a patient has metabolic acidosis and a higher anion gap, it suggests an acid-producing problem. When the anion gap is normal, it suggests a bicarbonate-wasting problem.	24

* This table summarizes factors covered in the physiologic anatomy section that have important clinical applications worth emphasizing.

ARDS = Adult respiratory distress syndrome

Table 1–5. SUMMARY OF CAUSES OF KEY PULMONARY PHYSICAL ASSESSMENT PHENOMENON (*pages 27–40*)

Phenomenon	Key Causes	Page No.
Dyspnea	Increased work of breathing Can be pulmonary or cardiac in origin	27, 28
Cough	Airway irritation Airway disease Can be pulmonary or cardiac in origin	28
Hemoptysis	Airway disease Parenchyma disease Vascular lesions	28, 29
Chest Wall Asymmetry	Pleural accumulations expanding one side Atelectasis or fibrosis collapsing one side	32
Inspiratory Strider	Upper or large airway obstruction	32
Paradoxical Breathing	Diaphragm fatigue	33
Clubbing of Fingers	Chronic hypoxia	33
Cyanosis	5 gm of desaturated Hgb Can be central (pulmonary in origin) or just peripheral (circulatory in origin) Will be absent if Hgb is partially saturated with carbon monoxide	34
Decreased Focal Fremitus	Decreased pulmonary density Increased distance between the examinee's hand and the patient's lung	35
Increased Vocal Fremitus	Increased pulmonary density	35, 36
Subcutaneous Emphysema	Air leak into space under skin	36
Percussion Notes Over Lung:		36, 37
Tympanic note	Air under pressure (tension pneumothorax)	
Hyperresonance	Hyperinflation, decreased density	
Resonance	Normal lungs	
Hyporesonance or dullness	Consolidation, increased density	
Bronchial Breath Sounds Over Lung Fields	Consolidation	38
Bronchovesicular Sounds Over Lung Fields (except right upper lobe)	Consolidation	38
Decreased Breath Sounds	Decreased airflow Decreased density Increased distance between stethoscope and lung	38, 39
Fine Crackles (rales)	Atelectasis or restrictive disease	39
Coarse Crackles	Mucus or fluid in airways	39
Wheeze	Airway narrowing	39
Pleural Friction Rub	Pleural inflammation with loss of pleural fluid	39
Mediastinal Crunch	Airway in mediastinum	40
Increased Conduction of Voice Sounds	Consolidation	40
Decreased Conduction of Voice Sounds	Decreased density Increased distance between stethoscope and lung	40

Table 1–6. COMPARISON OF PHYSICAL ASSESSMENT FINDINGS IN COMMON PATHOLOGIC CONDITIONS (*pages 27–40*)

Findings	↓ Density (air trapping)	↑ Density (consolidation)	Pleural Effusion	Pneumothorax
Tactile or Vocal Fremitus	Decreased	Increased	Decreased	Decreased
Position of Mediastinal Structures	Bilateral = normal Unilateral = deviate away	Airways filled = normal Airways collapsed = deviate toward	May deviate away	May deviate away
Chest Wall	May be less air movement or more work May have barrel chest	May be less movement in involved area or more work	May be less movement in involved area or more work	May be less movement in involved area or more work
Percussion	Hyperresonance or tympany	Hyporesonance or dullness	Hyporesonance or dullness	Hyperresonance or tympany
Breath Sounds	Decreased	Bronchialization of peripheral breath sounds	Decreased	Decreased
Voice Sound Transmission	Decreased	Increased	Decreased "E" to "A" at fluid level	Decreased

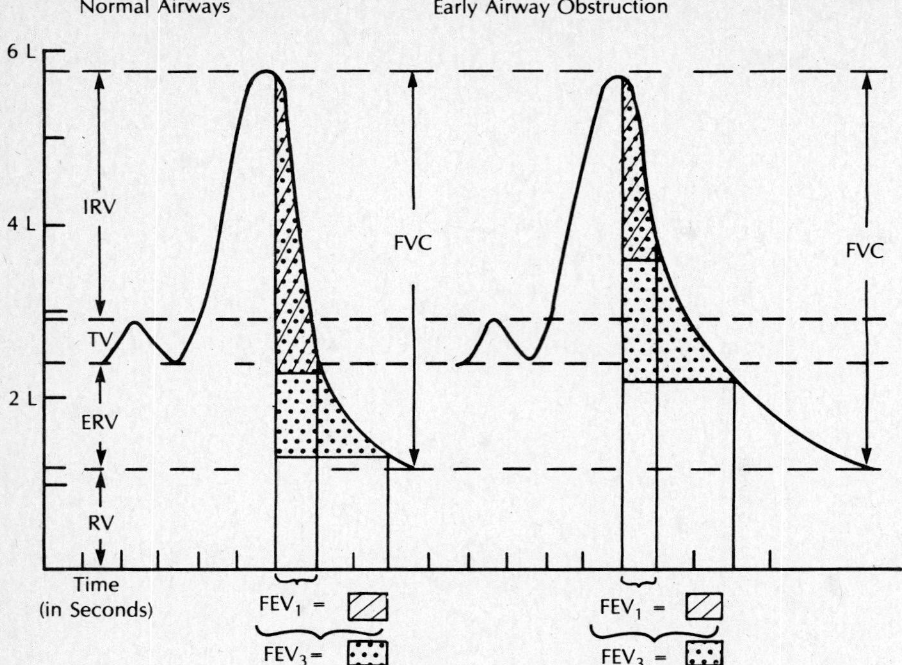

Figure 1–25. Comparison of forced flow studies in a patient with normal airways and a patient with early airway obstruction. Although the total forced vital capacities (FVC) are equal, the forced expiratory volumes in 1 second (FEV_1) and 3 seconds (FEV_3) are markedly different (*page 44*).

Table 1–7. COMPARISON OF TYPES OF COMPLIANCE (*page 45*)

Type	Formula	Comments
Static Compliance (C_{st})	$C_{st} = \frac{\text{Tidal Volume}}{\text{*Plateau Pressure}}$ Normal = 100 cc/cm H_2O	Assesses only distensibility of pulmonary tissues and chest wall
Dynamic Compliance (C_{dyn})	$C_{dyn} = \frac{\text{Tidal Volume}}{\text{*Peak Inspiratory Pressure}}$ Normal = 40–50 cc/cm H_2O	Includes pressure created by active airflow during inspiration

* Positive end-expiratory pressure (PEEP) must be subtracted.

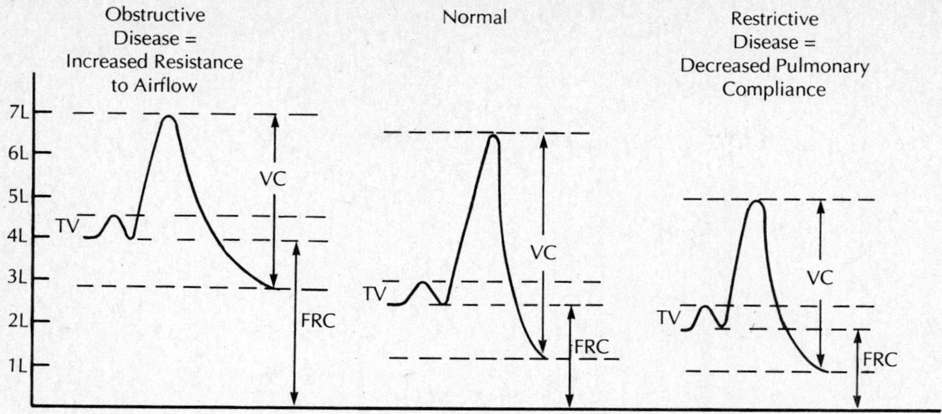

Figure 1–26. Comparison of pulmonary function studies in obstructive and restrictive pulmonary disorders (*pages 45–46*).

Table 1–8. MANIPULATION OF POSITIVE PRESSURE MECHANICAL VENTILATORS (*pages 55–61*)

Initiation of Inspiration	Manipulations of Inspiration	Ending of Inspiration	Manipulations of Expiration
Patient effort ("assisted")	Can alter flow patterns, flow rate, amount of O_2, temperature, humidification	Preset volume ("volume cycled")	May be delayed slightly ("inspiratory plateau")
Rate per minute ("controlled")		Preset pressure ("pressure cycled")	May not allow pressure to fall all the way to zero ("positive end-expiratory pressure")
Patient effort unless a time limit is exceeded ("assist/control")		Preset volume unless a maximum pressure is reached ("volume cycled/pressure limited")	
May allow patient to breathe spontaneously (intermittent mandatory ventilation)			

Table 1–9. SUMMARY OF MODES AND METHODS USED FOR POSITIVE PRESSURE MECHANICAL VENTILATION (*pages 57, 58*)

Type	Description	Comments
Controlled Mechanical Ventilation (CMV)	All breaths are machine-delivered at a set volume *and* rate; minute volume is therefore steady at a predetermined level	Cannot be triggered by patient. Some machines will allow patients to trigger but it requires excessive inspiratory force
Assist-Control (AC)	All breaths are machine-delivered at a preset volume with a minimal rate but the machine will also deliver a breath in response to patient effort or demand	Sets minimum but patient has ability to increase the minute ventilation
Intermittent-Mandatory Ventilation (IMV)	Allows patient to breathe spontaneously between breaths that are delivered by the machine at a preset volume and rate. Does not monitor patient-breathing activity	This system is easier for the patient to breathe spontaneously through than SIMV. The rate can be decreased during weaning.
Synchronized IMV (SIMV)	Same as IMV except it does monitor patient-breathing activity and synchronizes its delivery between or with patient efforts	This system requires a higher work of breathing on the part of the patient during spontaneous breaths. This must be kept in mind when used as a weaning technique.
Pressure Support Ventilation (PSV)	Patient must trigger the machine, which then reaches a preset pressure instantaneously and sustains it for the patient's entire inspiratory effort	This is another way to mechanically support patient's ventilatory activity. Can be gradually decreased as a means of weaning.

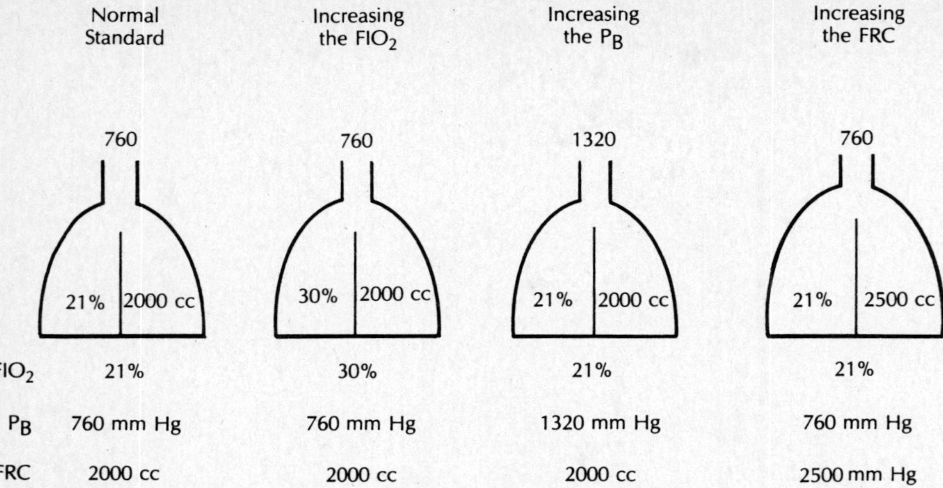

Figure 1–27. Alternatives for the treatment of hypoxemia are increasing the fraction of inspired oxygen or FIO_2 (*pages 61–65*), the barometric pressure or P_B (*page 65*), or the functional residual capacity or FRC (*pages 73–81*).

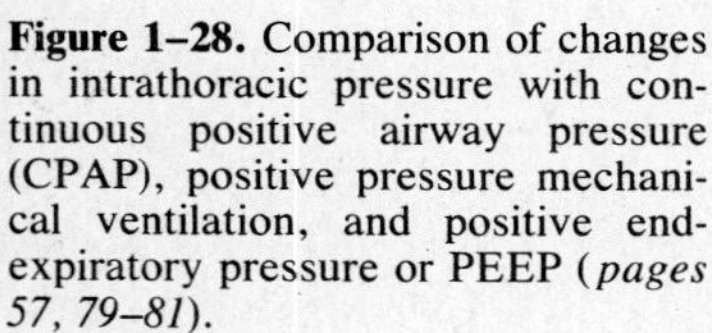
Figure 1–28. Comparison of changes in intrathoracic pressure with continuous positive airway pressure (CPAP), positive pressure mechanical ventilation, and positive end-expiratory pressure or PEEP (*pages 57, 79–81*).

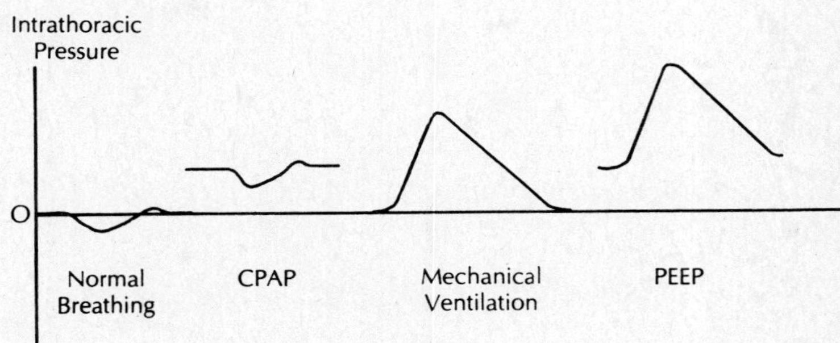

THE PULMONARY SYSTEM

Exercises

After reading the Pulmonary Section of the Core Curriculum, *fill in the blanks in the following statements. It can be done one topic at a time or all at once. The answers are at the end of the exercises.*

A. Physiologic Anatomy (*pages 1–27*)

1. Aerobic metabolism consumes the gas ______________________ and produces the gas ______________________.
2. Gas exchange between the cells and the bloodstream is called ______________________ respiration, whereas exchange in the lungs is called ______________________ respiration.
3. The vessel that brings oxygenated blood to the lung structures is the ______________________.
4. The anatomic dead space extends from the ______________________ to the ______________________.

5. Normal anatomic dead space is about ______________ cc per kilogram of body weight.
6. In a young child, the ______________ cartilage is a complete ring and a stricture that obviates the need for a cuff on an endotracheal tube.
7. The cough reflex is most sensitive at the ______________.
8. The ______________ nerves of the autonomic nervous system are responsible for bronchoconstriction.
9. Increasing carbon dioxide levels cause the terminal bronchiole in that area to ______________.
10. The alveolar cells that secrete surfactant are the ______________.
11. Surface tension reduction by surfactant has the following three effects:
    a. ______________
    b. ______________
    c. ______________
12. The minute ventilation can easily be assessed by multiplying the ______________ by the ______________.
13. The minute ventilation consists of the ______________ volume and the ______________ volume.
14. The two types of physiologic dead space are the ______________ and ______________ volume.
15. The ratio of the nonexchanging to the exchanging gas volume is called the ______________ and is normally ______________ %.
16. Effective alveolar ventilation is not easily measured but is inversely related to the ______________.
17. An elevated $paCO_2$ indicates that the effective alveolar ventilation is too ______________, possibly owing to ______________ in the dead space volume.
18. The pulmonary defense mechanisms that operate by transporting particles out of the lung are the ______________ and the ______________ systems.
19. The primary muscle for normal inspiration is the ______________, which is innervated through the ______________ spinal nerves.
20. The secondary muscles for normal inspiration are the ______________, which are innervated through the ______________ spinal nerves.
21. During spontaneous breathing, the intrathoracic volume goes ______________ while intrathoracic pressure goes ______________.
22. The normal intrapleural pressure is ______________ than the atmospheric pressure.
23. During a normal ventilatory cycle, the intrapulmonary pressures are ______________ during inspiration and ______________ during expiration.
24. The type of resistance created by tissue forces is called the ______________ or ______________.
25. The primary factor stimulating the medullary center to initiate inspiration is a drop in its extracellular ______________.
26. The Hering-Breuer reflex is the stimulation of ______________ receptors in the bronchi, which inhibit ______________.

27. Carbon dioxide is ____________ soluble and diffusible than oxygen.
28. Carbon dioxide normally has a ____________ pulmonary driving pressure for diffusion than oxygen.
29. The three factors than can cause a decrease in calculated alveolar oxygen tension are the following:
    a. ____________
    b. ____________
    c. ____________
30. The A-a gradient or the difference between the alveolar (pAO_2) and arterial oxygen tensions (paO_2) is obtained by first calculating the pAO_2 by the formula $pAO_2 = FIO_2\,(713) - \frac{paCO_2}{.8}$ and then subtracting the paO_2 from it. What is the A-a gradient in the following four patients?
    a. $FIO_2 = .21$, $paCO_2 = 40$, $paO_2 = 80$, $pAO_2 =$ ____ A-a = ____
    b. $FIO_2 = .30$, $paCO_2 = 40$, $paO_2 = 80$, $pAO_2 =$ ____ A-a = ____
    c. $FIO_2 = .21$, $paCO_2 = 80$, $paO_2 = 40$, $pAO_2 =$ ____ A-a = ____
    d. $FIO_2 = 1.00$, $paCO_2 = 40$, $paO_2 = 80$, $pAO_2 =$ ____ A-a = ____
31. Most of the oxygen transported in the bloodstream is found ____________.
32. On the normal oxyhemoglobin dissociation curve a paO_2 of 60 mm Hg causes a hemoglobin saturation of ____________ %.
33. List four factors that will shift the oxyhemoglobin dissociation curve to the right of normal.
    a. ____________
    b. ____________
    c. ____________
    d. ____________
34. The arterial oxygen content is calculated by the formula $CaO_2 = (Hgb \times 1.34 \times SaO_2) + (.0031 \times paO_2)$. What is the oxygen content in the following patients?

	paO_2	*Hgb*	*SaO_2*	*CaO_2*
a.	100 mm Hg	15 gm	99%	____________
b.	45 mm Hg	18 gm	75%	____________
c.	100 mm Hg	8 gm	99%	____________
d.	45 mm Hg	8 gm	75%	____________

35. Oxygen transport, or the amount of oxygen to the tissues per minute, is a product of the oxygen content per liter and the cardiac output: O_2 Trans = O_2 content × 10 × CO. Calculate the oxygen transport in the four patients listed in question 34 (a–d) at cardiac outputs of 3, 5, and 7 liters per minute.

	CaO_2	*CO of 3L*	*CO of 5L*	*CO of 7L*
a.	________	________	________	________
b.	________	________	________	________
c.	________	________	________	________
d.	________	________	________	________

36. The arterial-mixed venous oxygen content difference will rise if the tissue demand goes ____________ or the cardiac output goes ____________.
37. Most of carbon dioxide produced by the cells is transported by the bloodstream in the ____________.

38. Intrapulmonary blood volume goes ____________________ when the intrathoracic pressure falls.
39. Alveolar hypoxia causes the pulmonary arteriole to ____________________.
40. The mechanism described above in question 39 is (more/less) helpful in localized than in diffuse alveolar hypoxia.
41. The two mechanisms of hypoxemia that can occur in the presence of a normal alveolar-arterial oxygen gradient are ____________________ and ____________________.
42. The term used to refer to situations in which the air volume and blood volume presented to an alveolar-capillary unit are not proportionate is ____________________.
43. The mechanism of hypoxemia that is unresponsive to increased inspired oxygen tensions is ____________________.
44. As a solution becomes more acidic, the hydrogen ion concentration goes ____________________ and the pH goes ____________________.
45. The normal ratio of bicarbonate to carbon dioxide is ____________________.
46. Indicate what change, if any, has occurred in the carbon dioxide (pCO_2), bicarbonate (HCO_3^-), and pH levels for each of the four pure uncompensated acid-base imbalances.

	pCO_2	*HCO_3^-*	*pH*
a. Respiratory acidosis	______	______	______
b. Respiratory alkalosis	______	______	______
c. Metabolic acidosis	______	______	______
d. Metabolic alkalosis	______	______	______

47. Name the expected acid-base imbalances caused by each disorder listed.
    a. Hypoventilation ____________________
    b. Anxiety ____________________
    c. Shock ____________________
    d. Diabetic ketoacidosis ____________________
    e. Hypokalemia ____________________
    f. Nasogastric suction ____________________
48. List the expected compensation for each of the primary acid-base imbalances.
    a. Respiratory acidosis ____________________
    b. Respiratory alkalosis ____________________
    c. Metabolic acidosis ____________________
    d. Metabolic alkalosis ____________________
49. Describe the acid-base abnormalities found in each of the examples below.

	pO_2 (mm Hg)	*pH*	*pCO_2 (mm Hg)*	*HCO_3^- (mEq)*	*BE*	
a.	56	7.26	34	13	−12	______
b.	148	7.48	27	22	− 2	______
c.	35	7.52	30	32	+ 7	______
d.	104	7.21	30	8	−18	______
e.	31	7.05	65	14	−10	______
f.	239	7.37	23	13	−11	______
g.	90	7.26	72	33	+ 9	______
h.	72	7.49	22	20	− 4	______
i.	80	7.50	50	37	+12	______

B. Nursing Assessment Data Base (*pages 27–47*)

1. List three types of disorders that can result in dyspnea:
   a. ______________________
   b. ______________________
   c. ______________________
2. List three types of disorders or pathologic conditions that can result in cough:
   a. ______________________
   b. ______________________
   c. ______________________
3. Chest pain related to ______________________ is often well localized and increased with deep inspiration, whereas pain related to diaphragm inflammation is often referred to the ______________________.
4. Give two examples of pulmonary disorders that may have a familial tendency:
   a. ______________________
   b. ______________________
5. Quantifying the amount of smoking-related disease risk is done by multiplying the ______________________ times the ______________________ to determine the number of packs/years.
6. The junction on the manubrium and body of the sternum is called the ______________________.
7. An increase in the anterior-posterior diameter to more than the usual ______________________ of the transverse chest wall diameter results in a condition described as a ______________________.
8. ______________________ is a sign of respiratory muscle fatigue in which the abdomen falls instead of rises during inspiration.
9. Cyanosis is caused by ______________________.
10. The type of cyanosis associated with color changes in the mucous membranes is ______________________.
11. Carbon monoxide poisoning causes the patient's color to become ______________________.
12. In a right-sided tension pneumothorax, the trachea will deviate to the ______________________ side.
13. Emphysema will cause the amount of tactile or vocal fremitus to go ______________________.
14. Tactile or vocal fremitus is increased when lung density goes ______________________.
15. Percussion over a hemothorax will elicit a ______________________ note, whereas percussion over a normal lung will elicit a ______________________.
16. The type of normal breath sound in which inspiration is more audible than expiration is the ______________________ sound.
17. Name three areas where bronchovesicular breath sounds are normally heard.
    a. ______________________
    b. ______________________
    c. ______________________
18. Bronchial breath sounds over the lung parenchyma suggest an ______________________ in lung density.
19. The adventitious sound often related to restrictive disorders is ______________________.
20. The adventitious sound often related to obstructive disorders is ______________________.

21. The adventitious sound produced by secretions in the lung airways is ____________________.
22. Bronchophony, egophony, and whispered pectoriloquy occur in diseases that lead to ____________________ of the lung tissue.
23. The normal tidal volume in the adult is about ____________________ cc.
24. The maximum volume a patient can move in and out of the lungs in one breath is called the ____________________ (measured from end maximum inspiration to end maximum expiration) and the normal is ____________________ cc.
25. The volume of air contained in the lungs at the end of a normal expiration is called the ____________________.
26. One type of pulmonary function study that helps to evaluate obstruction to airflow in early obstructive diseases is the ____________________.
27. Pulmonary compliance is calculated to evaluate the ____________________ of the lungs.
28. Compliance goes ____________________ in patients with pneumonia or pulmonary edema.
29. In patients with increased airway resistance, the type of compliance that decreases the most is the ____________________ compliance.
30. In COPD, the compliance goes ____________________ and the functional residual capacity (FRC) goes ____________________.

C. Commonly Encountered Nursing Diagnoses (*pages 47–83*)

1. A properly placed endotracheal tube will end ____________________ as identified on the chest x-ray.
2. To limit damage to tracheal mucosa, endotracheal tube cuff pressures should be kept below ____________________ mm Hg.
3. List two possible complications for each of the following interventions:
   a. Esophageal airways ____________________ ____________________
   b. Endotracheal intubation
      (1) During insertion ____________________ ____________________
      (2) While in place ____________________ ____________________
      (3) Immediately following extubation ____________________ ____________________
   c. Mechanical ventilation ____________________ ____________________
   d. Oxygen therapy ____________________ ____________________
   e. Positive end-expiratory pressure ____________________ ____________________
4. Name three alterations in normal pulmonary protective mechanisms that are created by endotracheal intubation:
   a. ____________________
   b. ____________________
   c. ____________________
5. Occasionally, a patient may be mechanically ventilated by ____________________ techniques, which use very small volumes at very high rates.
6. When mechanically delivered inspiration is initiated by the patient's effort, the ventilator is said to be in the ____________________ mode.
7. The mode of mechanical ventilation that allows patients to breathe on

their own spontaneously between machine-delivered breaths is ____________________.

8. The mode of mechanical ventilation in which a preset pressure is reached quickly and then continues during each patient's breathing effort is called ____________________.
9. The main advantage of volume-cycled over pressure-cycled positive pressure ventilation is ____________________.
10. The absolute contraindications for intermittent positive pressure breathing (IPPB) include ____________________ and ____________________.
11. The volumes required for mechanical ventilation are ____________________ than the volumes required for spontaneous ventilation.
12. Positive pressure ventilators can ____________________ the venous return, one mechanism that may cause the cardiac output to go ____________________.
13. List possible adjustments in mechanical ventilation for the following blood gas results:
    a. paO_2 = 40 mm Hg, pH = 7.42, $paCO_2$ = 36 mm Hg ____________
    b. paO_2 = 80 mm Hg, pH = 7.25, $paCO_2$ = 62 mm Hg ____________
    c. paO_2 = 80 mm Hg, pH = 7.55, $paCO_2$ = 22 mm Hg ____________
14. The first intervention, after a rapid bedside check, in a patient who is "suddenly" fighting the ventilator is ____________________.
15. Give three examples of indications that a patient may be ready to wean from prolonged mechanical ventilation:
    a. ____________________
    b. ____________________
    c. ____________________
16. List three physical assessment findings that may indicate the patient is not tolerating weaning attempts:
    a. ____________________
    b. ____________________
    c. ____________________
17. List three mechanisms that may interfere with a patient's ability to be weaned from mechanical ventilation:
    a. ____________________
    b. ____________________
    c. ____________________
18. Indicate whether each of the following is a feature of assist/control (a/c) or intermittent mandatory ventilation (IMV) modes used in mechanical ventilators:
    a. Every breath is mechanically delivered ____________________
    b. Allows patient to breathe spontaneously ____________________
    c. Can be used as a weaning method ____________________
    d. Requires no active patient muscle activity ____________________
19. Medication classifications that may be considered for controlling patients on mechanical ventilators by inhibiting respiration include ____________________ or ____________________.
20. If paralyzing agents are used in conscious patients, they should also be ____________________, since these agents act only to ____________________.
21. The most commonly used bronchodilators act by stimulating the ____________________ receptors.

22. Indicate the pharmacologic classification of the following bronchodilators:
    a. isoproterenol ______
    b. aminophylline ______
    c. albuterol ______
23. Pulmonary patients often receive increased calories in the form of fat since they result in less production of ______.
24. Hypoxia is a decrease in ______ oxygenation, whereas hypoxemia is a decrease in ______.
25. Central nervous system changes that can result from hypoxia include ______ and ______.
26. Some patients with chronic hypercapnea may develop ______ if the paO_2 is raised to normal levels.
27. Two possible hazards of oxygen therapy in the adult are ______ and ______.
28. A goal in oxygen therapy that usually produces a SaO_2 of near 90% is a paO_2 of ______.
29. The type of face mask that delivers more precise oxygen concentrations is the ______.
30. Positive end-expiratory pressure treats some causes of hypoxemia by ______ the functional residual capacity.
31. Two possible major side effects of positive end-expiratory pressure are ______ and ______.
32. A technique used to increase functional residual capacity by maintaining a higher than ambient intrapulmonary pressure but allows the patient to breathe spontaneously without mechanically delivered breaths is ______.

D. Pathologic Conditions (*pages 71–96*)

1. Name two pathophysiologic mechanisms of hypoxemic acute respiratory failure:
   a. ______
   b. ______
2. List three manifestations of increased CO_2 with decreased pH:
   a. ______
   b. ______
   c. ______
3. List the arterial blood gas features of the following conditions:
   a. Hypoxemia respiratory failure ______
   b. Acute hypercapnic respiratory failure ______
   c. Chronic hypercapnic respiratory failure ______
4. In adult respiratory distress syndrome (ARDS), the pulmonary capillary permeability goes ______, surfactant production goes ______, and the functional residual capacity (FRC) goes ______.
5. The hypoxemia of ARDS is often refractory to ______ therapy but responsive to ______ therapy.
6. Arterial blood gasses in patients with early ARDS will typically reveal ______.
7. Diagnostic studies in a patient with ARDS may reveal ______ compliance, ______ % shunting, ______

__________ A-a gradient, and ____________________ pulmonary capillary wedge pressure.

8. The type of chronic airway obstruction associated with a chronic production cough followed by hypoxemia and cor pulmonale is ____________________.
9. The mechanisms of hypoxemia in chronic bronchitis are __________ __________ and ____________________.
10. The type of chronic airway obstruction that affects the respiratory bronchiole and the alveoli, causing loss of elastic properties and alveolar surface area, is ____________________.
11. The mechanisms of hypoxemia in emphysema are loss of __________ __________, which impairs diffusion, and ____________________.
12. The strongest risk factor for developing chronic obstructive airway disease in the United States is ____________________.
13. Indicate whether each of the following findings is more likely in chronic bronchitis or emphysema.
    a. Distended neck veins ____________________
    b. Barrel chest ____________________
    c. Cyanosis ____________________
    d. Pursed lip breathing ____________________
    e. Increased fremitus ____________________
    f. Hyperresonance ____________________
    g. Polycythemia ____________________
    h. Increased FRC ____________________
    i. Reduced FEV_1 nonresponsive to bronchodilators ____________________
14. An obstructive airway disease caused by airway hyperactivity is ____________________.
15. The mechanism of hypoxemia, if it occurs in the above condition, is ____________________.
16. Status asthmaticus can lead to (over/under) hydrated states, (increased/decreased) functional residual capacity, and (increased/decreased) density.
17. Two grave signs in patients with status asthmaticus are ____________________ and ____________________.
18. The triad of conditions described by Virchow that can lead to pulmonary emboli includes ____________________, ____________________, and ____________________.
19. Pulmonary infarction and abscess formation are (frequent/infrequent) complications of pulmonary emboli.
20. In acute pulmonary embolism, ventilation-perfusion ratios go ____________________, pulmonary vascular resistance goes ____________________, and the ____________________ ventricle may fail.
21. The most accurate diagnostic study for pulmonary emboli is ____________________.
22. Two nursing interventions that may help prevent pulmonary emboli are ____________________ and ____________________.
23. When rib sections are freed by fractures in at least two places and the chest wall moves paradoxically, it is called a ____________.
24. Signs of right-sided tension pneumothorax may include __________ __________ breath sounds and ____________________ percussion note over the right thorax, and deviation of the trachea to the ____________________.

25. Factors that increase the risk of developing pneumonia include impairment of both the ____________ and ____________ airway's defense system.
26. Pneumonia can lead to ____________ respiratory rate, ____________ breath sounds with ____________ superimposed, ____________ percussion note, and ____________ vocal fremitus.
27. Two general causes of pulmonary aspiration are ____________ and ____________.
28. Pathologic consequences of aspiration include ____________ functional residual capacity, ____________ compliance, and bronchial ____________.
29. The mechanism of hypoxemia in aspiration is ____________.
30. Indicate whether the following potential sequelae of near drowning are common or uncommon:
    a. Aspiration ____________
    b. Aspiration of large volume of fluid ____________
    c. Hypoxemia ____________
    d. Disseminated intravascular coagulation (DIC) ____________
31. Possible postoperative pulmonary changes include a ____________ in functional residual capacity, a ____________ in pulmonary compliance, and respirations that are more ____________ and ____________.
32. Preoperative teaching in patients with a high pulmonary risk profile should include ____________ and ____________.
33. A major problem with carbon monoxide inhalation is that it has a high affinity for ____________, which leads to tissue ____________.
34. The normal carboxyhemoglobin level, even in people who smoke, should not exceed ____________ %.
35. Name the type of neoplastic lung disease that fulfills each of the following descriptions:
    a. Has the best prognosis ____________
    b. Has the worst prognosis ____________
    c. Is the most common ____________
    d. Is most likely to metastasize early ____________
36. The most important risk factor for neoplastic lung disease is ____________.
37. Staging of cancer of the lung is based on these three factors:
    a. ____________
    b. ____________
    c. ____________

E. Summary of Patient Health Problems (*pages 84–124*)

After reading each disease, summarize the pathophysiology, etiology, nursing assessment data base, and nursing diagnoses. The certification examination holds you responsible for knowing the etiology and risk factors, the signs and symptoms, the collaborative diagnosis, the complications, and the management and the treatment goals. Those preparing to take it should also summarize these areas. If they are not clearly covered in the *Core,* a second resource may be necessary. The space allotted is purposefully limited to encourage concise descriptions of concepts and careful selection of key points. It is not as helpful to write the things you already know as it is to write those you need to study.

1. Acute Respiratory Failure

Pathophysiology	*Etiology/Risk Factors*	*Signs/Symptoms*

Collaborative Diagnosis	*Complications*	*Management/Goals*

2. Adult Respiratory Distress Syndrome

Pathophysiology	*Etiology/Risk Factors*	*Signs/Symptoms*

Collaborative Diagnosis	*Complications*	*Management/Goals*

3. Chronic Obstructive Pulmonary Disease

Pathophysiology	*Etiology/Risk Factors*	*Signs/Symptoms*

Collaborative Diagnosis	*Complications*	*Management/Goals*

4. Asthma and Severe Asthmatic Attack

Pathophysiology	*Etiology/Risk Factors*	*Signs/Symptoms*

Collaborative Diagnosis	*Complications*	*Management/Goals*

5. Pulmonary Embolism

Pathophysiology	*Etiology/Risk Factors*	*Signs/Symptoms*

Collaborative Diagnosis	*Complications*	*Management/Goals*

6. Chest Trauma

Pathophysiology	*Etiology/Risk Factors*	*Signs/Symptoms*

Collaborative Diagnosis	*Complications*	*Management/Goals*

7. Acute Pneumonia

Pathophysiology	*Etiology/Risk Factors*	*Signs/Symptoms*

Collaborative Diagnosis	*Complications*	*Management/Goals*

8. Pulmonary Aspiration

Pathophysiology	*Etiology/Risk Factors*	*Signs/Symptoms*

Collaborative Diagnosis	*Complications*	*Management/Goals*

9. Near Drowning

Pathophysiology	*Etiology/Risk Factors*	*Signs/Symptoms*

Collaborative Diagnosis	*Complications*	*Management/Goals*

10. Pulmonary Problems in Surgical Patients

Pathophysiology	*Etiology/Risk Factors*	*Signs/Symptoms*

Collaborative Diagnosis	*Complications*	*Management/Goals*

11. Acute Pulmonary Inhalation Injuries

Pathophysiology	*Etiology/Risk Factors*	*Signs/Symptoms*

Collaborative Diagnosis	*Complications*	*Management/Goals*

12. Neoplastic Lung Disease

Pathophysiology	*Etiology/Risk Factors*	*Signs/Symptoms*

Collaborative Diagnosis	*Complications*	*Management/Goals*

F. Application to Clinical Practice

Care for patients with pulmonary disease. Relate the anatomy, physiology, assessment, and pathophysiology found in this section to their individual clinical pictures. Make note of instances where they correlate and of those where they deviate from the expected presentation. Devise a care plan based on the data collected.

Answers to Pulmonary Exercises

A. Physiologic Anatomy

1. Oxygen, carbon dioxide (*page 1*)
2. Cellular, internal (*page 1*)
3. Bronchial artery (*page 1*)
4. Nose, start of the respiratory bronchiole or end of the terminal bronchiole (*page 2*)
5. 2 cc (*page 2*)
6. Cricoid (*page 3*)
7. Carina or bifurcation of the trachea (*page 3*)
8. Parasympathetic (*page 3*)
9. Dilate (*page 3*)
10. Type II alveolar cells (*page 4*)
11. a. Prevents alveolar collapse during expiration
    b. Decreases the work of breathing
    c. Acts as a defense against inhaled substances (*page 5*)
12. Respiratory rate, tidal volume (*page 5*)
13. Alveolar, dead space (*page 6*)
14. Anatomic, alveolar (*page 6*)
15. VD/VT, 20%–40% (*page 6*)
16. Arterial carbon dioxide tension (*page 6*)
17. Low, increase (*page 7*)
18. Mucociliary escalator, lymphatic (*page 8*)
19. Diaphragm, 3rd–5th cervical (*page 8*)
20. External intercostals, 1st-11th thoracic nerves (*page 8*)
21. Up, down (*page 9*)
22. Lower (*page 9*)
23. Below atmospheric, above atmospheric (*page 9*)
24. Elastic resistance, compliance (*pages 9, 10*)
25. pH (*page 11*)
26. Stretch, inspiration (*pages 11, 12*)
27. More (20 times more) (*page 12*)
28. Lower (*pages 12, 13*)
29. a. Decreased percent of inspired oxygen
    b. Decreased atmospheric pressure
    c. Increased levels of carbon dioxide (*page 13*)
30. *See answer below*
31. Bound to hemoglobin or in the red cell (*page 13*)
32. 90 (*page 14*)
33. a. Increased hydrogen ion concentration
    b. Increased carbon dioxide levels
    c. Increased temperature
    d. Increased 2,3-diphosphoglycerate levels (*pages 14, 15*)
34. *See answer below*
35. *See answer below*
36. Up, down (*page 16*)
37. Red cell (*page 17*)

30.

	pAO_2	*A-a*
a.	$.21\ (713) - \frac{40}{.8} = 100$	$100 - 80 = 20$
b.	$.30\ (713) - \frac{40}{.8} = 164$	$164 - 80 = 84$
c.	$.21\ (713) - \frac{80}{.8} = 50$	$50 - 40 = 10$
d.	$1.00\ (713) - \frac{40}{.8} = 663$	$663 - 80 = 583$ (*page 13*)

34. a. $(15 \times 1.34 \times .99) + (.0031 \times 100) = 20.21$ cc/100 cc blood
    b. $(18 \times 1.34 \times .75) + (.0031 \times 45) = 18.23$ cc/100 cc blood
    c. $(8 \times 1.34 \times .99) + (.0031 \times 100) = 10.92$ cc/100 cc blood
    d. $(8 \times 1.34 \times .75) + (.0031 \times 45) = 8.18$ cc/100 cc blood (*pages* 15, 16)

35.

	CaO_2	*CO of 3L*	*CO of 5L*	*CO of 7L*
a.	202 cc/liter	606 cc	1010 cc	1414 cc
b.	182 cc/liter	547 cc	911 cc	1276 cc
c.	108 cc/liter	324 cc	540 cc	756 cc
d.	84 cc/liter	252 cc	420 cc	588 cc (*page 16*)

38. Up (*page 17*)
39. Constrict (*page 18*)
40. More (*page 18*)
41. Low inspired oxygen tension, alveolar hypoventilation (*page 19*)
42. Ventilation to perfusion mismatch or $\dot{V}/\dot{Q}$ abnormalities (*pages 19–21*)
43. Shunting (or true shunting) (*page 21*)
44. Up, down (*page 22*)
45. 20:1 (*page 22*)
46. a. $\uparrow pCO_2$, $\leftrightarrow HCO_3^-$, $\downarrow$ pH
    b. $\downarrow pCO_2$, $\leftrightarrow HCO_3^-$, $\uparrow$ pH
    c. $\leftrightarrow pCO_2$, $\downarrow HCO_3^-$, $\downarrow$ pH
    d. $\leftrightarrow pCO_2$, $\uparrow HCO_3^-$, $\uparrow$ pH
47. a. Respiratory acidosis
    b. Respiratory alkalosis
    c. Metabolic acidosis
    d. Metabolic acidosis
    e. Metabolic alkalosis
    f. Metabolic alkalosis (*pages 23–25*)
48. a. Metabolic alkalosis
    b. Metabolic acidosis
    c. Respiratory alkalosis
    d. Respiratory acidosis (*page 25*)
49. a. Hypoxemia, acidemia due to metabolic acidosis with secondary respiratory alkalosis (poorly compensated).
    b. Hyperoxemia, alkalemia due to respiratory alkalosis without metabolic compensation.
    c. Hypoxemia, alkalemia due to both respiratory and metabolic alkalosis.
    d. Acidemia due to metabolic acidosis with secondary respiratory alkalosis (poorly compensated).
    e. Hypoxemia, acidemia due to both respiratory and metabolic acidosis.
    f. Hyperoxemia, metabolic acidosis with secondary respiratory alkalosis compensating pH.
    g. Acidemia due to respiratory acidosis with secondary metabolic alkalosis (poorly compensated).
    h. Alkalemia due to respiratory alkalosis with secondary metabolic acidosis.
    i. Alkalemia due to metabolic alkalosis with secondary respiratory acidosis (*pages 22–27*)

B. Nursing Assessment Data Base

1. Any three of these (*page 27*)
   a. Restrictive disease
   b. Obstructive disease
   c. Neuromuscular disease
   d. Chest wall disorders
2. Any three of these (*page 28*)
   a. Inhaled irritants
   b. Aspiration
   c. Airway disease
   d. Lung disease
   e. Left ventricular failure
3. Chest wall disorders, ipsilateral shoulder (*page 29*)
4. Any two of these (*page 30*)
   a. Asthma
   b. Cystic fibrosis
   c. Bronchiectasis
   d. Emphysema related to lack of α_1-antrypsin
5. Packs per day, years of smoking (*page 30*)
6. Angle of Louis or sternal notch (*page 31*)
7. One third, barrel chest (*page 32*)
8. Paradoxical breathing (*page 33*)
9. Increase in reduced hemoglobin or decreased hemoglobin saturation (*page 34*)
10. Central (*page 34*)
11. Cherry red (*page 34*)
12. Left (*page 35*)
13. Down (*page 35*)
14. Up (*page 35*)
15. Duller, resonant (*pages 36, 37*)
16. Vesicular (*page 32*)
17. a. Near sternum
    b. Between scapula
    c. Right upper lobe (*page 38*)
18. Increase (*page 39*)
19. Crackles (rales) (*page 39*)
20. Wheeze or rhonchi (*page 39*)
21. Rhonchi (*page 39*)
22. Consolidation or increased density (*page 40*)
23. 500–700 cc (*page 43*)
24. Vital capacity, 3000–5000 (*page 43*)
25. Functional residual capacity (*page 44*)
26. Forced expiratory volumes (*page 44*)
27. Distensibility (*page 45*)
28. Down (*page 45*)
29. Dynamic (*page 46*)
30. Up, up (*pages 45, 46*)

C. Commonly Encountered Nursing Diagnoses

1. 3 cm above the carina or at the sternal notch (*page 48*)
2. 20 (*page 49*)
3. There are many possible complications for each intervention listed. The pages are listed for reference.

a. (*page 48*)
b. (*page 48*)
(1) (*pages 51–52*)
(2) (*pages 52–53*)
(3) (*pages 53–54*)
c. (*pages 62–66*)
d. (*pages 76, 77*)
e. (*page 80*)

4. Any three of these (*page 51*)
a. Inadequate conditioning of inspired air
b. Increased mucus production
c. Decreased ciliary activity
d. Aphonia
e. Difficulty coughing and swallowing
5. High frequency (*page 56*)
6. Assist (*page 57*)
7. Intermittent mandatory ventilation (*page 57*)
8. Pressure support ventilation (*page 58*)
9. More reliable volume delivery (*page 58*)
10. Any two of these (*page 59*)
a. Massive pulmonary hemorrhage
b. Massive subcutaneous emphysema of unknown etiology
c. Pneumothorax
11. Larger (*page 60*)
12. Decrease, down (*page 62*)
13. a. Increase FIO_2 or add PEEP (*pages 66–81*)
b. Increase alveolar ventilation by either increasing the total volume or rate, or by decreasing dead space (*pages 66–81*)
c. Slowly decrease the alveolar ventilation by decreasing the total minute volume or by increasing the dead space (*pages 66–81*)
14. Disconnect the patient from the ventilator and ventilate manually with a self-inflating bag (*page 66*)
15. Any three of these (*page 67*)
a. Disease process improving
b. Adequate strength
c. Adequate nutritional status
d. PaO_2 above 55 or an FIO_2 .50 or below
e. Stable hemodynamic status
f. Adequate hemoglobin
g. Acceptable pulmonary function studies
h. Adequate level of consciousness
i. Psychologic preparedness
16. Any three of these (*pages 67–68*)
a. Decreased tidal volume
b. Increased respiratory rate
c. Increased apprehension
d. Diaphoresis
e. Fatigue
17. Any three of these (*page 68*)
a. Insufficient ventilatory drive
b. Hypoxemia
c. Respiratory muscle fatigue
d. Low compliance
e. High work of breathing
f. Many other nonpulmonary problems can contribute
18. a. Assist/control
b. Intermittent mandatory ventilation
c. Intermittent mandatory ventilation
d. Assist/control, and intermittent mandatory ventilation (*pages 57–58, 68–69*)
19. Any two of these (*page 70*)
a. Narcotics
b. Sedatives
c. Paralyzing agents
20. Sedated or narcotized, block motor activity (*page 70*)
21. Beta or Beta-2 (*page 71*)
22. a. Beta-1 and Beta-2
b. Methylxanthine
c. Beta-2 stimulant (*page 71*)
23. Carbon dioxide (*page 72*)
24. Tissue, arterial oxygen tension (*page 73*)
25. Any two of these (*page 74*)
a. Restlessness
b. Anxiety, apprehension
c. Headache
d. Confusion, disorientation
e. Impaired judgment
f. Yawning
26. Respiratory depression or hypoventilation (*pages 75, 76*)
27. Any two of these (*pages 76, 77*)
a. Hypoventilation
b. Microatelectasis
c. Oxygen toxicity
28. 50–60 mm Hg (*page 77*)
29. Air entrainment or venturi mask (*page 78*)
30. Increasing (*page 79*)
31. Decreased cardiac output, barotrauma (*page 80*)
32. Continuous positive airway pressure (CPAP) (*page 81*)

D. Pathologic Conditions

1. Any two of these (*pages 19–22, 84*)
a. Low inspired oxygen tension

b. Hypoventilation
c. Ventilation-perfusion mismatching
d. Shunting (true or absolute shunting)
e. Diffusion impairment

2. Any three of the following (*pages 85–86*):
   a. Central nervous system changes (headache, confusion, irritability, somnolence, dizziness)
   b. Muscle twitching, asterixis
   c. Miosis
   d. Papilledema, engorged fundal veins
   e. Diaphoresis
   f. Hypertension
3. a. ↓ pO_2
   b. ↓ pO_2, ↑ pCO_2, ↓ pH
   c. ↓ pO_2, ↑ pCO_2, ↑ HCO_3^-, ↓ pH (*pages 85–87*)
4. Up, down, down (*page 88*)
5. Oxygen, PEEP (*page 88*)
6. Progressive hypoxemia without hypercapnea (*page 90*)
7. Decreased, increased, increased, normal (*page 90*)
8. Bronchitis (*page 76*)
9. Ventilation-perfusion mismatching, hypoventilation (*page 91*)
10. Emphysema (*page 91*)
11. Alveolar surface area, ventilation-perfusion mismatching (*page 92*)
12. Smoking (*page 92*)
13. a. Chronic bronchitis
    b. Emphysema
    c. Chronic bronchitis
    d. Emphysema
    e. Chronic bronchitis
    f. Emphysema
    g. Chronic bronchitis
    h. Emphysema
    i. Emphysema (*pages 91–93*)
14. Asthma (*page 94*)
15. Ventilation-perfusion mismatching (*page 94*)
16. Under, increased, decreased (*pages 94–97*)
17. Diminished breath sounds, increased carbon dioxide levels (*page 97*)
18. a. Blood stasis
    b. Increased coagulability
    c. Change in blood vessel wall (*page 98*)
19. Infrequent (*page 98*)
20. Up, up, right (*pages 98, 99*)
21. Pulmonary angiography (*page 100*)
22. Any two of these (*page 101*)
    a. Early ambulation, exercise
    b. Turn, cough, deep breath
    c. Elastic stockings, pressure stockings
    d. Adequate hydration status
23. Flail chest (*pages 102, 103*)
24. Decreased or absent, hyperresonant or tympanic, left (*pages 103, 104*)
25. Upper, lower (*page 105*)
26. Increased, bronchial, crackles, duller, increased (*page 108*)
27. Vomiting, regurgitation (*page 109*)
28. Decreased, decreased, constriction or spasm (*pages 109–110*)
29. Shunting (or ventilation-perfusion mismatch) (*pages 109–110*)
30. a. Common
    b. Uncommon
    c. Common
    d. Uncommon (*pages 112–114*)
31. Decrease, decrease, rapid, shallow (*pages 115–116*)
32. Any two of these (*page 117*)
    a. Instruction to stop smoking 2 days before surgery
    b. Instruction in breathing, coughing, and activity exercises
    c. Instruction in range of motion
    d. Instruction in use of potential respiratory therapy equipment
33. Hemoglobin, hypoxia (*page 118*)
34. Ten (*page 119*)
35. a. Squamous-cell carcinoma
    b. Small-cell carcinoma
    c. Adenocarcinoma
    d. Small-cell carcinoma (*pages 120–121*)
36. Smoking (*page 122*)
37. a. Size, location, local complications
    b. Lymph-node involvement
    c. Distant metastasis (*page 124*)

E. Summary of Patient Health Problems

Refer to the following pages in the Core Curriculum

---

1. Acute Respiratory Failure (*pages 84–87*)
2. Adult Respiratory Distress Syndrome (*pages 87–90*)
3. Chronic Obstructive Pulmonary Disease (*pages 90–94*)
4. Asthma and Severe Asthmatic Attack (*pages 94–97*)
5. Pulmonary Embolism (*pages 98–101*)
6. Chest Trauma (*pages 101–105*)
7. Acute Pneumonia (*pages 105–109*)

THE PULMONARY SYSTEM

Post Quiz

The following questions are designed to test your understanding of some of the key points in the section. Select the one best answer for each. The correct answers appear at the end of the test.

---

1. The gas exchanging airways include the
   a. carina
   b. bronchi
   c. terminal bronchioles
   d. respiratory bronchioles
2. When doing an endotracheal intubation on a child under the age of 6,
   a. never inflate the cuff with more than 10 cc of air
   b. deflate the cuff for 5 minutes every hour
   c. remember that the left bronchus is easier to enter than the right
   d. because of the narrowing of the cricoid, it is not necessary to use a cuffed tube
3. Surfactant is synthesized mainly by
   a. alveolar type II cells
   b. bronchial glands
   c. macrophages
   d. alveolar type I cells
4. Pulmonary surfactant
   a. prevents the collapse of the bronchioles during expiration
   b. prevents the collapse of alveoli during expiration
   c. prevents the alveoli from overdistending during inspiration
   d. increases the work of breathing
5. One of the important pulmonary responses to hypoxia is
   a. vasoconstriction
   b. vasodilation
   c. bronchoconstriction
   d. bronchodilation
6. The vessel that carries oxygenated blood to the lungs is the
   a. pulmonary artery
   b. pulmonary vein
   c. bronchial artery
   d. bronchial vein
7. The pulmonary circulation
   a. is a relatively high-resistance circuit
   b. constricts in response to cholinergic stimulation
   c. contains 12% of the total blood volume
   d. has difficulty accommodating blood volume changes
8. The intrapulmonary pressure
   a. decreases as the chest wall expands
   b. is always subatmospheric

c. becomes more negative during expiration
d. is always lower than the intrapleural pressure

9. Expiration is due to
   a. the natural elastic recoil of the lungs
   b. contractions of the external intercostal muscles
   c. decreased atmospheric pressure
   d. contraction of the diaphragm
10. Early obstructive disease may be revealed by
   a. an increased VC
   b. a decreased FRC
   c. a decreased FEV_1
   d. decreased compliance
11. The tidal volume (V_T) is
   a. the amount of air left in the lungs at the end of a forced exhalation
   b. the sum of the inspiratory capacity and the functional residual volume
   c. the amount of air moved in and out with each breath
   d. the amount of air a patient can breathe in one minute
12. Alveolar ventilation is
   a. the respiratory rate multiplied by the tidal volume
   b. normally 5–6 L per minute
   c. the part of ventilation that is found in effective alveoli
   d. the sum of the anatomic and physiologic dead space
13. A parameter that is used to assess lung expansibility is
   a. compliance
   b. resistance
   c. FEV_1
   d. V_D/V_T
14. The alveolar oxygen tension is
   a. normally 80–100 mm Hg
   b. normally higher than the pIO_2
   c. affected by pCO_2 and H_2O vapor entering inspired gas
   d. not affected by hypo- or hyperventilation
15. Most carbon dioxide is transported as
   a. bicarbonate after a reaction involving water
   b. $paCO_2$
   c. combined with proteins
   d. carboxyhemoglobin
16. The oxygen-hemoglobin dissociation curve is
   a. the relationship between pO_2 and Hgb saturation
   b. the relationship between pO_2 and pCO_2
   c. the relationship between pO_2 and oxygen content
   d. a linear relationship
17. In the normal individual the strongest respiratory drive is based on changes in
   a. pO_2 of the alveoli
   b. pH of the medullary extracellular fluid
   c. pO_2 of blood in the aorta
   d. pH of venous blood
18. Compliance is
   a. the relationship between pressure and flow
   b. the relationship between pressure and volume
   c. increased with pneumonia
   d. not affected by the condition of the chest wall
19. Static compliance
   a. is the peak airway pressure divided by the tidal volume
   b. goes up in many lung diseases

c. is measured in liters per second
d. is usually higher than dynamic compliance
20. A shift in the oxygen-hemoglobin dissociation curve to the left
a. causes all the saturations to be lower than predicted from the pO_2
b. usually results in better oxygenation of the tissues
c. usually results in poorer oxygenation of the pulmonary capillary blood
d. may occur in hypothermia
21. An increased pCO_2 causes the oxygen-hemoglobin dissociation curve to
a. shift to the right
b. shift to the left
c. increase the RBC's affinity for O_2
d. increase the RBC's affinity for CO_2
22. The effect of 2,3-diphosphoglycerate is to
a. increase tissue oxygenation
b. increase oxygen-hemoglobin affinity
c. shift the oxygen-hemoglobin curve to the left
d. increase the venous oxygen content
23. An increased pCO_2 reflects
a. alveolar hypoventilation
b. alveolar hyperventilation
c. increased minute ventilation
d. compensation for metabolic acidosis
24. According to the Henderson-Hasselback equation, the ratio of base to acid is
a. 1:20
b. 1:1
c. 20:1
d. 7.45:7.35
25. A blood gas with the following values

pO_2 = 65 torr   pH = 7.25
pCO_2 = 50 torr HCO_3^- = 24

represents
a. acute respiratory acidosis
b. acute respiratory alkalosis
c. chronic respiratory acidosis
d. chronic respiratory alkalosis
26. A blood gas report for a patient in diabetic ketoacidosis would most likely show
a. metabolic alkalosis with partial respiratory compensation
b. respiratory alkalosis with partial metabolic compensation
c. metabolic acidosis with partial respiratory compensation
d. respiratory acidosis with partial metabolic compensation
27. Most of the oxygen is transported as
a. pCO_2
b. oxyhemoglobin
c. pO_2
d. H_2CO_3
28. Acetazolamide (Diamox) is given to
a. make the lungs blow off more CO_2
b. make the lungs retain more CO_2
c. make the kidneys excrete more HCO_3^-
d. make the kidneys excrete less HCO_3^-
29. Inhalation of carbon monoxide can result in
a. increased carboxyhemoglobin
b. increased oxyhemoglobin

c. increased oxygen transport
d. cyanosis

30. Continuous adventitious sounds caused by airway narrowing and usually heard best on expiration are
   a. crackles
   b. wheezes
   c. rubs
   d. bronchial sounds
31. Which of the following is *not* a sign of consolidation?
   a. whispering pectoriloquy (increased transmission of the whisper)
   b. bronchial sounds heard in the peripheral lung tissues
   c. bronchophony (increased transmission of the voice sounds)
   d. hyperresonance
32. Percussion of the chest will elicit hyperresonance in
   a. normal lung tissue
   b. atelectatic lung tissue
   c. pneumothorax
   d. pneumonia
33. Intracuff pressures of endotracheal tubes cause less necrosis and work best when maintained below
   a. 5 mm Hg
   b. 20 mm Hg
   c. 60 mm Hg
   d. 100 mm Hg
34. The sound normally heard between the scapulae is
   a. vesicular
   b. bronchial
   c. bronchovesicular
   d. bronchophony
35. Fine end-expiratory crackles that clear with coughing and deep breathing are most likely to be associated with
   a. restrictive disease
   b. emphysema
   c. secretions in the large airways
   d. pleuritis
36. Positive end-expiratory pressure
   a. decreases the FRC
   b. is used to treat hypoxemia and atelectasis
   c. will always increase cellular oxygenation
   d. is an alternative to mechanical ventilation
37. Possible complications of mechanical ventilation include
   a. high cardiac output
   b. barotrauma
   c. negative water balance
   d. polyuria
38. The mode of mechanical ventilation whereby the patient can trigger the ventilator but all breaths are machine-delivered is
   a. controlled
   b. assist-control
   c. synchronized intermittent mandatory (SIMV)
   d. continuous positive airway pressure (CPAP)
39. Potential complications of oxygen therapy include
   a. hyperventilation in patients with COPD
   b. atelectasis

c. retrolental fibroplasia in adults
d. increased compliance

40. In setting up a volume-cycled positive pressure ventilator on assist/control in a postoperative patient without lung disease,
a. the tidal volume is usually initially set at 10–15 cc/kg
b. the I:E ratio should be 2:1
c. the pressure limit is set 10–20 below the pressure observed when the tidal volume is delivered
d. no back-up rate is required

41. Cyanosis of the mucous membranes of the mouth can be most accurately attributed to
a. hypoxia
b. an abnormal amount of unsaturated hemoglobin
c. possible presence of carbon monoxide poisoning
d. peripheral rather than central cyanosis

42. Arterial blood gases with a pO_2 of 40 mm Hg, a pCO_2 of 36 mm Hg, and a pH of 7.15 are consistent with
a. hypoxemia with respiratory alkalosis
b. hypercapnea with respiratory alkalosis
c. hypoxemia with metabolic acidosis
d. hypercapnea with metabolic acidosis

43. Chronic hypoxia may result in
a. polycythemia
b. anemia
c. pulmonary vasodilation
d. metabolic acidosis

44. Signs of hypercarbia and acidemia would most likely include
a. central nervous system changes
b. decreased saturation on the pulse oximeter
c. cyanosis
d. bradycardia

45. Early clinical manifestations of ARDS include
a. tachypnea
b. hypoventilation
c. lethargy
d. increased compliance

46. Signs of tension pneumothorax include
a. a mediastinal shift toward the affected side
b. hyporesonance on the affected side
c. widening of the intercostal spaces on the affected side
d. rhonchi over the unaffected side

47. Diagnostic studies in patients with severe chronic airway obstruction may reveal
a. increased forced expiratory volumes
b. prolonged inspiratory phase
c. decreased functional residual capacity
d. hypoxemia during sleep

48. The prognosis for near drowning is predominantly dependent on
a. whether it was fresh or salt water aspiration
b. whether the victim is male or female
c. the length of the hypoxic episode
d. the occurrence of immediate reflex larnygospasm

49. The most reliable diagnostic tool for pulmonary emboli is
a. the physical examination
b. the chest x-ray study

c. the lung scan
d. pulmonary angiography

50. The initial treatment of status asthmaticus is most likely to be
    a. sedation
    b. bronchodilators
    c. mechanical ventilation
    d. diuretics

Answers to Pulmonary Post Quiz

1. **d** (*page 3*)
2. **d** (*page 3*)
3. **a** (*page 4*)
4. **b** (*page 5*)
5. **a** (*page 18*)
6. **c** (*page 2*)
7. **c** (*page 18*)
8. **a** (*page 9*)
9. **a** (*page 9*)
10. **c** (*page 44*)
11. **c** (*page 43*)
12. **c** (*page 5*)
13. **a** (*page 45*)
14. **c** (*page 13*)
15. **a** (*page 17*)
16. **a** (*page 14*)
17. **b** (*page 11*)
18. **b** (*page 10*)
19. **d** (*page 45*)
20. **d** (*page 15*)
21. **a** (*page 15*)
22. **a** (*page 15*)
23. **a** (*page 7*)
24. **c** (*page 22*)
25. **a** (*pages 23–25*)
26. **c** (*page 24*)
27. **b** (*page 15*)
28. **c** (*page 26*)
29. **a** (*page 119*)
30. **b** (*page 39*)
31. **d** (*pages 35–40*)
32. **c** (*page 36*)
33. **b** (*page 49*)
34. **c** (*page 38*)
35. **a** (*page 39*)
36. **b** (*pages 79, 80*)
37. **b** (*page 57*)
38. **b** (*pages 42, 43*)
39. **b** (*pages 76, 77*)
40. **a** (*pages 60, 61*)
41. **b** (*page 34*)
42. **c** (*pages 23–26*)
43. **a** (*pages 91–94*)
44. **a** (*page 85*)
45. **a** (*pages 87–90*)
46. **c** (*pages 103, 104*)
47. **d** (*pages 90–94*)
48. **c** (*pages 112–114*)
49. **d** (*page 100*)
50. **b** (*page 97*)

As explained in the instructions in the introduction to the book, these are primarily the comprehend or recall, and apply or analyze levels of questions. Examples of synthesis or evaluate questions can be found in the comprehensive examination at the end of the book on pages 278 to 293.

2

The Cardiovascular System

SECTION-RELATED TIPS FOR THOSE STUDYING TO TAKE THE CERTIFICATION EXAMINATION

There are two areas that are worth reviewing before studying this section: (1) determinants of flow and (2) determinants of myocardial oxygen supply and demand. They are the backbone of much of the physiologic principles that guide interventions in patients with cardiovascular disorders.

DETERMINANTS OF FLOW

The function of the cardiovascular system is to provide blood flow. Therefore, the factors that determine cardiovascular function can be examined by looking at the laws of the physics of flow. It can be shown that flow rate through tubes is directly related to the pressure gradient across its two ends. Flow, then, from the left ventricle through the systemic system into the right atrium is increased as the left ventricular systolic pressure increases or the right atrial pressure decreases. Obviously, the magnitude of change possible is much higher in the left ventricle.

Factors that are indirectly related to flow rate are collectively referred to as resistance or impedance forces. The most important resistance factor is the diameter of the lumen. Narrowing it decreases flow exponentially. A second determinant is the viscosity of the solution. The higher the viscosity, the slower the flow.

In the cardiovascular system, the arteriole controls resistance by dilating to increase flow and by constricting to decrease it. The reason the right ventricle can provide adequate flow through the pulmonary system with far less systolic pressure than the left ventricle is because the pulmonary vascular tree has far less resistance. Changes in blood viscosity are most often due to changes in the hematocrit. Small changes in the hematocrit can cause significant changes in resistance to flow.

The relationship between the three variables, flow rate (F), pressure gradient (ΔP), and resistance (R), can be stated mathematically by the formula:

$$F = \frac{\Delta P}{R}$$

Further mathematical manipulation can be used to solve for the other two variables, such as

$$R = \frac{\Delta P}{F}, \qquad \Delta P = F \times R$$

These interrelationships are the bases for reaching a working understanding of cardiovascular physiology.

DETERMINANTS OF MYOCARDIAL OXYGENATION

Myocardial Perfusion

Blood flow required to meet the demand resulting from repetitive myocardial muscle activity is delivered through the coronary arteries. Each coronary artery originates behind one of the cusps of the aortic valve. This facilitates their need for more flow during diastole than during systole because during diastole the cusps are bellowed out with blood and this directs flow into their ostia. Systole greatly restricts flow, especially to the left ventricle. Blood flows from the coronary arteries on the epicardial surface of the heart through perpendicular branches down to the endocardium. Most of the venous return is via surface veins.

Factors That Affect Oxygen Supply

Flow through the coronary circuit must meet the changing oxygen demands of the myocardium. The primary determinant of oxygen supply is the coronary blood flow affected by the pressure gradient and the resistance [$F = (\Delta P/R)$]. Normally, the coronary arteries dilate in response to increased demand much as the rest of the vascular beds do. Where flow to the heart is unique is in the pressure gradient. The heart is the only organ where the diastolic pressure is more important to perfusion than the systolic. In addition to right atrial pressure at the other end of the circuit, there is pressure around the perpendicular branches which increases during systole. Tachycardias both increase systolic time and decrease diastolic time to challenge perfusion. Pressure against subendocardial perfusion increases when patients have high ventricular diastolic pressures.

Other factors affecting oxygen supply are extraction and oxygen content. Extraction is normally increased to the extent that coronary venous saturation runs about 25% compared with other veins, which average 75% at rest. The heart routinely extracts three quarters of the oxygen available while the rest of the body only extracts one quarter. Oxygenation deficits, therefore, are more likely in the myocardium than in other organs during hypoxemic or anemic states, since others can benefit from increased extraction and increased cardiac output. The heart has to increase its demand to increase its supply via the latter mechanism.

Factors That Affect Oxygen Demand

The primary determinant of demand is heart rate, since all others are multiplied by it. Others include the force of contraction, the resistance to outflow, and wall tension. Laplace's law demonstrates that wall tension is a product of the diastolic pressure inside the ventricle and the surface area. It is not just how high the pulmonary artery wedge pressure or left ventricular filling pressure is, but also how large the intraventricular area is.

From these physiologic principles, it can be seen why the development of heart failure in patients with coronary artery disease is associated with a poor prognosis. The development of a compensatory tachycardia decreases supply and increases demand. Increased ventricular diastolic pressures also decrease supply and increase demand.

Please see the instructions at the beginning of the book for important general suggestions that are relevant to the bulk of the *Core Curriculum* content. They apply to this section as well as to all of the others.

Summary

Factors That Increase Supply	Factors That Increase Demand
↑ Coronary blood flow	↑ Heart rate
↑ Diastolic pressure	↑ Contractility
↑ Diastolic time	↑ Afterload
↑ Transmural gradient	↑ Wall tension
↑ Oxygen extraction	
↑ Oxygen content	

FIGURES AND TABLES

Refer to these figures and tables while reading the Cardiovascular Section of the Core Curriculum.

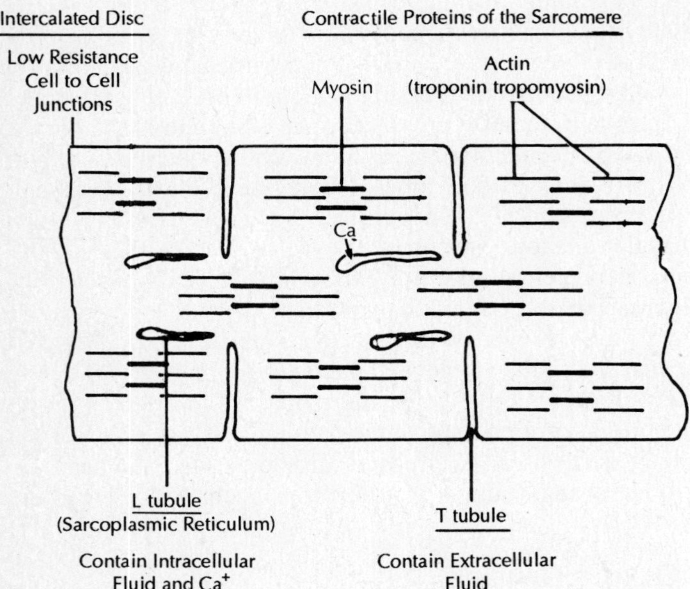

Figure 2–1. Specialized structure muscle cell (*pages 132–133*).

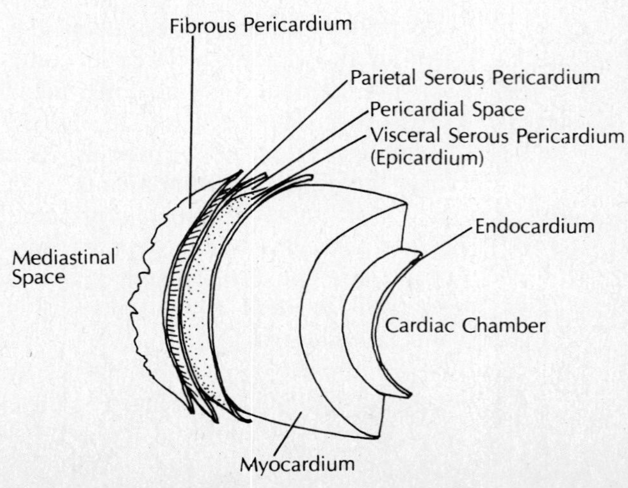

Figure 2–2. Cross-sectional anatomy of the cardiac wall (*pages 133–134*).

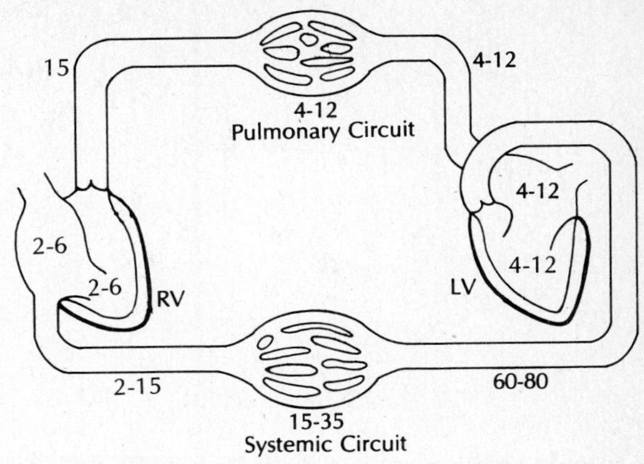

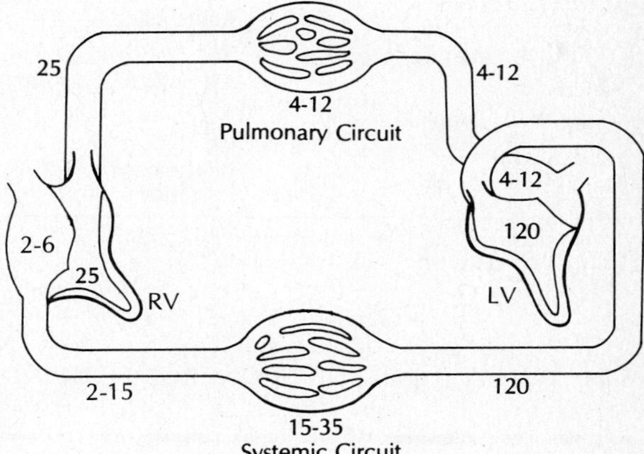

Figure 2–3. Comparison of the diastolic (*top*) and systolic (*bottom*) pressures and valve positions. Right and left ventricles are indicated *RV* and *LV*, respectively. All pressures are in mm Hg (*pages 134, 135, 149, 194–197*).

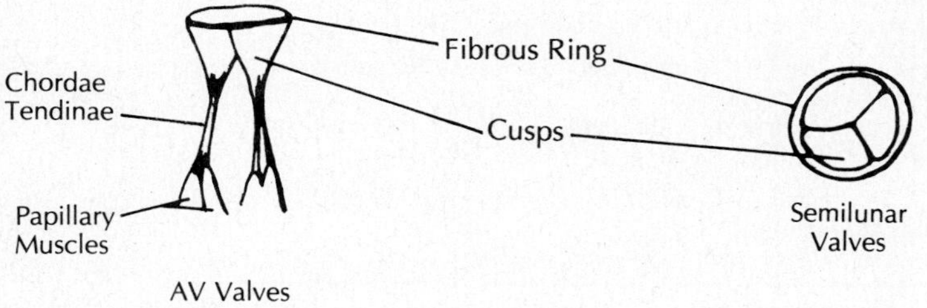

Figure 2–4. Structure of the atrioventricular (AV) and semilunar valves (*pages 134, 135*).

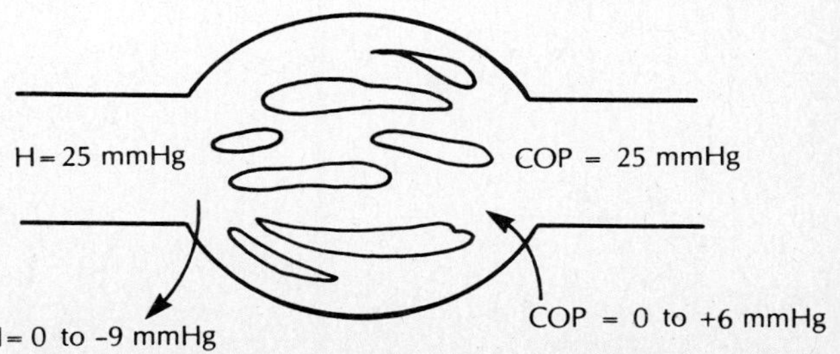

Figure 2–5. Factors affecting fluid movement across the systemic capillary membrane: hydrostatic pressure (H), which tends to push fluid from higher pressure areas, and colloid osmotic pressure (COP), which tends to draw fluid toward higher pressure areas. The overall balance of these pressures is no net fluid movement (*page 136*).

Table 2–1. COMPARISON OF RIGHT AND LEFT CORONARY ARTERIES (*pages 138, 139*)

	Right Coronary Artery	Left Coronary Artery
Branches	Posterior descending (80% of time) Acute marginal	Anterior descending Circumflex
Conduction Structures Supplied	SA node (55% of time) AV node (90% of time)	RBB Anterosuperior LBB
Muscle Walls Supplied	RA RV Inferoposterior LV Posterior septum	Anterior LV Anterior septum Lateral LV

SA indicates sinoatrial; AV, atrioventricular; RBB, right bundle branch; LBB, left bundle branch; RA, right atrium; RV, right ventricle; LV, left ventricle.

Table 2–2. FACTORS THAT CONTROL PERIPHERAL BLOOD VESSELS (*pages 140–142*)

Mechanism	Description
Local Control	Is dominant unless overridden by autonomic reflex mechanisms Designed so that blood flow matches tissue demand (↑ demand = arteriolar dilation; ↓ demand = arteriolar constriction)
Autonomic Regulation	Sympathetic stimulation = vasoconstriction in arteries and veins Parasympathetic = vasodilation in arteries and veins
Stretch Receptors	↑ Stretch of select arteries = ↓ sympathetic tone; ↓ stretch of select arteries = ↑ sympathetic tone ↑ Stretch of vena cava or atria = ↑ sympathetic tone; ↓ stretch of vena cava or atria = ↓ sympathetic tone
Vasomotor Center	Stimulation via ↓ BP, ↓ paO_2, ↑ $paCO_2$ or ↓ pH = ↑ HR, ↑ SV, ↑ BP, venoconstriction Inhibition (by reverse of above factors) = vasodilation, ↓ SV, ↓ BP

BP indicates blood pressure; HR, heart rate; SV, stroke volume.

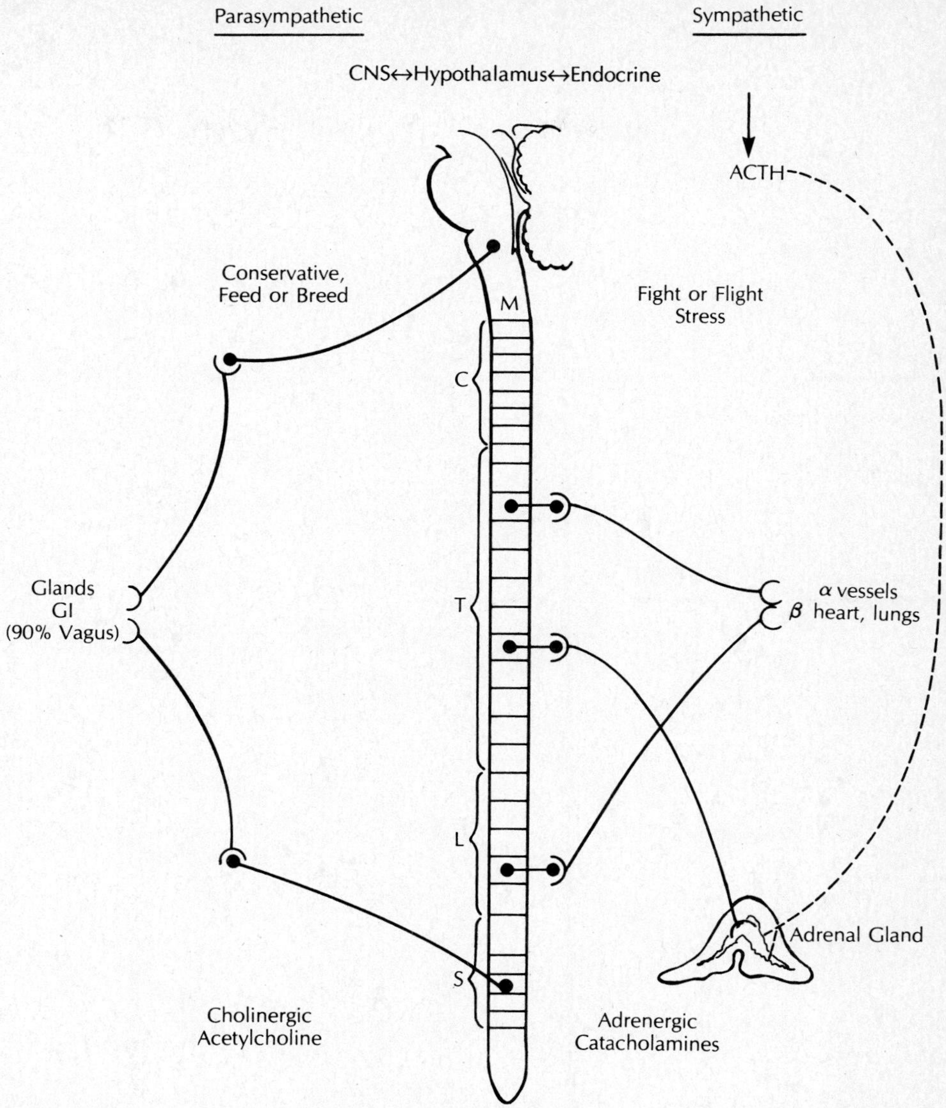

Parasympathetic
Sympathetic
CNS↔Hypothalamus↔Endocrine
ACTH
Conservative,
Feed or Breed
Fight or Flight
Stress
M
C
T
L
S
Glands
GI
(90% Vagus)
α vessels
β heart, lungs
Adrenal Gland
Cholinergic
Acetylcholine
Adrenergic
Catacholamines

Figure 2–6. Comparison of the parasympathetic and sympathetic aspects of the autonomic nervous system, including the origin of the peripheral nerves, the site of ganglions (—•), the major types of reactions caused, and the kind of nerve ending activity (*bottom*). The central nervous system (CNS) is depicted in center with medulla (*M*), and cervical (*C*), thoracic (*T*), lumbar (*L*), and sacral (*S*) cord segments indicated. Some of the anatomy is presented in the nervous system section (*pages 141, 144*).

K
Na
Ca
Polarized
(Resting)
Ca
Na
Depolarization
K
Repolarization

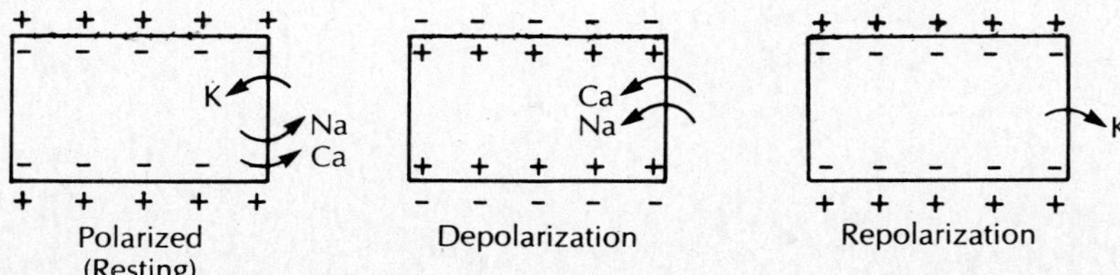

Figure 2–7. Ionic movement and changes in intracellular charge during phases of depolarization and repolarization (*pages 145–147*).

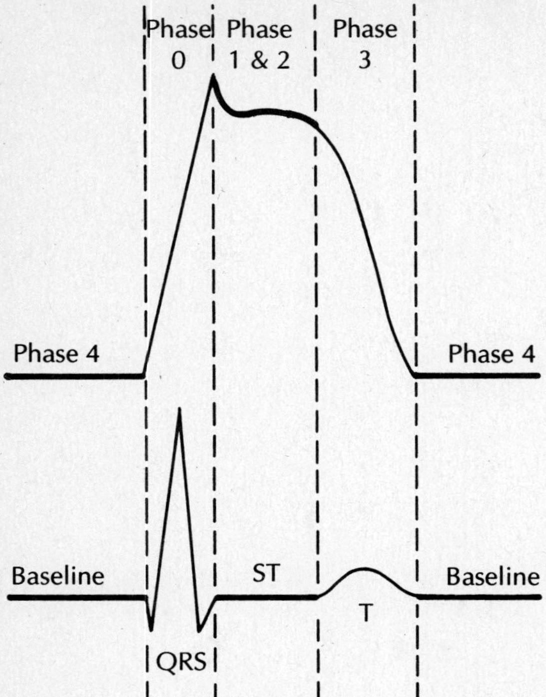

Figure 2–8. Comparison of electrical events in the ventricle myocardium as depicted by the action potential (*top*) and surface electrocardiogram (ECG) (*bottom*) (*pages 145–147*).

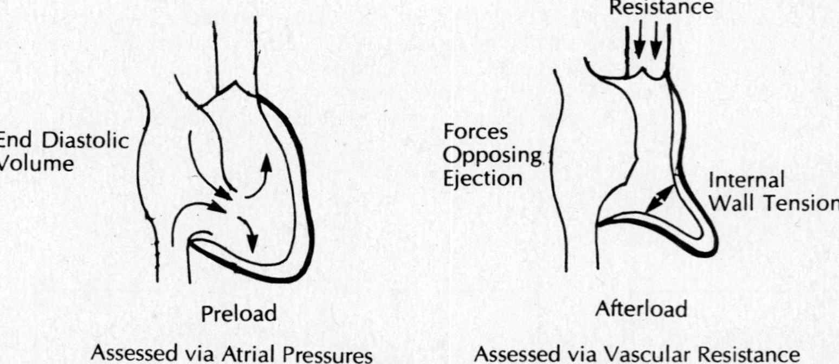

Figure 2–9. Comparison of preload and afterload SVR indicates systemic vascular resistance; LAP indicates left atrial pressure; RAP indicates right atrial pressure; PAW̄P indicates pulmonary artery wedge pressure (*pages 150–152*).

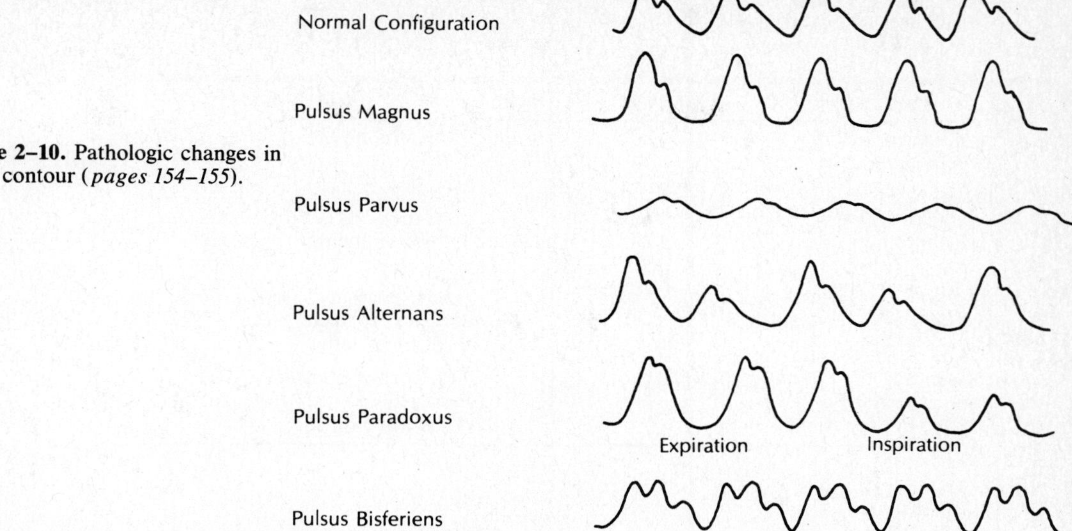

Figure 2–10. Pathologic changes in pulse contour (*pages 154–155*).

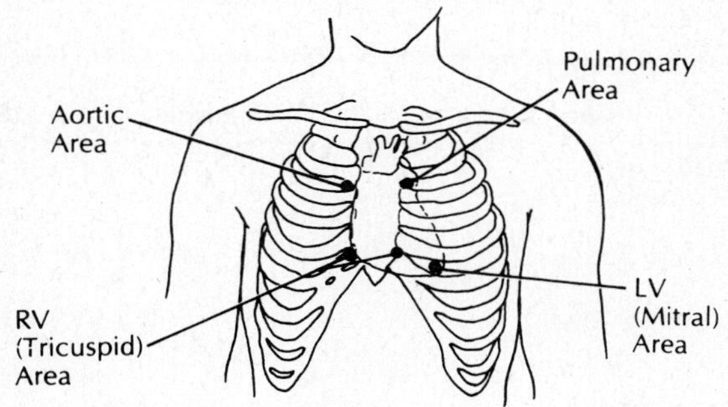

Figure 2–11. Primary areas used for inspection, palpation, and auscultation (*pages 156–157*).

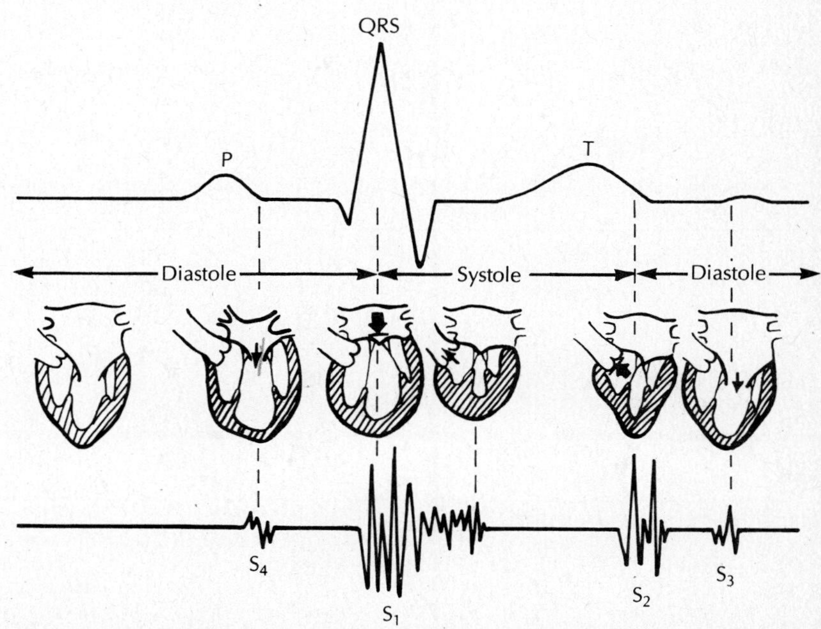

Figure 2–12. Relationship between electrical (*top*), mechanical (*middle*), and audible events (*bottom*) of a cardiac cycle. Heavier arrows indicate abrupt deceleration of blood flow due to valve closure. Thinner arrows indicate less abrupt phases of augmented blood flow (*pages 156–158*).

Table 2–3. COMPARISON OF TYPES OF SPLITTING OF THE SECOND HEART SOUND (S_2) INTO AORTIC (A) AND PULMONIC (P) COMPONENTS (*pages 158–159*)

Type	Expiration	Inspiration	Major Causes
Physiologic Splitting (only heard in inspiration)	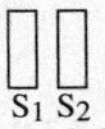 S_1 S_2	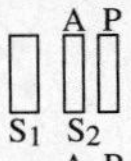 A P S_1 S_2	Occurs normally
Fixed Splitting (heard continuously with constant distance between A_2 and P_2)	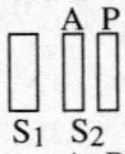 A P S_1 S_2	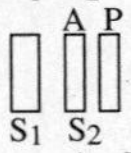 A P S_1 S_2	Atrial Septal Defect Disorders that lead to a constant load on the right ventricle
Wide Splitting of S_2 (heard continously with distance wider in inspiration)	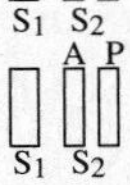 A P S_1 S_2	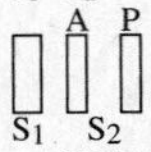 A P S_1 S_2	Disorders that cause the right ventricle to complete ejection after the left
Paradoxical Splitting (heard continuously with distance wider in expiration)	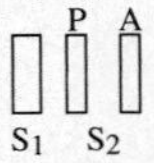 P A S_1 S_2	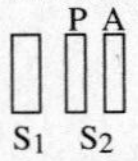 P A S_1 S_2	Disorders that cause the left ventricle to complete ejection after the right

Table 2–4. COMPARISON OF CHARACTERISTICS OF COMMON SYSTOLIC MURMURS (*pages 163–165*)

Murmur	Area (Radiation)	Timing	Comments
Mitral insufficiency	Apex (left axilla)	Pansystolic	Blowing, high pitched
Tricuspid insufficiency	Lower LSB (RSB)	Pansystolic	Harsh, ↑ on inspiration
Aortic stenosis			
Valvular	2nd ICS RSB (neck, back, apex)	Systolic ejection	Crescendo-decrescendo, harsh
Subvalvular	2nd, 3rd, 4th ICS at RSB (apex, LSB)	Systolic ejection	Crescendo-decrescendo, ↓ on expiration, ↑ with valsalva
Supravalvular	2nd ICS at RSB, Suprasternal notch (neck)	Systolic ejection	Crescendo-decrescendo, harsh
Pulmonary stenosis	2nd ICS at LSB (left neck)	Systolic ejection sound (click)	Crescendo-decrescendo, harsh, ↑ intensity and ↑ S_2 split on expiration
Intraventricular septal defect	LSB	Pansystolic	Heard all over
Coarctation of aorta	L midback between scapulae (neck)	Systolic ejection	Crescendo-decrescendo

LSB indicates left sternal border; RSB, right sternal border; ICS, intercostal space.

Table 2–5. COMPARISON OF CHARACTERISTICS OF COMMON DIASTOLIC MURMURS (*pages 165–166*)

Murmur	Area (Radiation)	Timing	Comments
Mitral stenosis	Apex	Mid-diastolic or presystolic	Faint, ↑ by lying on left side, not affected by inspiration, may have opening snap
Tricuspid stenosis	4th ICS at LSB (apex, xiphoid)	Protodiastolic	May ↑ on inspiration, rumbling decrescendo, may have opening snap
Aortic insufficiency	3rd, 4th ICS at LSB and 2nd ICS at RSB	Pandiastolic	Blowing, faint, high pitched, decrescendo
Pulmonary insufficiency	2nd ICS at LSB (toward apex)	Pandiastolic	Decrescendo, high pitched, blowing, may ↑ on inspiration
Patent ductus arteriosus	2nd ICS at LSB (neck)	Continuous	Harsh

Table 2–6. SUMMARY OF CAUSES OF KEY CARDIOVASCULAR PHYSICAL ASSESSMENT PHENOMENA (*pages 152–166*)

Sign or Symptom	Common Cause	Page
Neck Vein Distention	Increased in patients with high CVP Decreased in patients with low CVP	153
Hepatojugular Reflux	Presence indicates presence of right ventricular compromise or failure Absence does not rule it out and guarding by the patient invalidates the test	154
Bounding Pulses (Pulsus Magnus)	Correlates with disorders that lead to high stroke volumes or hyperdynamic states	154
Thready Pulses (Pulsus Parvus)	Correlates with disorders that lead to decreased stroke volume or decreased blood flow	154
Pulsus Alternans	Present in some patients with severe left ventricular failure	155
Pulsus Paradoxus	Present in disorders that prevent the heart from full diastolic relaxation (pressure around outside of heart) or in severe hypovolemic states	155
Pulsus Bisferiens	Present in some patients with aortic valvular disorders, cardiomyopathy, or pericarditis	155
S_3 or S_4 Gallop	Present in patients with decreased ventricular compliance and usually indicates heart failure. (Major exceptions are young patients in a hyperdynamic state for S_3 and patients with new myocardial infarction for S_4)	159, 160
Murmurs	Correlates with turbulance often related to valvular disorders. The site of maximal intensity indicates which valve is to blame. Whether it is diastolic or systolic indicates which function that valve cannot perform (open or close, i.e., stenosis or regurgitance)	157, 161–166

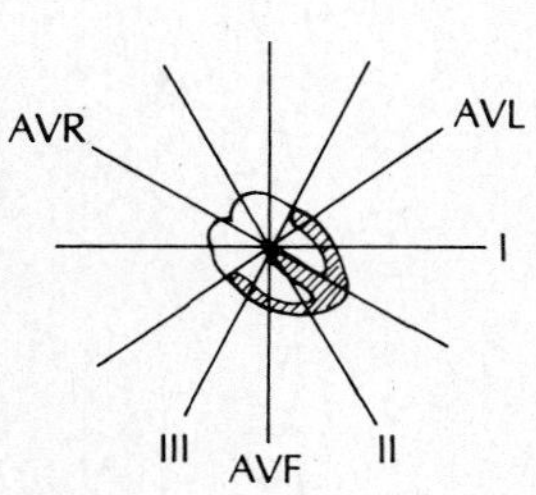

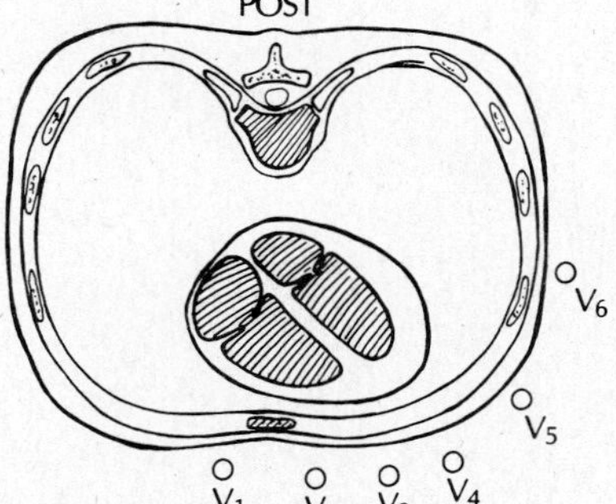

Figure 2–13. Normal position of the six limb leads (*left*) and six chest leads (*right*). The positive end of each lead is labeled (*pages 173–174*).

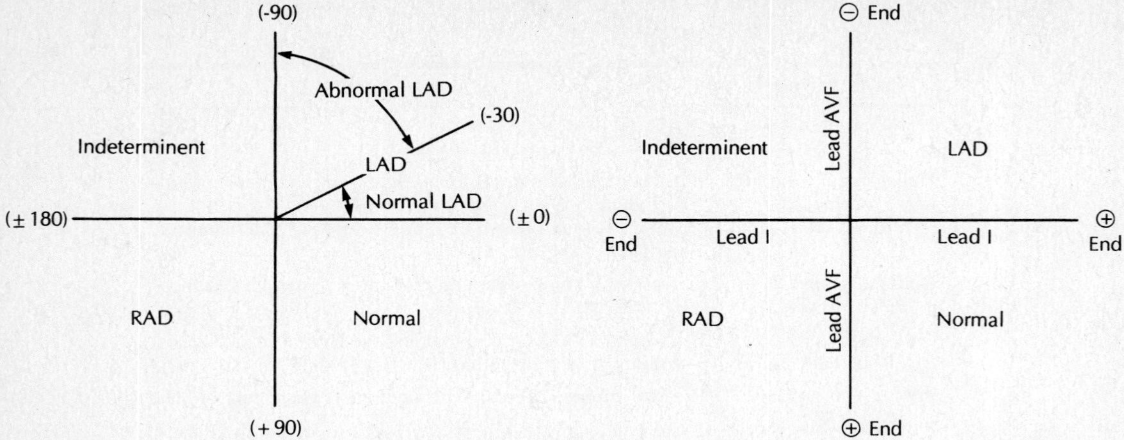

Figure 2–14. Left-hand diagram indicates borders of quadrants used to determine axis deviations to the right (right axis deviation, RAD) and left (left axis deviation, LAD). Right-hand diagram indicates the leads that correspond to those borders (*pages 175, 186*).

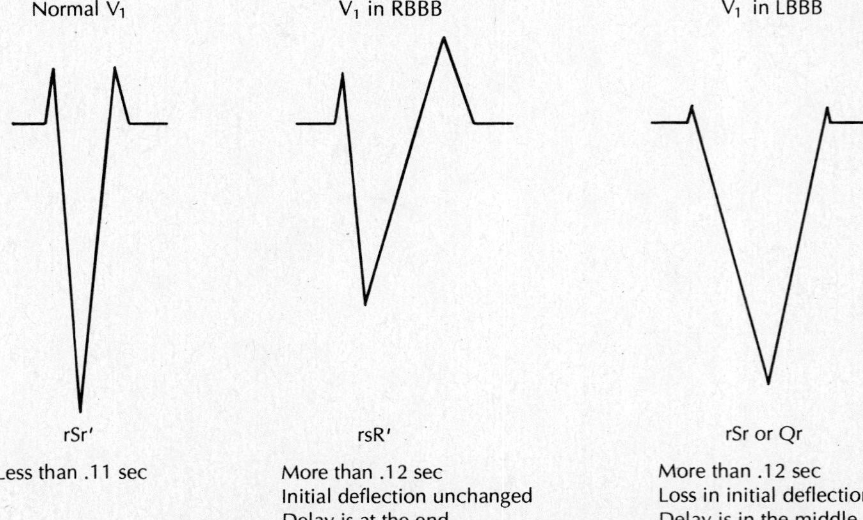

Figure 2–15. Classic changes in V_1 related to bundle branch block (*pages 185–186*).

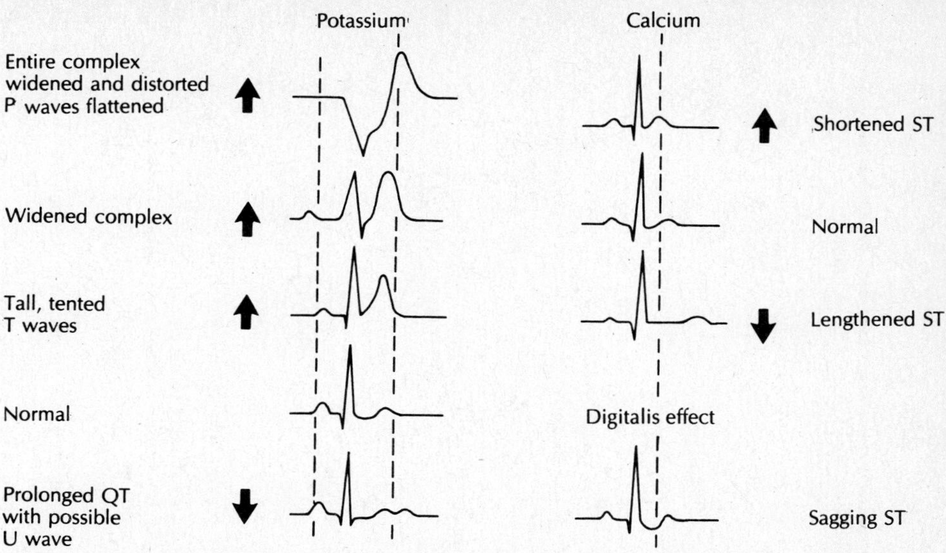

Figure 2–16. Comparison of ECG changes caused by increases (↑) and decreases (↓) in potassium and calcium levels. The effect of digitalis is also included (*pages 187–188*).

Table 2–7. SUMMARY OF SUSTAINED RHYTHMS (*pages 175–187*)

Rhythm	P Waves	QRS Waves	P : R Relationship	Comments
Sinus Rhythm	60–100/min Normal vector is −30° to 90°	60–100/min Normal vector is 0° to 90° (up to +120° in young pts, up to −30° in older pts) Normal duration is .08 to .10 sec	1 : 1 with PR .12 to .20 sec	Fairly regular; may vary with respiration and is then called sinus arrhythmia
Sinus Bradycardia	40–60/min Vector unchanged	40–60/min Vector and duration unchanged	1 : 1 with PR on the long side of normal	Fairly regular
Sinus Tachycardia	100–180/min Vector unchanged	100–180/min Vector and duration unchanged	1 : 1 with PR on the short side of normal	Fairly regular
Sinus Exit Block	60–100/min except when block occurs Pause is usually exactly twice the normal P to P interval	60–100/min except when block occurs Vector and duration unchanged	1 : 1 with normal PR	Suspect Wenckebach phenomenon when P waves appear to have group beating
Sinus Pause	60–100/min except when pause occurs Pause is not exactly twice the normal P to P interval Vector unchanged	60–100/min except when pause occurs Vector and duration unchanged	1 : 1 with normal PR interval	Becomes sinus arrest when the pause is excessive and asystole when persistent
Atrial Tachycardia	150–250/min Maintain typical P wave appearance Vector may change	200/min or less Vector and duration unchanged	May be 1 : 1 at lower rates AV becomes refractory to 1 : 1 conduction at higher rates and block down to 2 : 1 Treatment or conduction defects can result in higher degrees of AV block PR Interval tends to be constant unless the AV conducts with a Wenckebach phenomenon	Very regular P wave Regularity of QRS depends on the regularity of AV conduction Suspect Wenckebach phenomenon with group beating of QRS Suspect complete block if both atrial and ventricular rates are regular but do not have a fixed relationship

Multiformed Atrial Tachycardia	Above 100/min Atrial rate is irregular and there are 3 or more differently shaped P's. Each has its own rate and vector	Above 100/min Vector and duration unchanged	1 : 1 relationship May have a different PR for each P wave	May be called wandering atrial pacemaker at rates below 100/min
Atrial Flutter	250–350/min Continuous sawtooth appearance (called F wave) Very regular and predictable Will distort QRS, ST, and T wave	175/min or less Vector and duration unchanged	AV becomes refractory to 1 : 1 conduction and blocks down to 2 : 1 Treatment or conduction defects can result in higher degrees of AV block PR Interval tends to be constant unless the AV conducts with a Wenckebach phenomenon	Very regular F wave Regularity of QRS depends on the regularity of AV conduction Suspect Wenckebach phenomenon with group beating of QRS Suspect complete block if both atrial and ventricular rates are regular but do not have a fixed relationship
Atrial Fibrillation	Discrete activity replaced by chaotic depolarization Cannot be counted but known to vary 300–750/min Baseline constantly affected, even distorting ST and T waves Waves may be coarse and easily identified or fine and difficult to see at all	Up to 200/min Vector and duration unchanged	Chaotic, very irregular and unpredictable, depending on balance between AV stimulation and refractoriness Some may be conducted aberrantly Treatment and conduction defects may result in higher degrees of AV block	Typically irregular Suspect complete block if ventricular rate is regular
Junctional Rhythms	40–60/min if visible Vector reflects retrograde conduction May be just before or just after the QRS May be hidden in the QRS	40–60/min Vector and duration unchanged	1 : 1 with short PR interval in those that occur before QRS	Called accelerated junctional rhythm when the rate is 60–100/min Called junctional tachycardia when the rate is 100–160/min Called accelerated junctional tachycardia when the rate is 160–200/min

Table continued on following page

Table 2–7. SUMMARY OF SUSTAINED RHYTHMS (*pages 175–187*) *Continued*

Rhythm	P Waves	QRS Waves	P : R Relationship	Comments
Ventricular Tachycardia	60–100/min if sinus rhythm is present May not be visible	100–250/min Vector may change Duration is over .12 msec	Not related An occasional sinus may happen to hit a nonrefractory AV node and "capture" the ventricles with a supraventricular-looking QRS	Tends to be slightly irregular, especially at lower rates Called accelerated ventricular rhythm when the QRS rate is 60–100/min. Called idioventricular rhythm when the QRS rate is 20–60/min Called torsade de pointes when the QRS twists about the baseline
Ventricular Fibrillation	Cannot be seen	Cannot be seen Replaced by chaotic undulations May be coarse and obvious or fine and difficult to see	Not related	There is no pulse associated Called ventricular flutter when it has a more regular sawtooth pattern
Sinus Rhythm With 1° Block	60–100/min Vector unchanged	60–100/min Vector and duration unchanged	1 : 1 with PR over .20 sec	All P's conducted
Sinus Rhythm With 2° Block	60–100/min Vector unchanged	Less than P rate Vector and duration unchanged	Type I (Wenckebach): • PR's gradually prolong until P is finally not conducted • QRS is therefore predictably irregular resulting in group beating • Degree of PR prolongation gradually decreases (add most to first PR, least to last PR) • Therefore, the R to R interval gets shorter until the blocked P Type II (Mobitz II): • PR fixed when conducted	Some P's conducted Type I is a nodal block Type II is an infranodal block

			• Nonconducted P's interrupt the QRS rhythm Undifferentiated: • When the P : R relationship is a fixed 2 : 1, the type cannot be determined	
Sinus Rhythm With 3° or Complete AV Block	60–100/min Vector unchanged	Vector and direction unchanged if an escape junctional rhythm kicks in, typically at 40–60/min Vector may be changed and the duration will be lengthened if an escape idioventricular rhythm kicks in, typically below 40/min If no escape rhythm occurs, ventricular asystole will result	Not related	None of the P's are conducted This is one form of A-V dissociation
Wolff-Parkinson-White Syndrome	Normal	Duration increased due to delta wave, an early slurring of the usually vertical QRS onset	Normal	May be intermittent May be visible only in some leads Type A has a positive delta vector in V_1 through V_2 Type B has a negative delta vector in V_1 through V_3
Lown-Ganong-Levine Syndrome	Normal	Normal	The PR interval is shorter than normal	Like WPW, is due to congenital accessory A-V pathways

The term supraventricular tachycardia (SVT) may be used for any tachycardia with a QRS of origin above the ventricles. Called Paroxysmal SVT if it begins and ends abruptly.

Any rhythm of supraventricular origin could undergo 1st, 2nd (types I and II), or 3rd degree block in the AV node. For example, atrial tachycardia may coexist with AV disease. The degree of block can be determined by the same method, looking at the relationship between the P's and QRS's.

Table 2–8. SUMMARY OF PREMATURE BEATS (*pages 176–182*)

Rhythm	P Waves	QRS Waves	P:R Relationship	Comments
PAC's	Comes prematurely May have altered vector	Normal vector and duration if it occurs late enough to be conducted normally Abnormal duration and possibly vector when conducted aberrantly because only one bundle has recovered from its refractory period (80% have RBBB configuration) No QRS if it occurs so early that both bundles are still refractory	May or may not have a QRS	Look for nonconducted P's hidden on the T waves when sudden prolonged R to R intervals occur (May masquerade as a pause)
PJC's	Comes prematurely Vector reflects retrograde conduction	Normal vector and duration if it occurs late enough to be conducted normally Abnormal duration and possibly vector when conducted aberrantly because only one bundle has recovered from its refractory period (80% have RBBB configuration) No QRS if it occurs so early that both bundles are still refractory	May or may not have a P P may occur after the QRS, if conduction reaches the ventricles before the atria, P may be hidden in the QRS when both are depolarized simultaneously	Look for nonconducted inverted P's hidden on the T waves when sudden prolonged R to R intervals occur (May masquerade as a pause)
PVC's	None associated with this beat If sinus rhythm exists, P's may march through the premature beat eliminate without having their rhythm interrupted	Occurs prematurely Duration is over .12 sec Vector may be altered	Not related If it just barely precedes normal QRS, may occur after a normal P but the PR will be short and there still is not a real relationship between them	This is one form of AV dissociation Was considered dangerous to a vulnerable myocardium when (1) PVC occurs during T wave (2) 2 or more in a row (3) More than 6/min (4) More than one morphology These concepts are being challenged and under controversy

When ectopic beats occur during a pause or longer R to R interval instead of prematurely, they are called escape beats.

Table 2–9. DIFFERENTIAL DIAGNOSIS OF WIDE QRS TACHYCARDIAS (*pages 181–186*)

Criteria	Supraventricular with BBB	Ventricular Tachycardia
ECG Characteristics		
V_1 or MCL_1	If QRS is more positive, more likely to be triphasic If QRS is more negative, initial deflection is more likely to be a normal R or a distinct S May have typical right or left BBB appearance 80% of rate-related BBB have right BBB appearance	If QRS is more positive, more likely to be mono- or biphasic If QRS is more negative, initial deflection is more likely to be a broad R or a slurred S Not typical of either BBB
Initial Deflection	More likely the same as before in all leads if right BBB	More likely to be altered
QRS Duration	More likely to be less than .14 sec	More likely to be more than .14 sec
QRS Axis	Less likely to be changed, especially when V_1 is positive	More likely to be changed, especially when V_1 is positive
Capture Beats	Do not occur	May occur but are rare
Precordial Leads	Less likely to be in same direction (positive or negative) in all six leads	More likely to be in same direction (positive or negative) in all six leads
Other Characteristics		
Cannon Waves	Do not occur unless it is a junctional tachycardia in which case they may occur with each beat	Can occur randomly
Venous Waveforms	May have distinct a waves	No distinct a waves
History	More likely if history of PAC's	More likely if history of PVC's
Previous Rhythm Strips	May demonstrate PAC's with same QRS morphology	May demonstrate PVC's with same QRS morphology

Table 2–10. FACTORS AFFECTING CARDIAC OUTPUT (*pages 150–152, 190–192*)

Factor	Method of Assessing	Comments
Heart Rate	Pulse or ECG monitor	Can compromise if too low or if too high. Rates at which patients are symptomatic and need intervention vary greatly
Preload	Right atrial pressure for right ventricle Left atrial or pulmonary capillary wedge pressure	Is affected by: volume status venous tone ventricular function intrathoracic pressure
Afterload	Pulmonary vascular resistance for right ventricle Systemic vascular resistance for left ventricle	Is affected by: arteriolar tone arterial pressure obstruction to flow
Contractility	Direct assessment is difficult	Is affected by: autonomic tone drugs altered chemistry (acid-base and electrolytic imbalances) myocardial oxygenation

Table 2–11. ECG MANIFESTATIONS OF CHAMBER HYPERTROPHY (*pages 172–175*)

Chamber	Manifestation
Right Atria	Tall peaked P wave in II, III, avF
Left Atria	Wide notched P waves in limb leads and left V leads Biphasic with broad negative deflect in P wave in V_1
Right Ventricle	Large QRS's in right-sided V leads or V_3R Right axis deviation
Left Ventricle	Large QRS's in left-sided V leads or AVL Left axis deviation

Table 2–12. A SUMMARY OF FACTORS COVERED IN THE PHYSIOLOGIC AND ASSESSMENT SECTIONS THAT HAVE IMPORTANT CLINICAL APPLICATIONS WORTH EMPHASIZING (*pages 132–205*)

Factors	Clinical Applications	Page
T-tubules	Allow the wave of depolarization and Na and Ca entry to affect the whole cell interior	132
Sarcoplasmic Reticulum	Houses calcium necessary for contraction that if left free would be cytotoxic	132
Mitochondria	High concentration in the myocardium reflect the high demand for energy and explain the heart's high oxygen extraction (coronary venous blood is only 25%–30% saturated compared with 70%–75% in the rest of the body on average)	133
Arteries	Maintain pressure over great distances to provide the entire body with an equal opportunity to receive blood flow	135
Arterioles	Dilate and constrict in response to demand and autonomic control to distribute the blood flow appropriately. Drugs that alter resistance are drugs that affect the arterioles more than the veins	136
Capillary System	The microvasculature is permeable to fluid, the flux of which is determined by Starling's law of the capillary. Forces include hydrostatic pressures, colloid osmotic pressure, and vessel permeability	136
Venous System	These vessels are very compliant and accommodate changes in blood volume. Drugs that alter preload are drugs that affect the veins more than the arterioles	136–137
Stretch Receptors	Preload (atrial stretch) and afterload (arterial stretch) are monitored constantly in vivo and in response, autonomic tone is titrated moment to moment	141
Vasomotor Center	Acts in concert with the stretch receptors but responds to changes in blood gases (pH, pCO_2, pO_2) as well as blood flow	141–142
Factors Affecting Blood Pressure	Changes in pressure are directly related to blood flow and arterial resistance. $\Delta P = F \times R$ This simple relationship can be used to conceptualize both causes and treatment of problems in blood pressure	143
Action Potential	The numbers used to label the action potential are used as reference points to describe the effects of antiarrhythmic agents. They are easier to relate to if you can correlate these phases to their counterparts on the surface ECG	145–148
Role of Calcium in Myocardial Function	Extracellular Ca^+ plays a role in electrophysiology via the influx of calcium during depolarization, especially in pacing cells Intracellular Ca^+ from the sarcoplasmic reticulum plays a mechanical role by triggering sarcomere shortening. Both may be affected pharmacologically by calcium channel blockers	145–148
Indirect Monitoring of Ventricular Pressures	Direct monitoring of ventricular pressures can be avoided since the diastolic pressures are close to those of their atrial pressures, and the systolic pressures are close to those in their arteries. Incompetent valve function upsets these relationships and leads to abnormal pressure gradients	148–150
Heart Sounds	S_1 and S_2 are the sounds normally heard because they are due to valve closure (blood flow deceleration) and are both high pitched and high intensity. S_3 and S_4 are not normally heard because they are due to accelerations in diastolic filling and are both low pitched and low intensity	156–158

Table continued on following page

Table 2–12. A SUMMARY OF FACTORS COVERED IN THE PHYSIOLOGIC AND ASSESSMENT SECTIONS THAT HAVE IMPORTANT CLINICAL APPLICATIONS WORHT EMPHASIZING (*pages 132–205*) *Continued*

Factors	Clinical Applications	Page
Factors Affecting Cardiac Auscultation	Right ventricular gallops and murmurs are louder under conditions that increase venous return (inspiration and recumbent positions) Left ventricular gallops and murmurs are louder under conditions that increase resistance to left ventricular outflow (expiration or increased intrathoracic pressure)	158–163
MUGA Scans and 2-D Echocardiograms	Demonstrate size, position, and motion of the cardiac structures. Evaluation of relative systolic and diastolic size allows calculation of ejection fractions, a sensitive indicator of systolic ventricular function	167–169
Sudden Unexplained Axis Deviations	Suspect left anterior hemiblock if it deviates to the left; left posterior hemiblock if it deviates to the right. Other causes of axis deviation include myocardial infarction (deviates away), chamber hypertrophy (deviates toward) and displacement of the diaphragm up (to the left) or down (to the right).	187–188
Invasive Monitoring	Guidelines to optimize the risk/benefit ratio once a line has been inserted. (1) Make sure numbers used are accurate (2) Use the line for all that would be helpful to managing this patient (3) Prevent and monitor for complications (4) Remove the line as soon as the numbers are no longer needed	194–200
SvO_2 Monitoring	Trends the interaction between tissue's oxygen supply and demand. Increased when (1) Tissue supply increases (increased SaO_2, Hgb, or CO) (2) Tissue demand decreases (hypothermia, decreased metabolic rate)	198–199

MUGA indicates multiple gated acquisition.

Table 2–13. SYMPATHETIC AND PARASYMPATHETIC EFFECTS ON THE CARDIOPULMONARY SYSTEM WITH EXAMPLES OF DRUGS THAT INDUCE THEM (*pages 141, 144, 215, 216, 220–221*)

Type	Effect	Stimulators	Blockers
Sympathetic			
Alpha	Vasoconstriction	Neosynephrine Dopamine at ↑ 10 mcg/kg/min	Phentolamine
Beta B_1	↑ Heart rate ↑ Contractility ↑ Conduction ↑ Irritability	Isoproterenol Dopamine at 2–10 mcg/kg/min Dobutamine Aminophylline	Propranolol Nadolol Metoprolol Atenolol
B_2	Bronchodilation Vasodilation		Esmolol
Both alpha and beta		Epinephrine Norepinephrine Metaraminol (mainly alpha)	Labetolol
Parasympathetic	↓ SA Rate ↓ AV Conduction	Cholinergic drugs Digitalis Vagal stimulation	Atropine

Table 2–14. TYPES OF ANTIDYSRHYTHMIC AGENTS (*pages 219–222*)

Class	Characteristics		Examples
I	Fast Na Channel Blockers ↓ Rate of depolarization ↓ Conduction ↓ Excitability	A	Quinidine Prodainamide Disopyramide
		B	Lidocaine Phenytoin Tocainide Mexiletine
		C	Flecanide Encainide
II	Beta Blockers ↓ Contractility ↓ Conduction in AV node ↓ Sinus node rate		Propranolol Metoprolol Nadolol Timolol Atenolol
III	Prolong Refractory Period Little Effect on Conduction		Amiodarone Bretylium
IV	Ca Channel Blockers		Verapamil Nifedipine Diltiazem

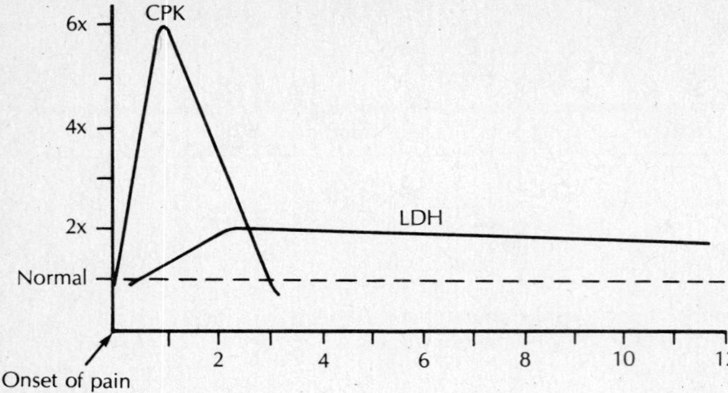

Figure 2–17. Relationship between rises in CPK, and LDH over time in days from the onset of chest pain in myocardial infarction (*pages 224, 225*).

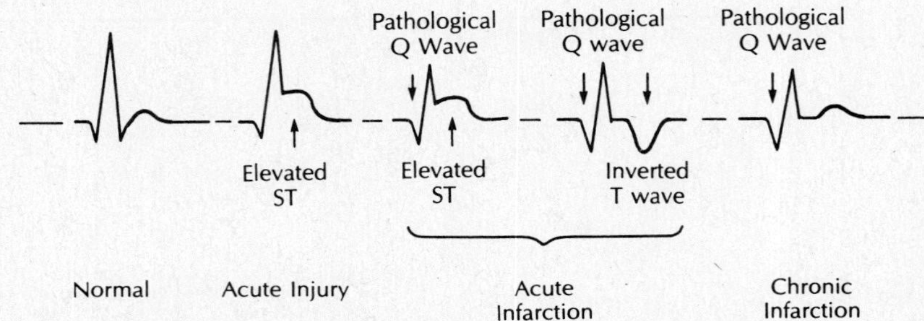

Figure 2–18. Evolution of ECG changes in transmural infarction (*page 226*).

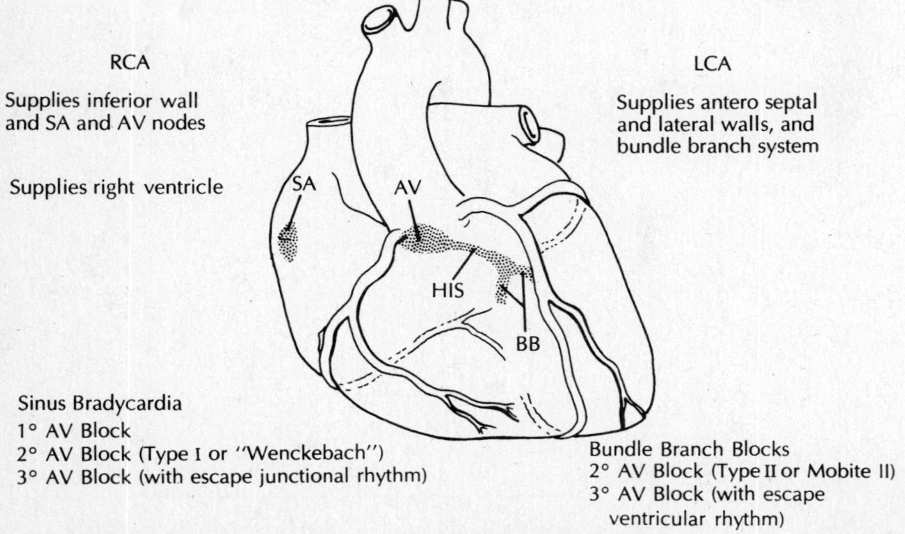

Figure 2–19. Comparison of structures damaged (*top*) and dysrhythmias expected (*bottom*) in obstruction of the right (RCA) and left (LCA) coronary arteries (*page 225*).

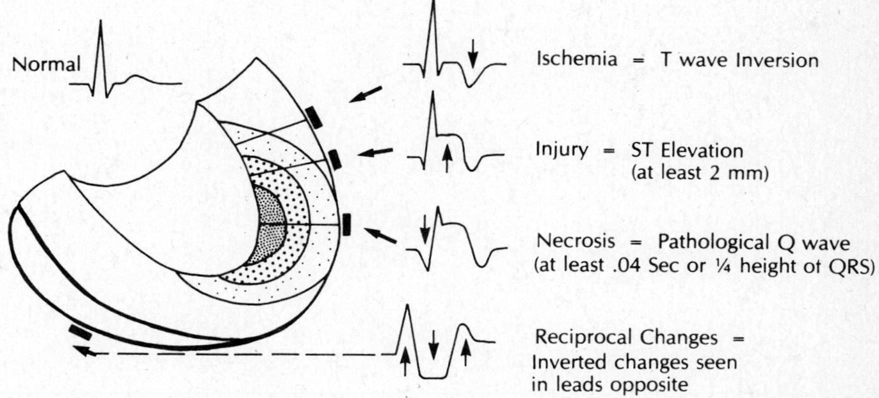

Figure 2–20. Summary of ECG patterns seen in transmural myocardial infarction (*page 226*).

Table 2–15. ECG CHANGES IN VARIOUS TYPES OF MYOCARDIAL INFARCTIONS (*pages 226, 227*)

Wall Infarcted	Leads That Monitor This Wall Directly	Leads That Reflect Changes Reciprocally
Anterior or Anteroseptal	V_1–V_4	II, III, AVF
Inferior or Diaphragmatic	II, III, AVF	V_1–V_4, I, AVL
Lateral	V_5, V_6, I, AVL	II, III, AVF
Posterior	None	V_1–V_3

Table 2–16. COMPARISON OF POTENTIAL INTERVENTIONS FOR PATIENTS WITH CAD (*pages 205–234*)

Intervention	Indications	Contraindications	Comments
Medical Therapy (risk reduction, nitrates, beta blockers, calcium channel blockers)	Control of progression and degree of symptoms by modifying balance of myocardial oxygen supply and demand	Specific to each agent	Important to monitor the side effects, drug interaction, and patient compliance
Percutaneous Transluminal Coronary Angioplasty	Angina or myocardial infarction with appropriate lesions causing greater than 50% stenosis in one or two vessels Patient should be a candidate for possible emergency surgery	Lesions at the aortic orifice or of the left main coronary artery Variant angina	Potential complications include: dissection or occlusion acutely, bleeding or decreased flow in cannulated peripheral artery, reactions to contrast, arrhythmias, reocclusion acutely or over time
Coronary Artery Bypass Grafting	Medically refractory angina due to lesions with more than 50% stenosis Left main or multivessel disease Emergency management of complications of PTCA or of acute myocardial infarction	Patients in whom the potential risk of surgery outweighs the benefits	Potential complications are numerous and are carefully monitored for and managed by specially trained nurses who usually care for these types of patients 1:1 the early post-operative period
Thrombolytic Therapy	New myocardial infarction	Patients at risk of bleeding (recent trauma, delivery, CVA, procedure, surgery, history of bleeding disorder) Streptokinase is contraindicated in patients who have received it before because of the potential for antibody reactions)	Potential complications in addition to bleeding include reperfusion arrhythmias and reocclusion Selection or exclusion criteria continue to be modified as studies are ongoing
Intra-Aortic Balloon Pump	Temporary support and stabilization of patients with preinfarction angina, cardiogenic shock due to acute myocardial infarction, or poor cardiac function immediately post-cardiac surgery	Aortic insufficiency Severe peripheral vascular disease	In general, this intervention is meant for short-term use in patients to buy time or to prevent further loss of functioning myocardium. VADs may be needed for more severe or prolonged dysfunction Potential complications include decreased flow distal to insertion site, aortic dissection, infection, sepsis, thrombocytopenia

Note: Other interventions are under investigation that may be used instead of or in conjunction with bypass grafting in some subsets. They include laser therapy, stents, endarderectomy, and high-speed rotary devices.

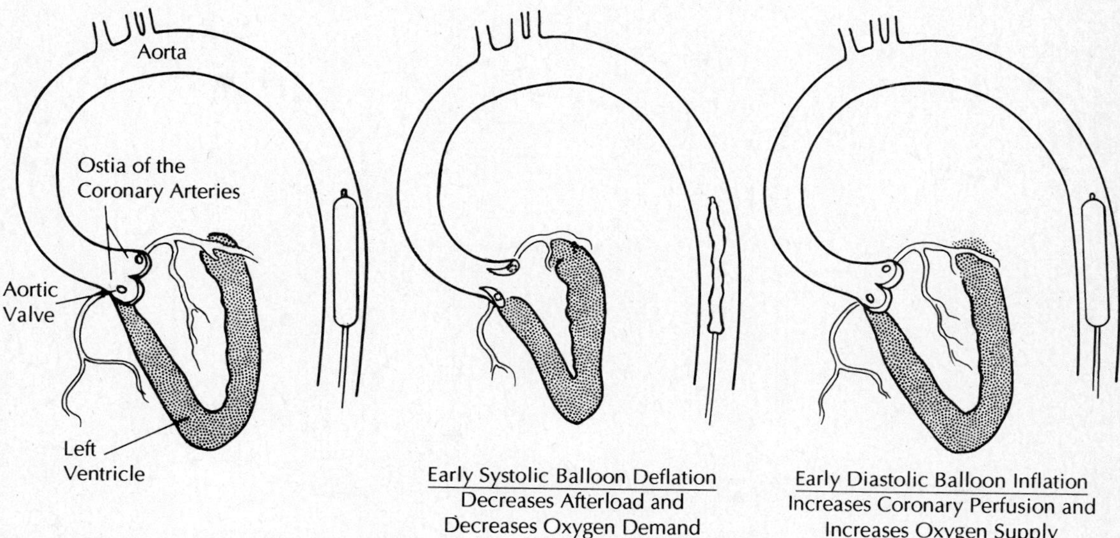

Figure 2–21. The systolic and diastolic effects of the intra-aortic balloon pump (*page 231*).

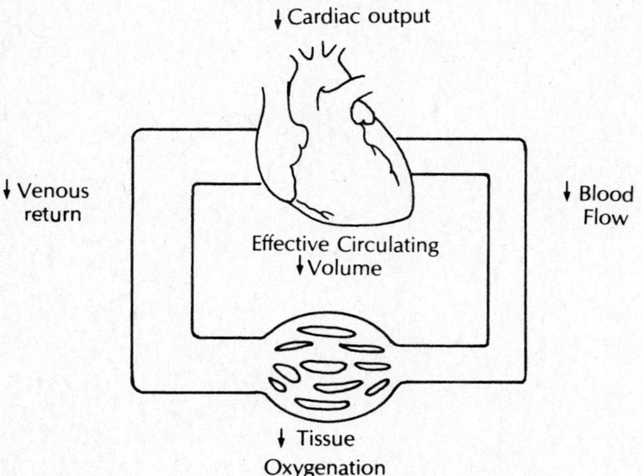

Figure 2–22. Hemodynamic mechanisms of shock (*pages 299–304*).

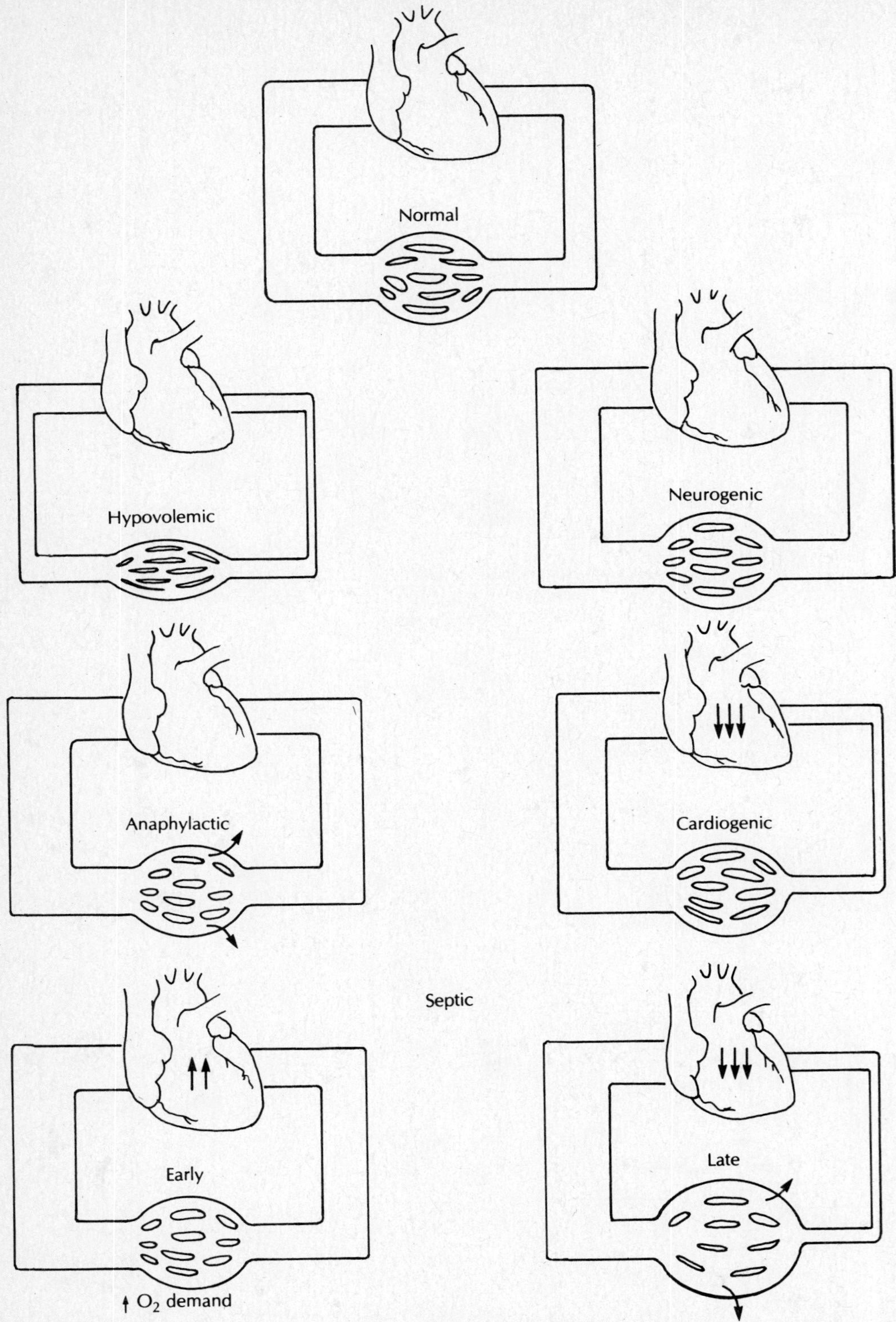

Figure 2–23. Comparison of hemodynamic changes in various categories of shock (*pages 304–306*).

Table 2–17. COMPARISON OF HEMODYNAMIC CHANGES IN THE VARIOUS FORMS OF SHOCK (*pages 304–306*)

Type	Volume	Preload	Afterload	Cardiac Output
Hypovolemic	↓	↓	↑	↓
Neurogenic	↔	↓	↓	↓
Anaphylactic	↓	↓	↓	↓
Cardiogenic	↔	↑	↑	↓
Septic				
Early	↔	↓	↓	↑ or ↔
Late	↔, ↓, or ↑	↔, ↓, or ↑	↑	↓

THE CARDIOVASCULAR SYSTEM

Exercises

After reading the Cardiovascular Section of the Core Curriculum, *fill in the blanks in the following statements. It can be done one topic at a time or all at once. The answers are at the end of the exercises.*

A. Physiologic Anatomy (*pages 132–152*)

1. The contractile unit of muscle cells is called the ______________.
2. The thick filament is made up of the contractile protein ______________.
3. To produce more adenosine triphosphate, the cardiac cell contains more ______________.
4. The outer layer of the heart or inner layer of the pericardium is called either the ______________ or the ______________.
5. More than ______________ % of blood flow from the atria to the ventricles is passive, whereas the rest is provided by the ______________.
6. The valves that must close against pressure during systole are the ______________ and ______________.
7. The semilunar valves are open during the ______________ phase of a cardiac cycle.
8. Two primary factors affecting resistance to blood flow are ______________ and ______________.
9. The major vessel controlling vascular resistance is the ______________.
10. When the capillary hydrostatic pressure falls, the amount of fluid leaving the bloodstream goes ______________.
11. The primary capacitance vessels are the ______________.
12. The role of the AV node is to ______________ conduction.
13. The part of the conduction system that directly depolarizes the ventricular muscle mass is the ______________.
14. Indicate which coronary artery supplies each of the following structures the majority of the time:
    a. Sinus node ______________
    b. Right bundle ______________
    c. Atrioventricular node ______________

d. Anterior wall ____________________
e. Inferior wall ____________________

15. Most of the coronary venous blood drains into the __________ __________ atrium through the ____________________.
16. Alpha sympathetic stimulation causes vessels to __________ __________.
17. When baroreceptors sense increased blood pressure, sympathetic tone goes ____________________.
18. When the vasomotor center senses increased blood pressure, the vasoconstrictor area is ____________________, venous volume goes ____________________, and the stroke volume goes __________ __________.
19. Calculate the pulse pressure (PP) and mean arterial pressure (MAP) in these three patients:
    a. BP = 210/120 PP = __________ MAP = __________
    b. BP = 90/60 PP = __________ MAP = __________
    c. BP = 140/80 PP = __________ MAP = __________
20. A positive inotropic agent increases the ____________________ of the myocardium.
21. Beta-adrenergic stimulation ____________________ the sinus node rate.
22. Parasympathetic stimulation ____________________ the sinus rate and possibly ____________________ atrioventricular conduction.
23. The atria or Bainbridge reflex ____________________ the heart rate when the atrial pressure rises.
24. The most abundant electrolytes are ____________________ intracellularly and ____________________ extracellularly.
25. The electrolytes that enter the cell during depolarization are __________ __________ and ____________________.
26. Return of the membrane potential to its normal state is called ____________________.
27. Major differences in the electrophysiology of pacing cells and myocardial cells are that the ____________________ cells have a lower resting membrane potential, and the ____________________ cells have a spontaneous phase 4 depolarization.
28. The primary electrolyte involved in excitation of the contractile process is ____________________.
29. Describe what causes the three waves seen in atrial pressure tracings.
    a. a wave ____________________
    b. c wave ____________________
    c. v wave ____________________
30. Isovolemic ventricular contraction occurs between __________ __________ and ____________________.
31. The term used to describe the end-diastolic volume or pressure is ____________________.
32. The more a muscle is stretched, the ____________________ it contracts, to a point.
33. Indicate whether the following will increase or decrease the preload:
    a. Hypovolemia ____________________
    b. Ventricular failure ____________________
    c. Vasodilation ____________________
34. Calculate the mean arterial pressure (MAP) and the systemic vascular

resistance (SVR) in both resistance units and dynes in the following patients:

	BP	*CVP*	*CO*	*MAP*	*SVR*			
a.	110/80	5	5.0	____	____	units	____	dynes
b.	210/120	10	3.5	____	____	units	____	dynes
c.	90/60	5	3.0	____	____	units	____	dynes

35. The higher the afterload, the ______________________ the myocardial oxygen demand.

B. Nursing Assessment Data Base (*pages 152–200*)

1. The junction of the manubrium to the body of the sternum is a reference point used to estimate the level of the atria, which lie ____________ ____________ below it.
2. On a scale of 0 to 3, normal pulses are ______________________.
3. Pulsus alternans is found in patients with ______________________, whereas pulsus paradoxus is a sign of ______________________.
4. If the apical area is found 9 cm from the left sternal border, the patient may have (right/left) ventricular hypertrophy, (upward/downward) displacement of the diaphragm, or a (right/left)-sided tension pneumothorax.
5. The aortic area for palpation and auscultation is located near the ______________________, and the pulmonic area is located near the ______________________.
6. The bell of the stethoscope is used for ______________________ pitched sounds.
7. The ______________________ heart sound is produced by closure of the mitral and tricuspid valves, and the ______________________ sound is produced by closure of the aortic and pulmonic.
8. The pulmonic component of the second heart sound is normally delayed during the ______________________ phase of respiration.
9. Left bundle branch block may lead to a ______________________ type of split in the second heart sound.
10. The ventricular gallop, or audible third heart sound, occurs during the ______________________ phase of the cardiac cycle.
11. A gallop heard best over the lower sternal border is likely to be due to ______________________ ventricular failure.
12. The atrial sound, or audible fourth sound, is due to increased resistance to ______________________.
13. A murmur due to mitral insufficiency is heard loudest with the stethoscope over the ______________________ during the ____________ ____________ phase of contraction.
14. A murmur due to aortic insufficiency is heard the loudest with the stethoscope over the ______________________ during the ____________ ____________ phase of contraction.
15. List a radiopharmaceutic test used to determine each of the following:
    a. Ejection fraction ______________________
    b. Ventricular wall motion ______________________
    c. Areas of ischemia ______________________
    d. Areas of recent necrosis ______________________
16. Taller than normal P waves may be found in ____________ ____________ atrial hypertrophy, whereas wider P waves occur with ______________________ atrial hypertrophy.

17. State the site of the positive pole in each of the following leads:
    a. Lead I: + = ______________________
    b. Lead II: + = ______________________
    c. V_1: + = ______________________
    d. aVR: + = ______________________
18. In the progression from V_1 to V_6, the R waves become ____________ ____________.
19. Indicate the most likely intraventricular conduction defect suggested by the following ECG changes:
    a. Loss of early septal depolarization with wide QRS ____________ ____________
    b. Left axis deviation ______________________
    c. Right axis deviation ______________________
20. Development of a u wave can be a sign of the electrolyte imbalance ______________________, whereas a prolonged ST can occur in ______________________.
21. The three major factors that affect the stroke volume are as follows:
    a. ______________________
    b. ______________________
    c. ______________________
22. The cardiac index is found by dividing the ______________________ by the ______________________ and is normally ______________ ____________ liters per minute per square meter.
23. Ventriculography is one method used to calculate the ____________ ____________, the proportion of the end-diastolic volume pumped by the ventricle.
24. As evaluated by coronary angiography, ______________________ % obstruction is considered significant in all of the coronary arteries except the left main where ______________________ % is considered significant.
25. Indicate whether the following will cause the right atrial pressure to increase or decrease:
    a. Right ventricular failure ______________________
    b. Hypovolemia ______________________
    c. Venodilator ______________________
    d. Cardiac tamponade ______________________
    e. Pulmonary hypertension ______________________
26. The phlebostatic axis is found at the junction of the ____________ ____________ and the ______________________.
27. Examples of disorders in which the pulmonary artery diastolic pressures do not correlate well with left ventricular filling pressures are ____________ ____________ and ______________________.
28. The pulmonary artery wedge or occluded pressure indirectly reflects the ______________________ pressure that goes ______________ ____________ in left ventricular failure, and ______________________ in hypovolemia.
29. Mixed venous oxygen saturation reflects the interaction between the amount of oxygen ______________________ and the amount ______________________ by the body.
30. List two things that may explain a mixed venous saturation of 90%.
    a. ______________________
    b. ______________________

C. Patient Health Problems (*pages 205–309*)

1. Three pathologies that may result from atherosclerosis of the coronary arteries are ______________________, ______________________, and ______________________.
2. Prinzmetal's, or atypical, angina occurs during ______________________.
3. Three types of drugs that may be used to treat exertional angina are ______________________, ______________________, and ______________________.
4. Of the first three available calcium-channel blockers, ______________________ has the most effect on heart rate, AV node conduction, and myocardial contractility, and ______________________ has the least.
5. The ideal candidate for transluminal coronary angioplasty has less than ______________________ vessels requiring intervention, and these lesions are ______________________ and ______________________.
6. Transluminal coronary angioplasty is relatively contraindicated in patients with ______________________ or ______________________.
7. Potential complications in patients undergoing transluminal coronary angioplasty include ______________________ and ______________________.
8. The primary advantage in using the internal mammary artery instead of the saphenous vein for coronary artery bypass is that it ______________________.
9. Elective coronary artery bypass grafting is the recommended treatment for angina that is refractory to ______________________, involves the ______________________ artery, or involves more than ______________________ vessels.
10. Emergency coronary artery bypass grafting may be necessary in patients with ______________________ or ______________________.
11. List three potential complications in the immediate postoperative period after coronary artery bypass grafting:
    a. ______________________
    b. ______________________
    c. ______________________
12. Indicate the action(s) of the following agents:
    a. Nitroprusside ______________________
    b. Nitroglycerin ______________________
    c. Dopamine at 2–10 mcg/kg/min ______________________
    d. Dopamine at over 10 mcg/kg/min ______________________
    e. Dobutamine ______________________
13. Class 1-A antidysrhythmic agents like quinidine or procainamide ______________________ the rate of depolarization by blocking ______________________ channels, and also ______________________ the myocardial contractility and conduction velocity.
14. Class II antidysrhythmic agents, or beta blockers, can both ______________________ the myocardial oxygen supply and ______________________ the demand.
15. Beta blockers are usually contraindicated in ______________________ and ______________________.
16. Class IV antidysrhythmic drugs, or calcium channel blockers, also ______________________ the afterload, one mechanism that ______________________ the myocardial oxygen demand.

17. Indicate the effect of digitalis glycosides on each of the following:
    a. Sinus node rate is ____________________
    b. Automaticity of myocardial muscle is ____________________
    c. AV conduction velocity is ____________________
    d. Contractility is ____________________
18. The likelihood of digitalis toxicity is increased by the presence of ____________________, ____________________, or ____________________.
19. Potential complications of myocardial infarction include ____________________ and ____________________.
20. Two examples of ways in which the pain of myocardial infarction differs from that of angina are ____________________ and ____________________.
21. The enzyme that rises the highest and fastest after the onset of pain in a myocardial infarction is ____________________.
22. Indicate whether the following are more likely to occur in right or left coronary artery thrombosis:
    a. Right ventricular infarction ____________________
    b. Anteroseptal wall infarction ____________________
    c. Inferior wall infarction ____________________
    d. Right bundle branch block ____________________
    e. Left anterior hemiblock ____________________
    f. Type I or Wenckebach AV block ____________________
    g. Bradycardia ____________________
23. Three cardinal signs of right ventricular infarction are ____________________, ____________________, and ____________________.
24. The ECG sign associated with myocardial necrosis is ____________________.
25. The anteroseptal wall is monitored by leads ____________________, the inferior wall by leads ____________________, and the lateral wall by leads ____________________.
26. Non-Q wave or subendocardial infarction is recognized by ST segment ____________________ and T wave ____________________ in the leads monitoring the epicardial surface.
27. Contraindicators for thrombolytic therapy include ____________________ and ____________________.
28. Potential complications of thrombolytic therapy include ____________________ and ____________________.
29. Deflation of the intra-aortic balloon during systole ____________________ the afterload and thereby ____________________ the myocardial oxygen demand.
30. Inflation of the intra-aortic balloon during diastole ____________________ the coronary perfusion and thereby ____________________ the myocardial oxygen supply.
31. Potential complications of the intra-aortic balloon pump include ____________________ and ____________________.
32. List three indications for cardiac pacing:
    a. ____________________
    b. ____________________
    c. ____________________
33. The five letters in the code used to describe pacemaker function refer to the following:
    a. First letter ____________________

b. Second letter ______________________
c. Third letter ______________________
d. Fourth letter ______________________
e. Fifth letter ______________________

34. The type of pacemaker malfunction that leads to competition with the patient's rhythm is ______________________.

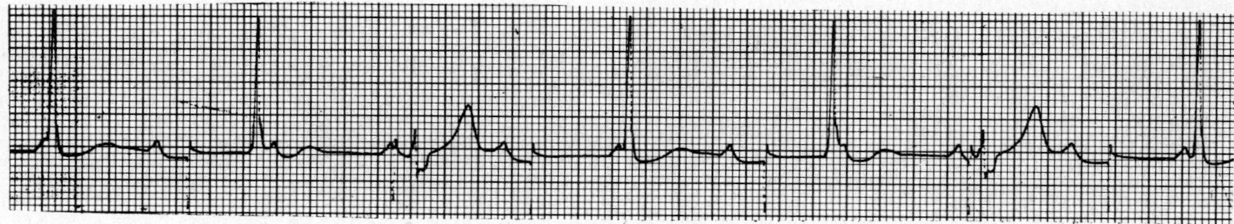

35. The rhythm strip above reveals a pacemaker that is failing to ______________________.

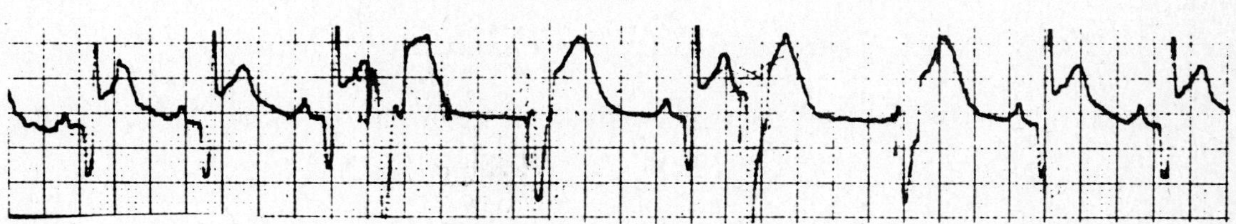

36. The rhythm strip above reveals a pacemaker that is failing to ______________________.
37. Pulmonary emboli or chronic lung disease can cause congestive heart failure, which begins in the ______________________ ventricle.
38. Dyspnea and rales will occur earliest from failure of the ______________________ ventricle.
39. Hepatosplenomegaly and distended neck veins will occur earliest from failure of the ______________________ ventricle.
40. Killip categorized ______________________ ventricular failure associated with myocardial infarction into classes ______________________ through ______________________, going from least to worst severity.
41. Amrinone causes ______________________ contractility, and ______________________ of peripheral vessels.
42. The roles of morphine in the treatment of heart failure include ______________________ and ______________________.
43. Fibrin deposits can cause ______________________ pericarditis, whereas effusions cause ______________________ pericarditis.
44. Dressler's syndrome is pericarditis associated with ______________________.
45. The pain of pericarditis increases when the patient ______________________ or ______________________.
46. The ECG in patients with pericarditis may first reveal ______________________.
47. Classic signs of cardiac tamponade include ______________________ and ______________________.
48. Infective endocarditis is one disease that can lead to Roth spots, which are ______________________; Janeway lesions, which are ______________________; or Osler's nodes, which are ______________________.
49. The embolic phenomenon associated with infective endocarditis is due to ______________________ and treated with ______________________.

50. The three classifications of cardiomyopathy are as follows:
    a. ______________________
    b. ______________________
    c. ______________________
51. The type of cardiomyopathy in which vasodilators are indicated but inotropic agents are contraindicated is ______________________.
52. End-stage cardiomyopathy is treated by ______________________ if the patient is an appropriate candidate.
53. Rupture of the left ventricular papillary muscle will lead to a murmur heard during ______________________, increased flow into the ______________________, and dilation of the ______________________ and the ______________________.
54. The valvular disease onset most likely to be associated with an enlarged left atrium, a hypertropied left ventricular, and a systolic apical murmur is ______________________.
55. Mitral stenosis is most likely to cause dilation of the ______________________ ventricle and ______________________ hypertension.
56. The type of valvular disease most likely to cause bounding pulses or water-hammer pulse is ______________________.
57. Aortic stenosis can lead to a ______________________ pulse pressure and a murmur heard during ______________________.
58. Two common presentations for patients with valvular disease include ______________________ and ______________________.
59. When a patient with atrial septal defect develops pulmonary hypertension, the shunt may reverse directions, turning from ______________________ to ______________________ into ______________________ to ______________________.
60. A child with atrial septal defect may appear cyanotic if there is a ______________________ to ______________________ shunt.
61. A cardiac catheterization in a patient with a ventricular septal defect may reveal increased oxygen saturation in the right ventricle in ______________________ to ______________________ shunt, or decreased saturated in the systemic artery in ______________________ to ______________________ shunt.
62. Patent ductus arteriosus is an abnormal communication between the pulmonary artery and the ______________________.
63. When patients with congenital defects reverse their shunts, it is called ______________________ syndrome.
64. The congenital disorder associated with a continuous machinery-like murmur at the left upper sternal border is ______________________.
65. The most common site for congenital coarctation of the aorta is just distal to the ______________________, which leads to hypotension in the ______________________ extremities and hypertension in the ______________________ extremities.
66. Sustained hypertension can cause vascular damage that leads to ______________________ blood flow to end organs.
67. Encephalopathy in patients with hypertensive crises occurs when loss of cerebral autoregulation leads to ______________________.
68. Although there are other signs and symptoms needed to complete the classification, in general, accelerated hypertension is the term used for diastolic pressures over ______________________ mm Hg; malignant hypertension, for diastolics over ______________________ mm Hg;

and hypertensive encephalopathy, for pressures over ____________ mm Hg.

69. Elevation in urinary vanillylmandelic acid occurs in hypertensive crisis caused by ____________.
70. The treatment of a hypertensive crisis may include drugs that ____________ the arterioles or ____________ sympathetic activity.
71. Describe the action of the following drugs used to treat hypertensive crises:
    a. Nitroprusside ____________
    b. Hydralazine ____________
    c. Methyldopa ____________
72. The most common site for an abdominal aortic aneurism is between the ____________ and ____________ arteries.
73. The pain associated with thoracic aortic aneurysms may start in the ____________ and radiate to the ____________ or ____________.
74. Acute occlusive disease leading to decreased blood flow to the lower extremities may lead to such signs and symptoms as ____________ or ____________.
75. Postoperative complications that should be monitored for after repair of aortic aneurysms include ____________, ____________, and ____________.
76. Compromised external respiration is called respiratory failure, whereas compromised internal or cellular respiration is called ____________.
77. The effects of shock on specific sites include ____________ of the veins, ____________ in glomerular filtration, release of renin from the ____________ cells, and shifting of fluid ____________ the capillary due to decreased capillary hydrostatic pressure.
78. Consequences of shock include ____________ sodium transport out of the cell, ____________ anaerobic metabolism, and accumulation of ____________ acid.
79. Cardiogenic shock can ensue after more than ____________ % of the left ventricular muscle mass has been damaged.
80. Shock induced by spinal cord injury is categorized as ____________ shock.
81. The type of shock most likely to be associated with an increased pulmonary capillary wedge pressure is ____________.
82. Septic shock may begin with a hyperdynamic phase during which the cardiac output goes ____________ and the vascular resistance goes ____________.
83. The initial acid-base change that occurs from shock is ____________ but eventually ____________ dominates.
84. Dopamine or dobutamine may be used in patients in shock to ____________, whereas nitroglycerin or nitroprusside may be used to ____________.

D. Summary of Patient Health Problems (*pages 205–309*)

After reading each disease, summarize the pathophysiology, nursing assessment data base, and nursing diagnoses. The certification examination holds you responsible for knowing the etiology and risk factors, the signs and symptoms, the collaborative diagnosis, the complications, and the management and treatment goals. Those preparing to take it should also summarize these areas. If they are not clearly covered in the *Core,* a second resource may be necessary. The space allotted is purposefully limited to encourage concise descriptions of concepts and careful selection of key points. It is not as helpful to write the things you already know as it is to write those you need to study.

1. Coronary Artery Disease

Pathophysiology	*Etiology/Risk Factors*	*Signs/Symptoms*

Collaborative Diagnosis	*Complications*	*Management/Goals*

2. Angina Pectoris

Pathophysiology	*Etiology/Risk Factors*	*Signs/Symptoms*

Collaborative Diagnosis	*Complications*	*Management/Goals*

3. Myocardial Infarction

Pathophysiology	*Etiology/Risk Factors*	*Signs/Symptoms*

Collaborative Diagnosis	*Complications*	*Management/Goals*

4. Congestive Heart Failure

Pathophysiology	*Etiology/Risk Factors*	*Signs/Symptoms*

Collaborative Diagnosis	*Complications*	*Management/Goals*

5. Pericarditis

Pathophysiology	*Etiology/Risk Factors*	*Signs/Symptoms*

Collaborative Diagnosis	*Complications*	*Management/Goals*

6. Infective Endocarditis

Pathophysiology	*Etiology/Risk Factors*	*Signs/Symptoms*

Collaborative Diagnosis	*Complications*	*Management/Goals*

7. Cardiomyopathy

Pathophysiology	*Etiology/Risk Factors*	*Signs/Symptoms*

Collaborative Diagnosis	*Complications*	*Management/Goals*

8. Mitral Insufficiency

Pathophysiology	*Etiology/Risk Factors*	*Signs/Symptoms*

Collaborative Diagnosis	*Complications*	*Management/Goals*

9. Mitral Stenosis

Pathophysiology	*Etiology/Risk Factors*	*Signs/Symptoms*

Collaborative Diagnosis	*Complications*	*Management/Goals*

10. Aortic Insufficiency

Pathophysiology	*Etiology/Risk Factors*	*Signs/Symptoms*

Collaborative Diagnosis	*Complications*	*Management/Goals*

11. Aortic Stenosis

Pathophysiology	*Etiology/Risk Factors*	*Signs/Symptoms*

Collaborative Diagnosis	*Complications*	*Management/Goals*

12. Atrial Septal Defect

Pathophysiology	*Etiology/Risk Factors*	*Signs/Symptoms*

Collaborative Diagnosis	*Complications*	*Management/Goals*

13. Ventricular Septal Defect

Pathophysiology	*Etiology/Risk Factors*	*Signs/Symptoms*

Collaborative Diagnosis	*Complications*	*Management/Goals*

14. Patent Ductus Arteriosus

Pathophysiology	*Etiology/Risk Factors*	*Signs/Symptoms*

Collaborative Diagnosis	*Complications*	*Management/Goals*

15. Coarctation of the Aorta

Pathophysiology	*Etiology/Risk Factors*	*Signs/Symptoms*

Collaborative Diagnosis	*Complications*	*Management/Goals*

16. Hypertensive Crisis

Pathophysiology	*Etiology/Risk Factors*	*Signs/Symptoms*

Collaborative Diagnosis	*Complications*	*Management/Goals*

17. Peripheral Vascular Disease

Pathophysiology	*Etiology/Risk Factors*	*Signs/Symptoms*

Collaborative Diagnosis	*Complications*	*Management/Goals*

18. Shock

Pathophysiology	*Etiology/Risk Factors*	*Signs/Symptoms*

Collaborative Diagnosis	*Complications*	*Management/Goals*

E. Application to Clinical Practice

Care for patients with cardiovascular disease. Relate the anatomy and physiology, assessment and pathophysiology found in this section to their individual clinical pictures. Make note of instances where they correlate and those where they deviate from the expected presentation. Devise a care plan based on the data collected.

Answers to Cardiovascular Exercises

A. Physiologic Anatomy

1. Sarcomere (*page 132*)
2. Myosin (*page 132*)
3. Mitochondria (*page 133*)
4. Visceral serous pericardium, epicardium (*page 133*)
5. 70, atrial contraction or kick (*page 134*)
6. Mitral, tricuspid (*pages 134, 135*)
7. Systolic or ejection (*page 135*)
8. Any two of these (*page 135*):
   a. Vessel diameter
   b. Blood viscosity
   c. Vessel's elastic recoil
9. Arteriole (*page 136*)
10. Down (*page 136*)
11. Veins and venules, or venous system (*page 136*)
12. Delay (*page 138*)
13. Purkinje system (*page 138*)
14. a. Right
    b. Left
    c. Right
    d. Left
    e. Right (*pages 138, 139*)
15. Right, coronary sinus (*page 140*)
16. Constrict (*page 141*)
17. Down (*page 141*)
18. Inhibited, up, down (*page 142*)
19. *See answer below*
20. Contractility (*page 144*)
21. Increases (*page 144*)
22. Decreases, slows (*page 144*)
23. Increases (*page 144*)
24. Potassium, sodium (*page 145*)
25. Sodium, calcium (*page 145*)
26. Repolarization (*page 146*)
27. Myocardial, pacing (*pages 145–147*)
28. Calcium (*pages 147, 148*)
29. a. a wave = atrial contraction
    b. c wave = closure of the A-V valves
    c. v wave = increasing atrial volume during ventricular systole (until A-V valves open) (*pages 148–150*)
30. Closing of the A-V valves, opening of the semilunar valves (*page 149*)
31. Preload (*page 150*)
32. More (*page 150*)
33. a. Decrease
    b. Increase
    c. Decrease (*pages 150, 151*)
34. *See answer below*
35. Higher (*page 151*)

B. Nursing Assessment Data Base

1. 5 cm (*page 153*)
2. 2+ (*page 154*)
3. Severe left ventricular failure; pericardial effusion or constriction, severe emphysema, cardiac tamponade, or hemorrhagic shock (*page 155*)
4. Left, upward, right (*page 156*)
5. Right upper sternal border, left upper sternal border (*pages 156, 157*)
6. Low (*page 157*)
7. First, second (*page 157*)
8. Inspiratory (*page 157*)
9. Paradoxical (*page 159*)
10. Diastolic (*page 159*)
11. Right (*page 159*)

19.

	BP	*PP = S − D*	*MAP = ⅓PP + D*
a.	210/120	90	⅓(90) + 120 = 150
b.	90/60	30	⅓(30) + 60 = 70
c.	140/80	60	⅓(60) + 80 = 100 (*pages 143, 144*)

34.

MAP = ⅓PP + DP	*SVR units* = $\frac{MAP - CVP}{CO}$	*SVR dynes = units × 80*
a. ⅓(30) + 80 = 90	$\frac{90 - 5}{5}$ = 17 units	17 × 80 = 1360 dynes
b. ⅓(90) + 120 = 150	$\frac{150 - 10}{3.5}$ = 40 units	40 × 80 = 3200 dynes
c. ⅓(30) + 60 = 70	$\frac{70 - 5}{3}$ = 21.7 units	21.7 × 80 = 1736 dynes

(*page 151*)

12. Atrial contraction or atrial kick (*page 160*)
13. Apex, systolic (*page 163*)
14. 3rd-4th intercostal spaces at left sternal border or 2nd intercostal space at right sternal border, diastolic (*page 165*)
15. a. Multiple-gated acquisition scans (MUGAs)
    b. Multiple-gated acquisition scans (MUGAs)
    c. Thallium imaging
    d. Technetium pyrophosphate imaging (*pages 167–168*)
16. Right, left (*page 172*)
17. a. Left arm
    b. Left leg
    c. 4th intercostal space, right sternal border
    d. Right arm (*pages 173–174*)
18. Progressively larger (*page 174*)
19. a. Left bundle branch block
    b. Left anterior fascicular block
    c. Left posterior fascicular block (*pages 185–186*)
20. Hypokalemia, hypocalcemia (*pages 187–188*)
21. a. Contractility
    b. Preload
    c. Afterload (*page 191*)
22. Cardiac output, body surface area, 2.5–4.0 (*page 192*)
23. Ejection fraction (*pages 167, 193*)
24. 75, 50 (*page 193*)
25. a. Increase
    b. Decrease
    c. Decrease
    d. Increase
    e. Increase (*page 195*)
26. A line drawn from the 4th intercostal space at the sternal border, a line drawn at the middle anterior-posterior diameter (*page 196*)
27. Any two of these (*page 197*):
    a. Chronic obstructive pulmonary disease
    b. Adult respiratory distress syndrome
    c. Pulmonary emboli
    d. Heart rates above 125/min
    e. Mitral valve disease
28. Left atrial or left ventricular end-diastolic pressure, up, down (*page 197*)
29. Demanded, supplied (*page 198*)
30. a. Sepsis
    b. Hypothermia (*page 198*)

C. Patient Health Problems

1. Any three of these (*page 206*):
   a. Angina
   b. Myocardial infarction
   c. Congestive heart failure
   d. Sudden death
   e. Dysrhythmias
   f. Cardiomegaly
   g. Mitral insufficiency
   h. Ventricular aneurysm/rupture
   i. Cardiogenic shock
2. Rest (*page 208*)
3. Nitrates, beta blockers, calcium channel blockers (*page 209*)
4. Verapamil, nifedipine (*page 209*)
5. Three, discrete or proximal or non-calcified or concentric or away from bifurcations (*page 210*)
6. Any two of these (*page 211*):
   a. Left main disease
   b. Variant angina
   c. Lesions near coronary orifice
   d. Valvular disease
   e. Unacceptable risk for cardiac surgery
7. Any two of these (*page 211*):
   a. Dissection or spasm of the coronary artery
   b. Myocardial infarction
   c. Cardiac tamponade
   d. Hypotension
   e. Bleeding or decreased blood flow in cannulated artery
   f. Vasovagal reaction
   g. Restenosis
8. Is likely to remain patent longer (*page 213*)
9. Medical therapy, left main, two (*page 213*)
10. Any two of these (*page 213*):
    a. Preinfarction angina
    b. Complicated acute myocardial infarction
    c. Complications of angiography or transluminal angioplasty
11. Any three of these (*pages 213, 214*):
    a. Low cardiac output
    b. Bleeding
    c. Hypertension
    d. Cardiac tamponade
    e. Dysrhythmias
    f. Myocardial infarction
    g. Respiratory failure
    h. Renal failure
    i. Electrolyte imbalances
12. a. Vasodilation
    b. Vasodilation
    c. Beta-1 stimulation, increased urinary output
    d. Alpha stimulation, Beta-1 stimulation

e. Beta-1 stimulation (*pages 209–217*)
13. Decrease, sodium, decrease (*page 219*)
14. Increase, decrease (*page 220*)
15. Any two of these (*page 220*):
    a. Heart failure
    b. Cardiogenic shock
    c. Asthma
    d. Sinus bradycardia
    e. Insulin-dependent diabetes
    f. Greater than first-degree block
16. Decrease, decreases (*page 221*)
17. a. Decreased
    b. Increased
    c. Decreased
    d. Increased (*page 222*)
18. Any three of these (*page 222*):
    a. Renal failure
    b. Liver failure
    c. Hypokalemia
    d. Hypomagnesemia
    e. Hypercalcemia
    f. Alkalemia
    g. Hypoxemia
19. Any two of these (*page 223*):
    a. Dysrhythmias
    b. Heart failure
    c. Shock
    d. Embolism
    e. Papillary muscle rupture
    f. Dressler's syndrome
    g. Ventricular aneurysm or rupture
    h. Ventricular septal defect
20. Any two of these (*page 224*):
    a. Longer duration
    b. Not relieved by rest or nitroglycerin
    c. Pain is more severe
21. CPK (*page 225*)
22. a. Right
    b. Left
    c. Right
    d. Left
    e. Left
    f. Right
    g. Right (*page 225*)
23. High CVP, low cardiac output, minimal or absent pulmonary congestion (*page 225*)
24. A wide (> .04 seconds) or deep (> 25% of the QRS) Q wave (*pages 225–227*)
25. V_1 through V_4; II, III avF; V_5, V_6, I avL (*pages 226–227*)
26. Depression, inversion (*page 227*)
27. Any two of these (*pages 228, 229*):
    a. Recent surgery (within 2 weeks)
    b. Pregnancy or recent delivery
    c. History of recent cerebral vascular disease (within 3 months)
    d. Uncontrolled hypertension
    e. Recent major trauma (within 6 months)
    f. Bleeding disorder or recent bleed
    g. Prolonged CPR
    h. Severe advanced illness
    i. Severe renal or liver disease
28. Any two of these (*pages 228–230*):
    a. Reperfusion dysrhythmias
    b. Bleeding
    c. Reocclusion
    d. Allergic reaction only for streptokinase or eminase after previous exposure
29. Decreases, decreases (*page 231*)
30. Increases, increases (*page 231*)
31. Any two of these (*page 230*):
    a. Ischemia of cannulated limb
    b. Aortic dissection
    c. Thrombocytopenia
    d. Septicemia
    e. Local infection
32. Any three of these (*page 235*):
    a. Sick sinus syndrome
    b. Symptomatic bradyarrhythmias
    c. Second-degree A-V block
    d. Third-degree A-V block
    e. Tachyarrhythmias
    f. Sensitive carotid sinus syndrome
    g. Post cardiac surgery
33. a. Chamber paced
    b. Chamber sensed
    c. Response to sensing
    d. Programmable functions
    e. Antitachyarrhythmic functions (*page 238*)
34. A failure to sense (*page 239*)
35. Capture (*page 239*)
36. Sense (*page 239*)
37. Right (*page 243*)
38. Left (*page 243*)
39. Right (*page 243*)
40. Left, one (I), four (IV) (*page 243*)
41. Increased, dilation (*pages 245–246*)
42. Any two of these (*page 246*):
    a. Vasodilation
    b. Reduce pain
    c. Reduce anxiety
    d. Decrease myocardial oxygen consumption
43. Constrictive, restrictive (*page 247*)
44. Myocardial infarction (*page 247*)
45. Any two of these (*page 248*):
    a. Inspires
    b. Lies down
    c. Turns the thorax
46. ST segment elevation in many leads with the exception of V_1 and avR (*page 248*)
47. Any two of these (*page 249*):
    a. Right- and left-sided filling pressures rise and equalize
    b. Decreased blood pressure and cardiac output

c. Decreased pulse pressure
d. Pulsus paradoxus

48. White spots on the retina, vascular lesions on palms or soles, vascular lesions on digits (*page 252*)
49. Vegetations on the valves, antimicrobials (*page 255*)
50. a. Dilated or congestive
b. Hypertrophic
c. Restrictive (*page 256*)
51. Hypertrophic (*page 259*)
52. Cardiac transplantation (*page 260*)
53. Systole, left atrium, left atrium, left ventricle (*pages 261–264*)
54. Mitral insufficiency (*pages 261–264*)
55. Right, pulmonary (*page 265*)
56. Aortic insufficiency (*page 269*)
57. Narrow, systole (*page 271*)
58. Any two of these (*pages 261–272*):
a. Heart failure
b. Embolic phenomenon
c. Palpations or arrhythmias
d. Murmurs heard on physical exam
59. Left to right, right to left (*pages 272, 273*)
60. Right, left (*page 273*)
61. Left to right, right to left (*page 278*)
62. Aorta (*page 279*)
63. Eisenmenger's (*pages 276, 279*)
64. Patent ductus arteriosus (*pages 279, 280*)
65. Left subclavian artery, lower, upper (*pages 282–283*)
66. Decreased (*page 284*)
67. Increased cerebral blood flow or cerebral edema and hemorrhage (*page 285*)
68. 120, 140, 250/150 (*page 286*)
69. Increased catacholamines or pheochromocytoma (*page 287*)
70. Dilate, inhibit (*page 288*)
71. a. Vasodilator
b. Vasodilator
c. Sympathetic blocking agent (*page 288*)
72. Renal, iliac (*page 292*)
73. Chest, shoulders or neck or back (*page 291*)
74. Any two of these (*page 292*):
a. Pain
b. Pallor
c. Decreased pulses
d. Paresthesias
e. Weakness or paralysis
75. Any three of these (*pages 296–298*):
a. Hypertension
b. Decreased distal peripheral pulses
c. Central nervous system dysfunction
d. Cardiac ischemia or injury
e. Dysrhythmias
f. Hemorrhage, hypotension
g. Renal failure
h. Temperature changes
i. Respiratory compromise
j. Bowel ischemia
k. Spinal cord ischemia
76. Perfusion failure or shock (*page 299*)
77. Constriction, decrease, juxtoglomerular, into (*page 300*)
78. Decreased, increased, lactic (*page 302*)
79. 40 (*page 302*)
80. Neurogenic (*page 303*)
81. Cardiogenic (*page 304*)
82. Up, down (*page 305*)
83. Respiratory alkalosis, metabolic acidosis (*page 306*)
84. Increase cardiac output, decrease resistance or afterload (*page 307*)

D. Summary of Patient Health Problems

Refer to the following pages in the Core Curriculum

THE CARDIOVASCULAR SYSTEM

Post Quiz

The following questions are designed to test understanding of some of the key points in the section. Select the one best answer for each of the following. The correct answers are at the end of the test.

1. Stimulation of the vagus nerve causes
   a. increased coronary blood flow
   b. decreased A-V node conduction
   c. increased atrial contractility
   d. all of the above
2. All of the following apply to papillary muscles *except*
   a. they assist the semilunear valves
   b. the valve leaflets may prolapse during systole if they do not function adequately
   c. they are attached to chordea tendinae
   d. they contract during ventricular systole
3. The vessels with the most blood volume are the
   a. arteries
   b. arterioles
   c. capillaries
   d. veins
4. The coronary venous return drains primarily into the
   a. right atrium
   b. right ventricle
   c. left atrium
   d. left ventricle
5. The systemic veins hold about ______________________ % of the circulating blood volume.
   a. 18
   b. 5–10
   c. 40–50
   d. 60–70
6. A form of angina in which pain develops at rest but does not usually occur with exertion is
   a. preinfarction angina
   b. accelerated angina
   c. crescendo angina
   d. Prinzmetal's angina
7. Manifestations of mitral insufficiency include
   a. increased ejection fraction
   b. increased left atrial pressure
   c. right to left shunting
   d. increased pulse pressure
8. Pulsus alternans is
   a. associated with increased intracranial pressure
   b. associated with cor pulmonale
   c. often seen in patients with hypothyroidism
   d. a pulse that is regular in rate but alternates in amplitude from beat to beat
9. The aortic area is found in the
   a. 5th ICS to the left of the sternum
   b. 4th ICS to the right of the sternum

c. 2nd ICS to the right of the sternum
d. area just above the apical pulse

10. The fourth heart sound (S_4)
 a. is found just before the first sound (S_1)
 b. can be heard well with the diaphragm of the stethoscope
 c. is associated with aortic stenosis
 d. occurs at the beginning of ventricular diastole
11. In the majority of patients, the right coronary artery supplies the
 a. right bundle branch
 b. left anterior fascicle
 c. posterior septum
 d. anterior septum
12. Pulsus paradoxus is a sign of
 a. cardiac tamponade
 b. Prinzmetal's angina
 c. acute bacterial endocarditis
 d. left ventricular failure
13. Which of the following is more likely to cause a murmur heard best between S_2 and the next S_1 in the 2nd right ICS?
 a. ventricular septal defect
 b. aortic insufficiency
 c. aortic stenosis
 d. mitral stenosis
14. An earlier sign of left ventricular failure is
 a. hypotension
 b. distended neck veins
 c. an S_3 gallop over the apex
 d. liver engorgement
15. A patient in cardiogenic shock with a low cardiac output and high vascular resistance may be given
 a. dopamine and norepinephrine
 b. isoproterenol and corticosteroids
 c. norepinephrine and corticosteroids
 d. dopamine and nitroglycerin
16. Leukocytosis and disseminated intravascular coagulation are more likely to occur as complications of
 a. hypovolemic shock
 b. cardiogenic shock
 c. septic shock
 d. neurogenic shock
17. The form of shock that often presents with urticaria and laryngeal edema is
 a. hypovolemic
 b. cardiogenic
 c. septic
 d. anaphylaxis
18. Cellular consequences of poor perfusion include
 a. decrease in intracellular sodium
 b. increase in adenosine triphosphate (ATP)
 c. decreased metabolic capability
 d. alkalosis
19. The v wave on the atrial pressure tracing occurs during
 a. early ventricular diastole
 b. late ventricular diastole
 c. ventricular systole
 d. atrial systole

20. Loss of capture in a patient with a pacemaker
    a. indicates the stimulus is not depolarizing the myocardium
    b. indicates the pacemaker is not recognizing the patient's own intrinsic rhythm
    c. cannot occur in synchronized pacemakers
    d. indicates loss of contraction despite electrical activity (a spike and QRS but no pulse)
21. The most frequent cause of right ventricular failure is
    a. cor pulmonale
    b. pulmonary emboli
    c. left ventricular failure
    d. valvular heart disease
22. In right bundle branch block
    a. the QRS is less than .10 seconds
    b. there is early activation of the septum
    c. there are often deep Qs in II and III
    d. there is often an rSR′ in V_1
23. The lead in which the left arm is negative and the left leg is positive is
    a. lead I
    b. lead II
    c. lead III
    d. lead avL
24. The intranodal pathway that sends the wave of depolarization preferentially to the left atrium is
    a. Bachman's tract
    b. Thorel's tract
    c. Wenckebach's tract
    d. the Bundle of Kent
25. Wide-notched P waves in lead I and avL is a sign of
    a. mitral stenosis
    b. P pulmonale
    c. right atrial hypertrophy
    d. left ventricular strain
26. The normal action potential graph of a myocardial cell reveals that
    a. the resting membrane potential is +40 millivolts
    b. the threshold potential is −80 to −90 millivolts
    c. the inside of the cell becomes less negative during depolarization
    d. repolarization is faster than depolarization
27. Which of the following has a negative inotropic effect?
    a. isoproterenol (Isuprel)
    b. dopamine (Intropin)
    c. dobutamine (Dobutrex)
    d. propranolol (Inderal)
28. The beta-adrenergic effects include
    a. negative chronotropism
    b. negative inotropism
    c. increased cardiac output
    d. bronchoconstriction
29. Mechanisms that can raise the systemic blood pressure include
    a. stimulation of a cholinergic response
    b. inhibition of the vasoconstrictor area of the vasomotor center
    c. hypoxemic stimulation of the carotid chemoreceptors
    d. alpha-adrenergic blockade
30. Liver function studies are more likely to be abnormal in
    a. pericarditis

b. left ventricular failure
c. right ventricular failure
d. hypertensive crisis

31. The auscultatory finding associated with left bundle branch block is an S_2 that is split
a. on inspiration only
b. continuously but is more widely split on inspiration
c. on expiration but the split decreases or disappears on inspiration
d. continuously and is not affected by respiration

32. Causes of elevated preloads include
a. hypovolemia
b. vasodilation
c. cardiac tamponade
d. spontaneous breaths

33. The classic ECG sign of exercise-induced ischemia in patients with coronary artery disease is
a. ST segment depression
b. development of a u wave
c. prolongation of the QT interval
d. development of deep wide Q waves

34. The subcellular contractile unit of the myocardium is the
a. synctium
b. sinus node
c. sarcoplasmic reticulum
d. sarcomere

35. Frank-Starling's law of the heart
a. is not applicable in patients with heart failure
b. states the relationship between fiber stretch and contractility
c. states the relationship between preload and afterload
d. shows us why the preload should not be allowed to exceed the normal ranges in any patient

36. The term preload refers to the
a. end-diastolic ventricular volume or pressure
b. forces opposing ventricular ejection
c. systemic vascular resistance
d. inotropic state of the heart

37. Pure left ventricular failure will result in
a. right ventricular hypertrophy
b. hepatosplenomegaly
c. increased pulmonary wedge pressure
d. increased renal perfusion

38. Which of the following would not decrease pulmonary vascular congestion in pulmonary edema?
a. diuretics
b. high Fowler's position
c. morphine sulfate
d. propranolol (Inderal)

39. Dopamine at high doses (over 10 mcg/kg/min) will begin to
a. increase urinary output
b. increase contractility
c. cause vasoconstriction
d. increase the cardiac output

40. Effects of intravenous nitroglycerin include
a. decreased systemic vascular resistance
b. increased left ventricular work

c. increased left ventricular oxygen demand
d. increased preloads

41. Which of the following is not part of the pathophysiology of shock?
a. decreased effective circulating blood volume
b. decreased cardiac output
c. decreased peripheral perfusion
d. decreased anaerobic metabolism

42. The compensatory mechanisms of shock include
a. vasodilation
b. increased parasympathetic response
c. increased sodium retention and oliguria
d. shifting of fluid from the capillaries to the interstitial space

43. The most reliable noninvasive test for pericardial effusion is the
a. ECG
b. chest x-ray
c. echocardiogram
d. phonocardiogram

44. Pulmonary wedge pressure
a. is usually slightly below the pulmonary diastolic pressure
b. indicates right atrial pressure
c. is normally between 35 and 45 torr
d. can be directly assessed by evaluation of the neck veins

45. Verapamil's effects include
a. decreased A-V conduction
b. increased heart rate
c. increased contractility
d. vasoconstriction

46. Shock associated with high preloads is most likely to be
a. hypovolemic shock
b. neurogenic shock
c. septic shock
d. cardiogenic shock

47. When there are elevated ST segments and deep wide Q waves in leads II, III, and avF, the patient has
a. an acute inferior wall MI
b. a chronic inferior wall MI
c. anterior wall ischemia
d. subendocardial ischemia without necrosis

48. A posterior wall MI is diagnosed by
a. tall R waves in V_5 and V_6
b. deep wide Q waves in the anterior leads
c. ST segment elevation in V_1, V_2, and V_3
d. reciprocal changes in V_1, V_2, and V_3

49. Hypokalemia causes what changes in the ECG?
a. tall peaked T waves
b. prolongation of the QRS interval
c. prolongation of the QTU interval
d. shortening of the ST segment

50. Indications for pacing include
a. sick sinus syndrome
b. right bundle branch block
c. left anterior hemiblock
d. type I second-degree block

Answers to Cardiovascular Post Quiz

1. **b** (*page 144*)
2. **a** (*pages 134–135*)
3. **d** (*page 156*)
4. **a** (*page 140*)
5. **d** (*page 136*)
6. **d** (*page 207*)
7. **b** (*pages 262–264*)
8. **d** (*page 155*)
9. **c** (*page 157*)
10. **a** (*pages 157–158*)
11. **c** (*pages 138–139*)
12. **a** (*page 155*)
13. **b** (*page 165*)
14. **c** (*pages 159–160*)
15. **d** (*pages 307–308*)
16. **c** (*pages 306–307*)
17. **d** (*page 305*)
18. **c** (*pages 300, 302*)
19. **c** (*page 150*)
20. **a** (*pages 238–239*)
21. **c** (*pages 242–243*)
22. **d** (*page 186*)
23. **c** (*page 173*)
24. **a** (*page 138*)
25. **a** (*page 172*)
26. **c** (*pages 145–147*)
27. **d** (*page 152*)
28. **c** (*pages 144, 215–216*)
29. **c** (*pages 140–144*)
30. **c** (*pages 243, 245*)
31. **c** (*pages 243, 245*)
32. **c** (*pages 151, 197*)
33. **a** (*page 189*)
34. **d** (*page 132*)
35. **b** (*page 150*)
36. **a** (*page 150*)
37. **c** (*pages 242–244*)
38. **d** (*pages 152, 245–246*)
39. **c** (*page 215*)
40. **a** (*pages 163, 216–217*)
41. **d** (*pages 299–302*)
42. **c** (*pages 208, 299–302*)
43. **c** (*pages 169, 184, 249*)
44. **a** (*pages 195–198*)
45. **a** (*page 209*)
46. **d** (*pages 304–306*)
47. **a** (*pages 226–227*)
48. **d** (*page 227*)
49. **c** (*page 187*)
50. **a** (*page 230*)

These are primarily the comprehend or recall, and apply or analyze levels of questions. Examples of synthesis or evaluate questions can be found in the comprehensive examination at the end of the book on pages 278 to 293.

3

The Neurologic System

SECTION-RELATED TIPS FOR THOSE STUDYING TO TAKE THE CERTIFICATION EXAMINATION

This section is often difficult, even for the advanced practitioner, for two reasons. First, the labels for nervous system structures are often long Latin or Greek names that are not easy to relate to. Second, critically ill patients with primary diseases or injury of the central nervous system are often taken to centers that have specialized intensive care units (ICUs). The nurses who work in the ICUs are very proficient and have an important impact on patient outcome; those who do not, have far less contact or experience with these patients.

If the nervous system is not one of your strengths, I strongly recommend that you memorize names of key structures before you begin studying this section of the *Core*. Figures 3–1 through 3–3 and Table 3–1 are a good place to start. Once you have a handle on these, you will have a frame of reference for the material presented in this section.

OTHER RECOMMENDATIONS

1. The first part of this section covers a great deal of detailed anatomy that is not asked for on the examination. Do not worry about memorizing it just for test-taking purposes.
2. On the other hand, the names for clinical assessment phenomena are worth memorizing. They may be used on the examination and may often come up clinically.
3. Remember, there are often questions on the examination related to structures or phenomena named after people. The neurologic section has several names to remember (see Appendix A).

Please see the instructions at the beginning of the book for important general suggestions that are relevant to the bulk of the *Core Curriculum* content. They apply to this section as well as to all the others.

FIGURES AND TABLES

Refer to these figures and tables while reading the neurologic section of the Core Curriculum. *For this system, there are more diagrams in the* Core *so fewer were required for the* Study Guide.

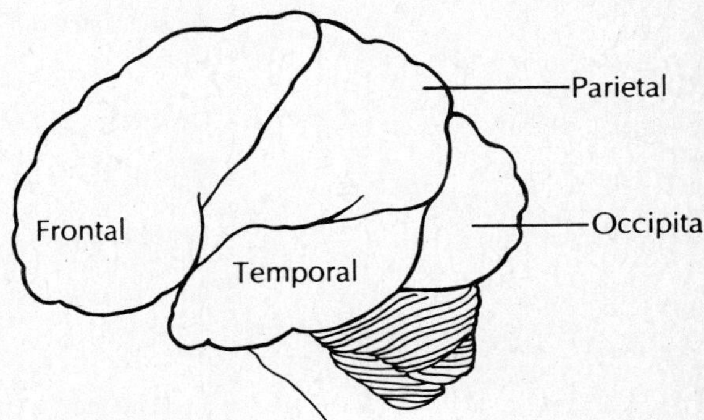

Figure 3–1. Right lateral view of the cerebral cortex (*pages 315–318*).

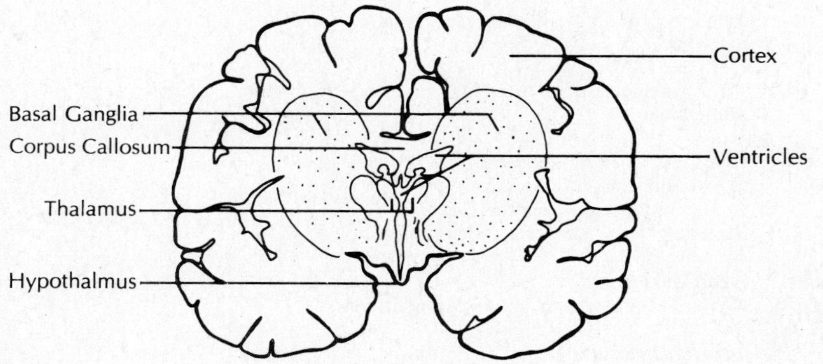

Figure 3–2. Sagittal cross-sectional view of the brain (*pages 318–320*).

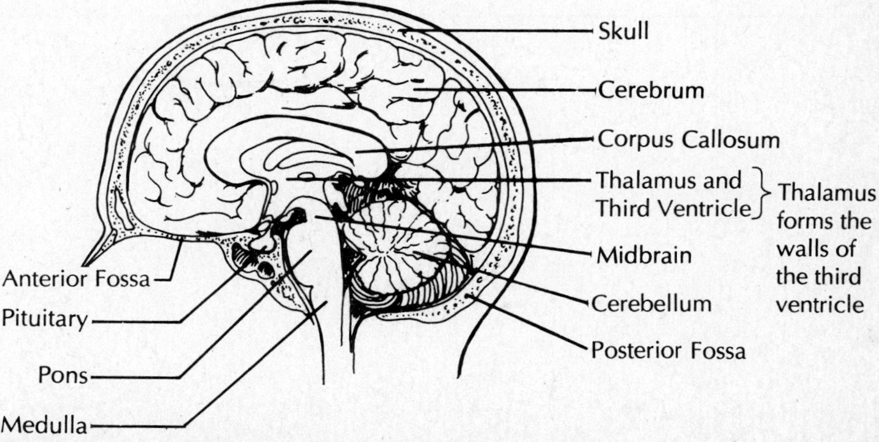

Figure 3–3. Lateral cross-sectional view of the brain (*pages 315–323*).

Table 3–1. SUMMARY OF FUNCTIONS OF THE DIVISIONS OF THE BRAIN (*pages 318–323*)

Structure	Functions
Cerebral Cortex	
Frontal lobe	Motor (expressive) speech Voluntary motor activity (pyramidal or corticospinal tract) Higher mental functions
Temporal lobe	Hearing Balance Sensory (cognitive) speech Emotion, behavior
Parietal lobe	Sensation Sensory integration and processing
Occipital lobe	Vision
Right Hemisphere	Geometric, spatial, visual, and musical functions
Left Hemisphere	Verbal, mathematical, and analytic functions
Basal Ganglia	Motor integration Muscle-tone control Postural reflexes } extrapyramidal tract center
Thalamus	Sensory relay
Hypothalamus	Regulation of temperature Regulation of food and water intake Behavior, especially sleep and aggressive or sexual behavior Regulation of autonomic nervous system Regulation of pituitary function
Limbic System	Affective and visceral aspects of emotional behavior Some memory
Brainstem	Gives rise to cranial nerves III–XII Motor and sensory pathways Connecting tracts to cerebellum Respiratory and cardiovascular centers
Ascending Reticular Activating System	Sleep-wake center Required for alertness and focusing attention
Cerebellum	Controls muscle tone and equilibrium Controls posture Controls nonstereotyped movements Coordinates motor activity

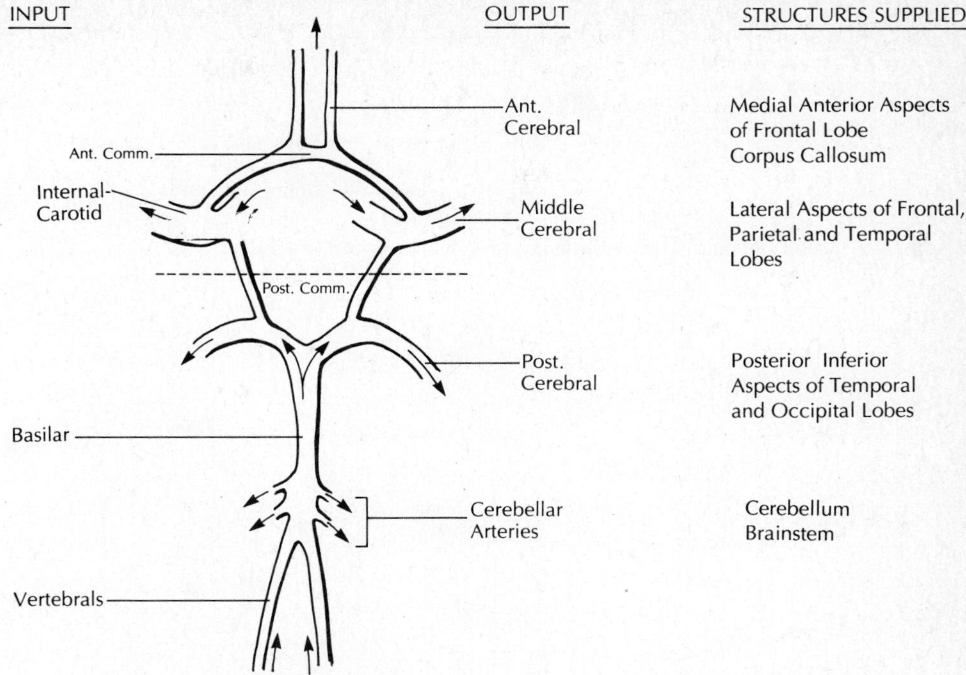

Figure 3–4. Major vessels going to and from the Circle of Willis. Dotted line indicates division between the internal carotid system (*above*) and the vertebral system (*below*) and the arrows indicate the direction of blood flow (*pages 323, 324*).

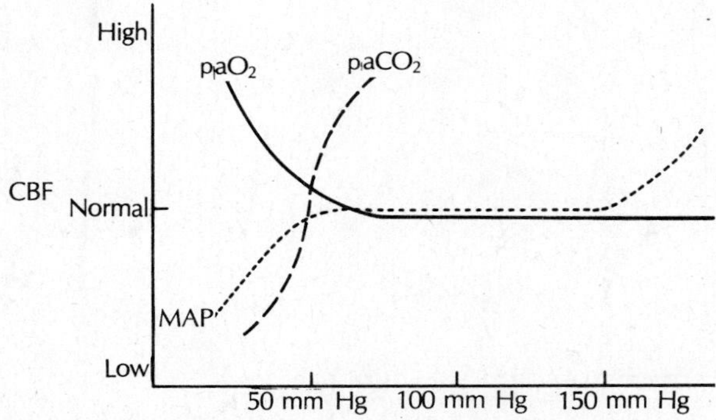

Figure 3–5. Effects of arterial oxygen tension (paO_2), arterial carbon dioxide tension ($paCO_2$), and mean arterial pressure (MAP) on cerebral blood flow (CBF) (*pages 324–325*).

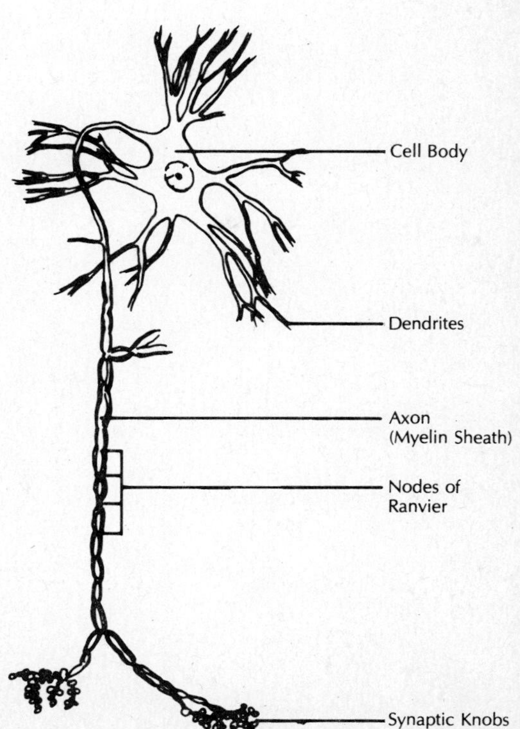

Figure 3–6. Anatomy of a typical neuron (*pages 328, 329*).

Factors Influencing___
Intracellular Na concentration
Summation of excitatory stimuli
Level of excitation (or refractoriness)
Level of inhibition (hyperpolarization)

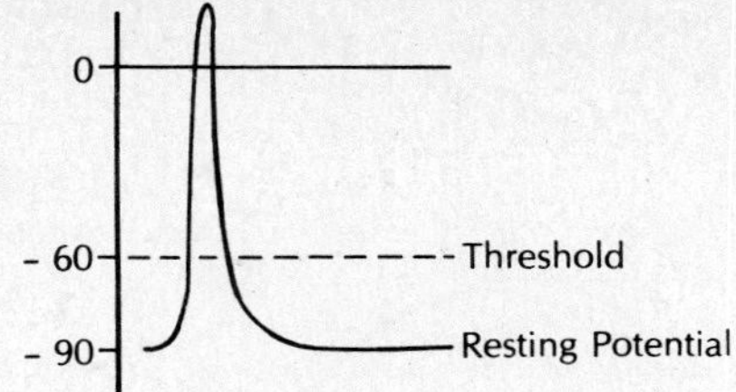

Figure 3–7. Action potential of the nerve and factors that influence it (*pages 332, 333*).

Figure 3–8. Major divisions of the spinal cord (*pages 334–341*).

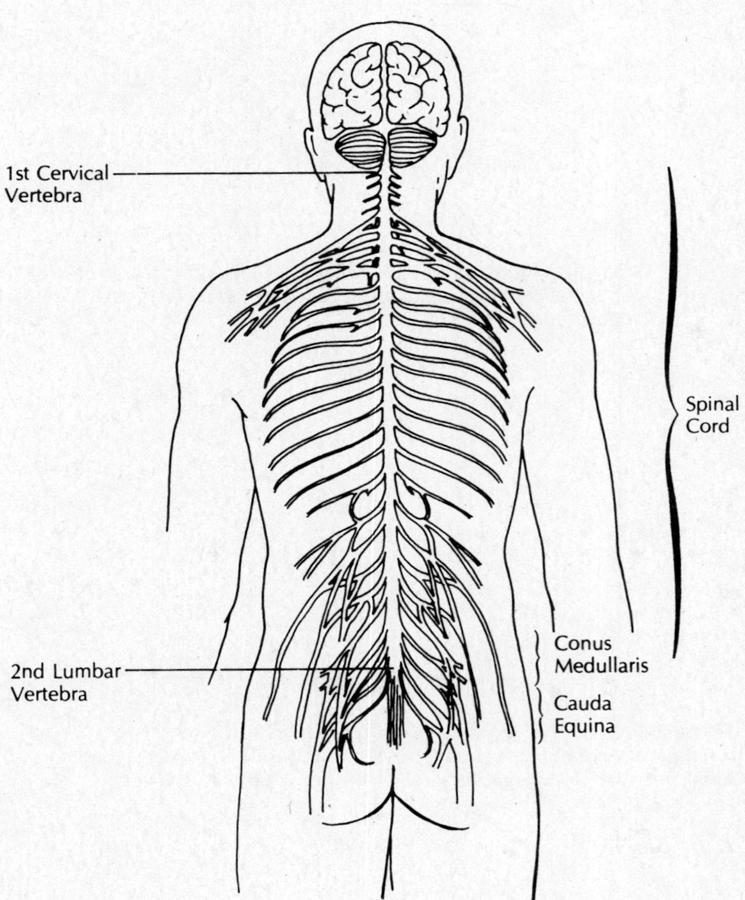

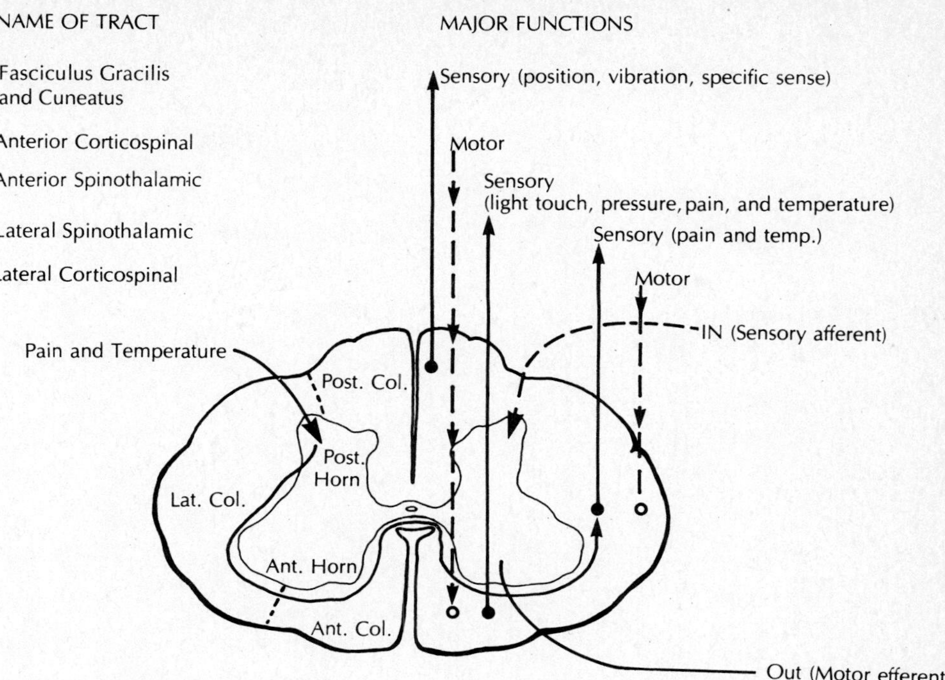

Figure 3–9. Anatomy of the spinal cord. The left half indicates the division of the gray matter (*dotted*) into horns and the white matter into columns (*Col.*). The right half indicates major afferent (*in*), efferent (*out*), ascending (*sensory*), and descending (*motor*) nerve tracts. Although most tracts cross above at the bottom of the medulla, the pain and temperature tracts cross just after entry (*pages 334–338*).

Table 3–2. SUMMARY OF MAJOR ASCENDING AND DESCENDING TRACTS (*pages 336–338*)

Tract	Origin and Column	Destination	Type of Impulse
Ascending			
Fasciculus Gracilis and Cuneatus	Posterior horn Posterior column	Thalamus	Tactile localization, position, vibration, joint, 2 point discrimination
Lateral spinothalamic	Posterior horn Contralateral anterolateral column	Thalamus	Pain and temperature
Anterior spinothalamic	Posterior horn Contralateral anterolateral column	Thalamus	Superficial touch and pressure, pain, temperature
Spinocerebellar	Posterior horn Lateral column	Cerebellum	Proprioceptive data
Spinotectal	Posterior horn	Midbrain	General sensation
Descending			
Rubrospinal	Midbrain Lateral column	Anterior horn	Controls muscle tone and synergy
Corticospinal	Cerebral cortex Lateral and anterior columns	Anterior horn	Voluntary movement
Tectospinal	Midbrain Anterior columns	Cranial nerve nuclei	Cephalic responses to general sensation

Superficial or Somatic Areas Innervated

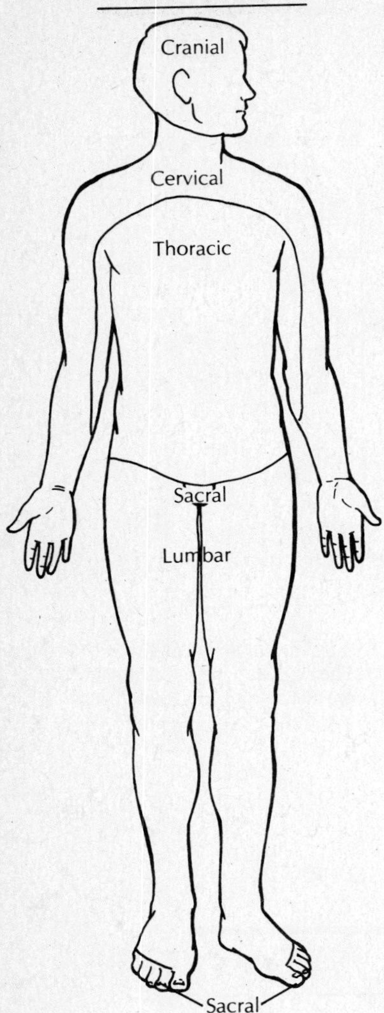

Internal and Visceral Structures Innervated

= diaphragm movement

= sympathetic tone

= bowel & bladder control

= sexual function

Figure 3–10. Summary of the functions of the peripheral nerves (*pages 340, 341, 354, 355, 397, 398*).

Table 3–3. SUMMARY OF CRANIAL NERVE FUNCTIONS (*pages 342–345*).

	Nerve	Central Origin and/or Destination	Functions
I	Olfactory	Multiple connections from nose	Sensory for smell
II	Optic	Retina to occipital lobe	Sensory for vision
III	Oculomotor	Midbrain to eye	Motor for moving eye, lifting lid, and constricting pupil
IV	Trochlear	Midbrain to eye muscles	Motor for moving eyes
V	Trigeminal	Pons to face	Sensory for face Motor for chewing
VI	Abducens	Pons to eye muscle	Motor for moving eye
VII	Facial	Junction of pons and medulla to and from face and mouth	Motor for moving face Sensory for taste
VIII	Acoustic	Junction of pons and medulla from ear	Sensory for hearing and equilibrium
IX	Glossopharyngeal	Medulla to and from back of mouth and throat	Motor and sensory for posterior oral (taste) and pharyngeal cavities
X	Vagus	Medulla to and from multiple cranial, thoracic, and abdominal structures	Main nerve of the parasympathetic nervous system Also overlaps with function of IX
XI	Spinal Accessory	Medulla to neck muscles	Motor for moving head and shoulders with neck muscles
XII	Hypoglossal	Medulla to tongue	Motor for moving tongue

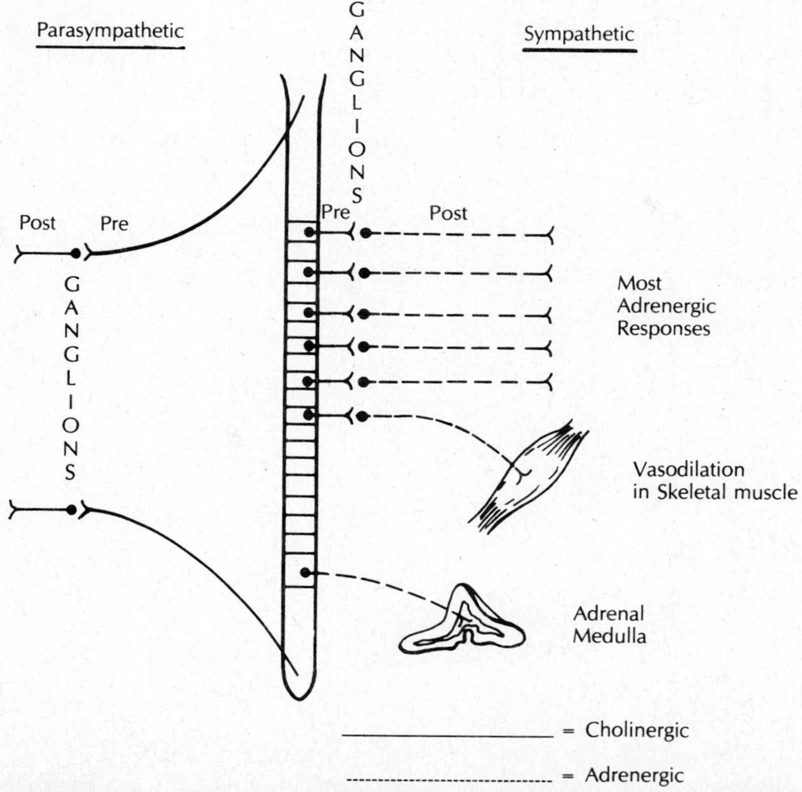

Figure 3–11. Comparison of the peripheral nerves of the parasympathetic and sympathetic nervous systems (*pages 345–348*).

Table 3–4. FACTORS COVERED IN THE PHYSIOLOGIC ANATOMY SECTION THAT HAVE IMPORTANT CLINICAL APPLICATIONS WORTH EMPHASIZING (*pages 315–348*)

Factor	*Clinical Application*	*Page*
Scalp Vessels Contract Poorly	Hypovolemia in a trauma patient is occasionally due to large volumes of blood loss in the field from large scalp wounds	315
Vessels Between Skull and Brain Tissue	The high vascularity of the superficial structures surrounding the brain put the patient with head injury at risk of hematomas. Examples include: (1) Large venous sinuses that lie between the dura (2) Branches of the Circle of Willis (cerebral arteries) that lie with the pia on the surface of the cortex in the subarachnoid space (3) Branches of the external carotid that penetrate the skull and ride along the dura (meningeal arteries)	315–318
Tentorium Cerebelli (often called tentorium)	Rigid layer of dural tissue that divides the bony cranial vault into two compartments, supratentorial and infratentorial or posterior fossa. It is an incomplete barrier that is open around the area of the brainstem. Herniation syndromes are often related to this anatomy.	316
Divisions of the Brain	Understanding the functions of these structures helps to relate symptoms and neurologic deficits to pathology or causes.	318–323
Relationship Between Brainstem and Cranial Nerves	Evaluation of cranial nerves is often part of the work-up for brainstem function. It is also part of the diagnosis of brain death.	321, 322
CSF Characteristics	The CSF is altered by certain disorders. For example: (1) Bacterial processes cause increased white cells, proteins, and turbidity with decreased glucose (2) Guillain-Barré may cause increased protein without an increase in white cells (3) Brain tumors may cause decreased glucose with positive cytology (4) Hyperglycemia may cause the glucose to rise to $> 60\%$ of the blood level	327
CSF-Filled Structures	CSF acts as a natural contrast to other cranial structures, which is helpful when interpreting many noninvasive diagnostic studies.	327
CSF Circulation	Visualizing the pathway taken by circulating CSF is useful when differentiating the type of hydrocephalus and the site of obstruction. For example: (1) Obstruction of the aqueduct of Sylvius leads to increased size of the third and lateral ventricles (2) Obstruction at the foramina of Luschka and Magendie leads to increased size of all four ventricles	327, 328
Neuroglial Cells	In addition to performing many supportive functions for the neurons, they make up the majority of brain tumors.	329
Brain Metabolism	Because the brain is dependent on a constant supply of oxygen and glucose to meet its high energy requirements, there are many cardiovascular, respiratory, and endocrine physiologic responses when the supply is diminished. Neurologic symptoms result when these compensatory mechanisms fail.	330
Cerebral Arteries	The portions of the cortex supplied by these arteries determine the most likely symptoms to occur when disease disrupts flow through them. (1) The anterior cerebral artery syndrome often includes loss of motor and sensory functions of the contralateral lower extremity as well as changes in memory, emotions, and personality (2) The middle artery syndrome often includes loss of motor and sensory functions to the contralateral side with less involvement of the lower extremities, transient deviation of the head and eyes toward the lesion, and partial visual-field deficit (3) The posterior cerebral artery syndrome classically results in a variety of visual deficits	323

Cerebral Blood Flow	The physiologic effects of arterial pressure, pCO_2, and pO_2 are the rationale behind some of the management principles in patients with increased intracranial pressure. They include: (1) Optimizing arterial pressure and therefore cerebral perfusion pressure (2) Prevention of hypoxemia (3) Use of hyperventilation	324
Dural Venous Sinuses	The size and distensibility of these vessels are the rationale behind some of the other management principles in patients with increased intracranial pressures. Distention of these veins due to patient position, increased intrathoracic pressure, or increased central venous pressure could cause a further increase in pressure.	325
Blood-Brain Barrier	The free permeability of these capillaries to water explains the neurologic manifestation of water intoxication. Their free permeability to gases explains the respiratory center's quick response to changes in pCO_2. The limited permeability to ions protects the brain from earlier manifestations of electrolyte disturbances.	330
Neurotransmission	This complex physiology and biochemistry explains why alterations in neurologic function can be the result of problems in nutrition, neurotransmitters, or electrolyte balance.	331–334
Spinal Cord	Motor and sensory impulses are structurally separated in the spinal cord. The gray matter is where all impulses enter (sensory) or exit (motor) the cord. The white matter is where the impulses ascend (sensory) or descend (motor) the cord.	334–336
Major Tracts	It is useful to remember that many tracts are named after their origin and destination when learning their functions. For example: (1) The spinothalamic tracts ascend from the spinal cord to the thalamus and therefore must have to do with sensation (2) The corticospinal tracts descend from cortex to spinal cord and therefore must have to do with motor function	335
Sensory Tracts	This diagram pulls together the structures involved in sensation and the potential sites of causes of sensory symptoms.	337 (Fig. 3–13 in *Core*)
Motor Pathways	This diagram pulls together the structures involved in motor function and the potential sites of causes of motor symptoms.	339 (Fig. 3–14 in *Core*)
Neuromuscular Transmitters	Understanding this complex physiology helps in understanding the many causes of altered neuromuscular transmission. They include: (1) Disease or damage of involved structures (2) Effects of drugs (3) Changes in electrolytes	341, 342
Cranial Nerves	Knowledge of cranial nerve anatomy and function helps when learning the causes of many of the clinical findings. For example: (1) Changes in III and IV may be associated with midbrain dysfunction since they originate there (2) Changes in V, VI, VII, and VIII may be associated with pontine dysfunction since they originate there (3) Changes in IX, X, XI, and XII may be associated with medullary dysfunction since they originate there (4) I–VIII travel along the base of the skull, not brain, with the meninges and therefore may be affected in basilar skull fractures or meningitis (5) IX–XII travel around the neck and/or mediastinum and may be affected in patients with disorders of that area	342–345

Table 3–5. STRUCTURES EVALUATED BY SELECTED NEUROASSESSMENT TECHNIQUES (*pages 349–362*)

Test	Structures
Pupillary reaction to light	Cranial nerves II and III
Range of ocular movements	Cranial nerves III, IV, VI
Corneal reflex	Cranial nerves V, VII
Doll's eyes (oculocephalic reflex)	Cranial nerves III, VI, VIII
Caloric test (oculovestibular reflex)	Cranial nerves III, IV, VIII, Frontal lobes
Gag reflex	Cranial nerves IX, X
Deep-tendon reflexes	Sensory and motor nerves
Tests for dystaxia, hypotonia, nystagmus, and dysarthria	Cerebellar function
Tests for stereognosis, topognosia, graphognosia and tactile inattention	Cortical discrimination

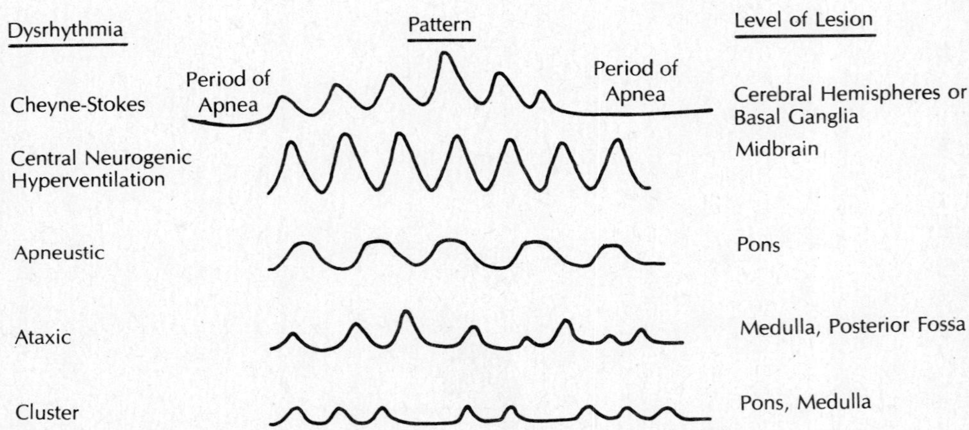

Figure 3–12. Respiratory dysrhythmias and the level of lesion involved (*page 360*).

Table 3–6. GENERAL GOALS IN INTERVENTIONS IN PATIENTS WITH CNS DISORDERS (*pages 366–375*)

Goal	Rationale
Prevent hypoxemia	May cause cerebral edema or vasodilation
Prevent hypoventilation	May cause cerebral vasodilation and ↑ ICP
Prevent severe hyperventilation	May cause cerebral vasoconstriction or impaired oxygen delivery
Recognize hypovolemia	May decrease cerebral perfusion
Recognize water loss or diabetes insipidus leading to hypernatremia	May decrease cerebral perfusion or lead to cerebral cellular dehydration
Recognize syndrome of inappropriate ADH	May cause increased cerebral edema

ADH indicates antidiuretic hormone

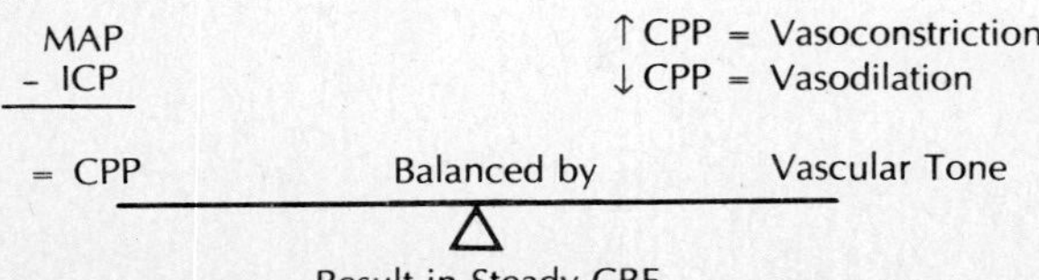

Figure 3–13. Mechanisms by which the brain autoregulates to maintain a constant cerebral blood flow (CBF). Relationship between cerebral perfusion pressure (CPP), intracranial pressure (ICP), and mean arterial pressure (MAP) and vascular tone are shown (*pages 375–386*).

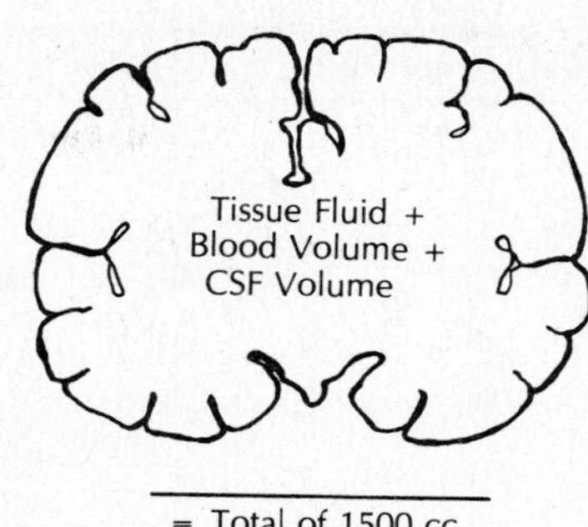

= Total of 1500 cc

↑ Volume = ↑ Pressure

High ICV
↓
Attempts to compensate
↓
Decompensation and Higher ICP
↓
Low CPP and CBF
↓
Vasodilation and Higher ICV
↓
Higher ICP and Lower CPP
↓
Low pO_2 and High pCO_2
↓
Vasodilation and Higher ICV

Figure 3–14. Pathologic consequences of increased intracranial volume (ICV) and pressure (ICP). Effects on cerebral perfusion pressure (CPP) and cerebral blood flow (CBF) are included (*pages 375–386*).

Table 3–7. COMPARISON OF TYPES OF INTRACRANIAL HEMORRHAGE (*pages 393–395, 412–418*)

Site	Common Causes	Common Clinical Characteristics
Subdural Hematoma	Venous bleeding after trauma Can occur spontaneously in patients with coagulation disorders	Acute, subacute, or chronic onset Signs of increased intracranial pressure
Epidural Hematoma	Arterial bleeding after trauma (except for posterior fossa hematomas, which are often venous) Often associated with skull fractures and middle meningeal artery damage	Classic presentation: (1) Short period of unconsciousness (2) Lucid interval (3) Rapid deterioration Signs of increased intracranial pressure Posterior fossa hematoma may cause signs of cardiopulmonary instability before signs of increased intracranial pressure
Intracerebral Hematoma	Traumatic rupture of vessels	Signs vary by size and area of involvement
Ruptured Intracranial Aneurysm	Spontaneous rupture of aneurysm of vessel in or near Circle of Willis Can cause intracerebral hematoma (above) or hemorrhage into subarachnoid space	Signs of meningeal irritation Signs of increased intracranial pressure Severity graded by symptoms (Grade I to VI) May develop vasospasm or rebleed
Arteriovenous Malformations	Congenital anomaly that may enlarge over time	Signs of increased intracranial pressure Seizures common in larger ones

Table 3–8. COMPARISON OF POSSIBLE SYMPTOMS OF CEREBROVASCULAR ACCIDENTS OF THE RIGHT AND LEFT HEMISPHERES (*pages 407–412*)

Symptom	Damage to Right Hemisphere	Damage to Left Hemisphere
Homonymous Hemianopsia	Left sided	Right sided
Hemiparesis or Hemiplegia	Left sided	Right sided
Special Sensory Losses	Astereognosia Astatoagnosia Anosognosia Constructional apraxia Dressing apraxia Inattention to visual and auditory stimuli on left side (Note: Last four are related to specialized functions of the right cerebral cortex)	Astereognosia Astatoagnosia Finger agnosia Right-left confusion Aphasia (Note: Last three are related to specialized functions of the left cerebral cortex)
Head and Eye Deviation	To right side	To left side

THE NEUROLOGIC SYSTEM

Exercises

After reading the neurology section of the Core Curriculum, *fill in the blanks in the following statements. It can be done one topic at a time or all at once. The answers are at the end of the exercises.*

A. Physiologic Anatomy (*pages 315–348*)

1. The normal cranial volume in the adult is ________________ cc.
2. The two intracranial structures formed by the dural layer of the meninges are called the ________________ and ________________.
3. The tough outer covering of the brain that contains the meningeal arteries and large venous sinuses is the ________________.
4. Cerebrospinal fluid lies between the ________________ and ________________ meninges.
5. Cerebrospinal fluid is reabsorbed back into the venous system through the ________________ villi.
6. The vessels of the plexus come from the arteries along the ________________ mater.
7. The tract responsible for voluntary motor activity is called the ________________ and it originates in the ________________ lobe.
8. The ________________ cerebral lobe is responsible for judgment, the ________________ lobe for hearing, the ________________ lobe for sensory association, and the ________________ lobe for vision.
9. In most people the right hemisphere is dominant for ________________ and ________________; the left for ________________ and ________________.

10. The central nervous system structure that regulates motor activity and influences tone and reflexes along with the cerebellum is the ________________________.
11. The central nervous system structure that serves as a major sensory relay station between the brainstem and cortex is the ____________ ________.
12. The central nervous system structure that serves as a major center of regulation is the ______________________.
13. The limbic system is responsible for ______________________ and ________________________.
14. The nuclei of the 3rd and 4th cranial nerves are in the ________ ______________; the 5th, 6th, 7th in the ____________________; the 9th, 10th, 11th, 12th from the ______________________; the 8th from both the ______________________ and ______________________.
15. The ascending reticular activating system is responsible for__________ __________.
16. The central nervous system structure responsible for equilibrium, posture, and nonstereotypic movements is the ______________________.
17. The blood flow through the Circle of Willis comes from the ___________ ___________ and the ______________________ arteries.
18. The ______________________ cerebral artery supplies more of the cerebral cortex than the other two cerebral arteries.
19. The cerebellum and brainstem receive their blood flow from the ______________________ system.
20. The collateral circuit that connects the basilar to the internal carotids is the ______________________.
21. The meningeal arteries receive their flow from the ____________ _________ and supply the ______________________.
22. The cerebral perfusion pressure is the difference between the _________ ____________ and the ______________________ and it should be above ______________________ mm Hg.
23. List the three factors that affect cerebral blood flow.
    a. ______________________
    b. ______________________
    c. ______________________
24. Normal cerebrospinal fluid pressure is ______________________ and its normal glucose is ______________________.
25. Most of the cerebrospinal fluid is made in the ______________ _____ and the total production rate is about ______________________.
26. Trace the pathway of cerebrospinal fluid flow from the choroid plexus to the venous sinuses.
    ____
    ____
    ____
27. Extensions that usually carry impulses away from the cell body are the ______________________.
28. Axon transmission rate is increased by the presence of the nodes of ______________________.
29. The most abundant type of cell in the central nervous system is the ______________________.
30. The main energy substrate used by the brain is ____________ _________.

31. The brain's consumption of oxygen is constant at about ______ ______ % of the body's total resting consumption.
32. The blood-brain barrier is more permeable to ______ ______, ______, and ______ than normal capillary walls.
33. The main transmitter across the neuromuscular junction is ______ ______.
34. An example of a cerebral neurotransmitter that acts as an inhibitor is the ______.
35. When a nerve is stimulated to a subthreshold level and therefore is not excited, it is said to be ______.
36. When the resting membrane potential of a nerve is made more negative, its ability to depolarize is ______.
37. The most moveable vertebrae are the ______; the most numerous are the ______; and the largest are the ______.
38. The spinal cord extends from the ______ vertebra to the top of the ______ vertebra.
39. Descending or efferent motor impulses exit the spinal cord via the ______ horns, whereas the ascending or afferent impulses enter via the ______ horns.
40. The ______ matter consists of columns or ______ ______, carrying impulses up and down the spinal cord, in many tracts or ______.
41. By convention, it can be surmised that a tract called the corticospinal tract begins in the ______ and ends in the ______ ______, therefore transmitting impulses in a ______ ______ direction.
42. A tract called the spinothalamic tract must begin in the ______ ______ and end in the ______, therefore transmitting impulses in a ______ direction.
43. Pain and temperature impulses enter the cord through the ______ ______ horn, travel to white columns on the ______ ______ side, then ascend to the ______.
44. Trace a vibration sensation's pathway from the leg to the cortex.
______
______
______
45. Lesions of the ______ motor neurons can eventually result in spastic paralysis and hyperreflexia.
46. Trace a voluntary motor impulse's pathway in the corticospinal tract.
______
______
______
47. Peripheral sympathetic fibers originate in the ______ ______ and ______ areas of the spinal cord; whereas the parasympathetic fibers originate in the ______ ______ and ______ areas.
48. A ______ is an area of skin innervated by a single peripheral nerve.
49. The ______ is the label for the nerves found in the lumbar cistern.

50. Acetylcholine is broken down by ____________ at the neuromuscular junction.
51. The ____________ cranial nerve is responsible for vision and the ____________ cranial nerve is responsible for hearing.
52. The cranial nerves that move the eye are the ____________, ____________, and ____________.
53. Facial sensation is mediated via the ____________ cranial nerve; facial motion by the ____________ cranial nerve.
54. The cranial nerves that overlap in function to innervate the pharynx are the ____________ and ____________.
55. The ____________ cranial nerve is responsible for innervating the neck muscles, whereas the ____________ cranial nerve moves the tongue.
56. Draw a large circle and use numbers or Roman numerals to indicate where each cranial nerve innervates and to create a cartoon face.

57. The predominant type of autonomic postganglionic nerve fibers that secrete acetylcholine are ____________.
58. The nerves that cause the vessels in skeletal muscles to constrict secrete ____________.

B. Nursing Assessment Data Base (*pages 348–366*)

1. Difficulty articulating is called ____________.
2. Loss of sense of smell is called ____________.
3. Bitemporal hemianopsia is caused by lesions of the ____________, whereas homonymous hemianopsia is caused by lesions of the ____________.
4. The ability to move the eyes to gaze in all the various directions requires the function of the ____________, ____________, and ____________ cranial nerves.
5. The corneal reflex is sensed by the ____________ cranial nerve and the resultant movement is caused by the ____________ cranial nerve.
6. The gag reflex is a function of the ____________ and ____________ cranial nerves.
7. Babinski's response to stroking the plantar surface of the foot is ____________ of the great toe, and it indicates disease of the ____________ motor neurons.
8. Two of the major clinical signs of cerebellar dysfunction are ____________ and ____________.
9. The capeline is the dermatomic landmark for the ____________ spinal nerves, the nipple line for ____________, the

umbilicis for ____________________, and the little toe for ____________________ nerve.

10. Two of the tests for higher order sensory interpretation and integration in the cerebral cortex are those for ____________________ and ____________________.
11. Indicate whether or not the following lesions can lead to loss of consciousness:
    a. Bilateral cerebral lesions ____________________
    b. Unilateral cerebral lesions ____________________
    c. Spinal cord lesions ____________________
    d. Widespread injury of the reticular formation system ____________________
12. List the three categories tested in the Glasgow Coma Scale:
    a. ____________________
    b. ____________________
    c. ____________________
13. An oval-shaped pupil may indicate ____________________.
14. The pupil will ____________________ with disruption of parasympathetic innervation via the ____________________ cranial nerve, and the pupil will ____________________ with disruption of its sympathetic innervation.
15. The pupillary reflex is a test of the sensory function of the ____________________ cranial nerve, and the motor function of the ____________________ cranial nerve.
16. State the type of lesion most likely to produce the following:
    a. Paratonia ____________________
    b. Flexor posturing ____________________
    c. Extensor posturing ____________________
17. The normal response of a comatose patient to caloric irrigation or testing of the oculovestibular reflex is ____________________ and ____________________.
18. The doll's eyes test or oculocephalic reflex is a test of the ____________________, ____________________, and ____________________ cranial nerves.
19. Rank the following respiratory dysrhythmias from highest to lowest level of central nervous system involvement by putting a number after each (1 for highest, 2 for intermediate, 3 for lowest).
    a. Cheyne-Stokes ____________________
    b. Central neurogenic hyperventilation ____________________
    c. Cluster ____________________
20. Cushing's reflex is an increase in the ____________________ sometimes associated with a ____________________ in heart rate in response to a rise in intracranial pressure.
21. Testing of deep-tendon reflexes in patients with upper motor neuron disease is likely to reveal ____________________, whereas those with a lower motor neuron disease exhibit ____________________.
22. The main limitation of computerized tomography is in the diagnosis of ____________________ lesions of the cranium.
23. If contrast is used to enhance computerized tomography scans, the volume and concentration of urine may be ____________________ for several hours.
24. Lumbar puncture is contraindicated in the patient with increased ____________________.

C. Commonly Encountered Nursing Diagnoses (*pages 366–375*)

1. Expected outcomes for a patient with increased intracranial pressure include a cerebral perfusion pressure above ______________________ and an intracranial pressure below ______________________.
2. Expected outcomes in a neuro patient with a potential for altered oxygen supply include a paO_2 above ______________________ and a hemoglobin above ______________________.
3. Signs that a fluid volume deficit in a neuro patient may be due to diabetes insipidus include ______________________ urinary output and ______________________ urine specific gravity.
4. List three commonly encountered nursing diagnoses in the patient with neurologic disorders:
   a. ______________________
   b. ______________________
   c. ______________________

D. Patient Health Problems (*pages 375–462*)

1. The Monro-Kellie doctrine states that when one component of the intracranial volume goes up, another must go ______________________ or the pressure will ______________________.
2. Mechanisms that compensate for an increasing intracranial pressure act by decreasing the cranial volume of ______________________ and ______________________.
3. As intracranial compliance falls, intracranial elastance ______________________.
4. The cerebral perfusion pressure is calculated by finding the difference between the ______________________ and the ______________________.
5. When the intracranial pressure rises, the cerebral vessels ______________________ to prevent a fall in cerebral blood flow.
6. Two blood gas changes that may cause cerebral arteries to dilate are ______________________ and ______________________.
7. The herniation syndrome where a unilateral cerebral lesion forces the uncus of the temporal lobe downward and medial is called ______________________; the one in which the posterior fossa structures are forced through the foramen magnum is called ______________________.
8. Three causes of increased brain volume are ______________________, ______________________, and ______________________.
9. The cerebral edema that results from dysfunction of the blood-brain barrier is categorized as ______________________, and the type that results from cerebral hypoxia as ______________________.
10. Indicate whether each of the following is more likely to increase or decrease the intracranial pressure:
    a. Water intoxication ______________________
    b. Hyperflexion of the neck ______________________
    c. Valsalva maneuver ______________________
    d. Loss of autoregulation ______________________
    e. Obstruction of CSF flow ______________________
    f. Hyperventilation ______________________
    g. Lowering the head of the bed ______________________
    h. Drainage of CSF ______________________
11. Key areas of nursing assessment in patients with potential for increased

intracranial pressure include ______________ and ______________.

12. The normal intracranial pressure is less than ______________ mm Hg.
13. The four most common techniques used to monitor intracranial pressure are ______________, ______________, ______________, and ______________.
14. The pathologic wave form seen in patients undergoing intracranial pressure monitoring is called ______________.
15. List three interventions that may be considered to control intracranial hypertension, depending on the severity and cause:
    a. ______________
    b. ______________
    c. ______________
16. The two types of hydrocephalus are ______________ and ______________.
17. Hydrocephalus may occur as a complication of ______________ or ______________.
18. The scalp has a ______________ tendency to bleed than most other areas of the body.
19. The type of skull fracture most likely to damage the cranial nerves or cause a leak of cerebrospinal fluid is ______________.
20. Anosmia may occur as a result of fractures of the ______________ or ______________.
21. Fractures of the ______________ fossa may result in rhinorrhea or "owl's" eyes.
22. Battle's sign can result from fracture of the ______________ fossa.
23. Posterior fossa hemorrhage can cause dysfunction of two important structures of the brain: the ______________ and the ______________.
24. Treatment of an uncomplicated basal skull fracture with a cerebrospinal fluid leak is directed toward the prevention of ______________ and ______________.
25. Transient loss of cerebral function following a blow to the head is called a ______________.
26. Closed head injuries are categorized into four levels: levels ______________ are associated with loss of consciousness lasting less than 24 hours, and levels ______________ are associated with loss of consciousness lasting more than 24 hours.
27. Symptoms of cerebral concussion ______________ within 12 hours, whereas symptoms of cerebral contusion can ______________ for 72 hours.
28. The main goal in the treatment of patients with cerebral contusions is to recognize and prevent or control ______________.
29. Subdural and posterior fossa epidural hematomas are usually related to ______________ bleeds.
30. Traumatic injury to the middle meningeal artery is a common cause of ______________ hematomas.
31. A patient with ______________ hematoma may present without a history of trauma and a very slow onset of symptoms.
32. A patient with a (an) ______________ hematoma may

present with a short period of unconsciousness followed by a lucid interval.

33. Patients with cerebral subdural or epidural hematomas are more likely to lose oculomotor function on the ______ side of the lesion, and motor function on the ______ side when the intracranial pressure rises.
34. In order of easiest to hardest, list three types of motor tasks the patient may be asked to do to evaluate the corticospinal tract:
    a. ______
    b. ______
    c. ______
35. Tests for proprioception and vibration assess function of the ______ tracts.
36. Injury to the ______ tracts of the spinal cord leads to loss of the sensations of light touch, pain, and temperature.
37. Central cord syndrome results in loss of motor function, which is more pronounced in the ______ than in the ______ extremities.
38. The type of spinal cord lesion that results in ipsilateral loss of motor function with contralateral loss of sensations for pain and temperature is ______.
39. A spinal cord injured patient may lose function of the diaphragm when the spinal cord involvement is above ______.
40. The term spinal shock is used to refer to loss of ______ and ______, which can occur in the acute phase of spinal cord injuries.
41. Hypotension and bradycardia may occur in the acute phase of spinal cord injury owing to loss of ______ nerve function in lesions above ______.
42. Poikilothermism may lead to alterations in ______ in spinal cord patients.
43. Measures to reduce the risk of venous thrombosis in spinal cord injured patients include ______ and ______.
44. Two potential gastrointestinal complications in patients with acute spinal cord injury are ______, which can lead to fluid loss, and ______, which can lead to blood loss.
45. The most common type of stroke is due to vascular ______, whereas only 25% are due to ______.
46. Cerebral vascular events in which symptoms resolve in less than 24 hours are called ______, whereas those in which it takes more than 24 hours to resolve are called ______.
47. Indicate whether the following are more likely to occur in strokes of the right or left hemisphere:
    a. Right hemiplegia ______
    b. Left homonymous hemianopsia ______
    c. Deviation of the head and eyes to right ______
    d. Dysphasia ______
    e. Right-left confusion ______
48. Because strokes are a disorder of the upper motor neuron, deep-tendon reflexes eventually become ______.
49. The most frequent site for intracranial aneurysms is vessels of or near the ______.

50. A patient with an intracranial aneurysm who is unconscious is at least a grade ______.
51. Two vascular complications of cerebral aneurysms are ______ and ______.
52. Medical management of vasospasm in patients with intracranial aneurysms may include ______ and ______.
53. Patients with small arteriovenous malformations often present with ______, whereas patients with larger ones most often present with ______.
54. Complications of brain tumors include ______ and ______.
55. The most common types of brain tumors are ______.
56. The most common presenting symptom of brain tumors is ______.
57. Indicate the most likely site of a brain tumor for each of the following symptoms:
    a. Expressive aphasia ______
    b. Unilateral neglect ______
    c. Psychomotor seizures ______
    d. Hyperesthesia ______
    e. Seizures with a visual aura ______
    f. Nystagmus ______
    g. Receptive aphasia ______
    h. Motor weakness ______
    i. Loss of self-restraint ______
58. List three signs of meningismus or meningeal irritation:
    a. ______
    b. ______
    c. ______
59. Petechiae or purpura are more likely to occur in patients with ______ meningitis.
60. Patients with meningitis may develop signs such as photophobia, diplopia, or facial paresis when the ______ are irritated.
61. A complication of meningitis that is caused by adrenal hemorrhage is called ______ syndrome.
62. Cerebrospinal fluid changes seen in patients with bacterial meningitis include ______ protein, ______ glucose, and ______ white blood cells.
63. Seizures are more likely to be primary in ______ patients and secondary in ______ patients.
64. Two examples of generalized seizures are ______ and ______.
65. Partial focal motor seizures that progress to involve more of the body are called ______.
66. Seizures that consist of elaborate purposeful-looking behavior and amnesia for it are called ______.
67. During seizures cerebral metabolism goes ______ and cerebral blood flow goes ______.
68. Status epilepticus may be caused by withdrawal from ______, ______, or ______.

69. Laboratory studies in the patient with status grand mal seizures reveal ______________ serum glucose, ______________ pO_2, ______________ pCO_2, ______________ pH, and ______________CPK.
70. Severe status grand mal can result in myoglobinuria, which can cause ______________ failure.
71. Phenytoin causes ______________ masking of neurologic signs than phenobarbital.
72. Polyneuritis or Guillain-Barré syndrome is related to ______________ of the nerves, causing a ______________ in transmission, which usually begins in the ______________ nerves and progresses ______________ the body.
73. The primary type of symptom of polyneuritis is ______________.
74. The cerebrospinal fluid change often seen in patients with Guillain-Barré syndrome is ______________.
75. The two common manifestations of autonomic dysfunction are fluctuations in the ______________ and ______________.
76. Myasthenia gravis is thought to be an autoimmune disease that results in a decrease in the number of ______________.
77. The clinical manifestations of myasthenia gravis usually involve the ______________ parts of the body.
78. Muscle weakness in patients with myasthenia gravis gets worse with ______________ activity.
79. The short-acting anticholinesterase agent used to diagnose myasthenia gravis is ______________.
80. Complications of myasthenia gravis include an exacerbation of the disease called ______________ crisis, and overtreatment causing ______________ crisis.
81. Severe myasthenia gravis may be treated by ______________ and ______________.
82. The pupillary sign seen in patients who overdose on opiates is ______________.
83. Severe alcohol intoxication may cause ______________ temperature, ______________ blood glucose, ______________ respiration, and ______________ reflexes.
84. Cocaine overdose causes the blood pressure, heart rate, and temperature to go ______________ and also causes a variety of symptoms of the ______________ and ______________ systems.
85. Salicylate overdose can cause the cerebral vessels to ______________, the $paCO_2$ to ______________, and bleeding times to be ______________.
86. Acetaminophen overdose is especially toxic to the ______________.
87. In patients with drug overdose, absorption can be diminished by ______________ or ______________, depending on the agent, the timing, and the patient's symptoms.
88. Rank the following according to the order in which they return in patients recovering from anesthesia:

a. Consciousness ____________________
b. Cough reflex ____________________
c. Swallowing and vomiting reflexes ____________________

89. Recovery from anesthesia may be hastened by administering ____________________ to reverse the effects of neuromuscular blockers, or ____________________ to reverse the effects of opiates.
90. Techniques that may be of value in removing certain drugs in patients who have overdosed are ____________________ and ____________________.
91. Malignant hyperthermia in a patient emerging from general anesthesia may be associated with ____________________ potassium, ____________________ CPK, ____________________pH, and skeletal muscle ____________________.
92. The drug used to treat malignant hyperthermia is ____________________.

E. Summary of Patient Health Problems (*pages 375–462*)

After reading each disease, summarize the pathophysiology, nursing assessment data base, and nursing diagnoses. Since the certification examination holds you responsible for knowing the etiology and risk factors, the signs and symptoms, the collaborative diagnosis, the complications, and the management and treatment goals, those preparing to take it should also summarize these areas. If they are not clearly covered in the Core*, a second resource may be necessary. The space allotted is purposefully limited to encourage concise descriptions of concepts and careful selection of key points. It is not as helpful to write the things you already know as it is to write those you need to study.*

1. Increased Intracranial Pressure

Pathophysiology	*Etiology/Risk Factors*	*Signs/Symptoms*

Collaborative Diagnosis	*Complications*	*Management/Goals*

2. Hydrocephalus

Pathophysiology	*Etiology/Risk Factors*	*Signs/Symptoms*

Collaborative Diagnosis	*Complications*	*Management/Goals*

3. Scalp Lacerations

Pathophysiology	*Etiology/Risk Factors*	*Signs/Symptoms*

Collaborative Diagnosis	*Complications*	*Management/Goals*

4. Skull Fractures

Pathophysiology	*Etiology/Risk Factors*	*Signs/Symptoms*

Collaborative Diagnosis	*Complications*	*Management/Goals*

5. Closed-Head Injuries

Pathophysiology	*Etiology/Risk Factors*	*Signs/Symptoms*

Collaborative Diagnosis	*Complications*	*Management/Goals*

6. Intracranial Hematomas

Pathophysiology	*Etiology/Risk Factors*	*Signs/Symptoms*

Collaborative Diagnosis	*Complications*	*Management/Goals*

7. Acute Spinal Cord Injuries

Pathophysiology	*Etiology/Risk Factors*	*Signs/Symptoms*

Collaborative Diagnosis	*Complications*	*Management/Goals*

8. Stroke

Pathophysiology	*Etiology/Risk Factors*	*Signs/Symptoms*

Collaborative Diagnosis	*Complications*	*Management/Goals*

9. Intracranial Aneurysms

Pathophysiology	*Etiology/Risk Factors*	*Signs/Symptoms*

Collaborative Diagnosis	*Complications*	*Management/Goals*

10. Arteriovenous Malformations

Pathophysiology	*Etiology/Risk Factors*	*Signs/Symptoms*

Collaborative Diagnosis	*Complications*	*Management/Goals*

11. Brain Tumors

Pathophysiology	*Etiology/Risk Factors*	*Signs/Symptoms*

Collaborative Diagnosis	*Complications*	*Management/Goals*

12. Meningitis

Pathophysiology	*Etiology/Risk Factors*	*Signs/Symptoms*

Collaborative Diagnosis	*Complications*	*Management/Goals*

13. Seizures

Pathophysiology	*Etiology/Risk Factors*	*Signs/Symptoms*

Collaborative Diagnosis	*Complications*	*Management/Goals*

14. Status Epilepticus

Pathophysiology	*Etiology/Risk Factors*	*Signs/Symptoms*

Collaborative Diagnosis	*Complications*	*Management/Goals*

15. Guillain-Barré Syndrome

Pathophysiology	*Etiology/Risk Factors*	*Signs/Symptoms*

Collaborative Diagnosis	*Complications*	*Management/Goals*

16. Myasthenia Gravis

Pathophysiology	*Etiology/Risk Factors*	*Signs/Symptoms*

Collaborative Diagnosis	*Complications*	*Management/Goals*

17. Drug Intoxication

Pathophysiology	*Etiology/Risk Factors*	*Signs/Symptoms*

Collaborative Diagnosis	*Complications*	*Management/Goals*

18. Recovery from Anesthesia

Pathophysiology	*Etiology/Risk Factors*	*Signs/Symptoms*

Collaborative Diagnosis	*Complications*	*Management/Goals*

F. Application to Clinical Practice

Care for patients with nervous system disease. Relate anatomy and physiology, assessment, and pathophysiology found in this section to their individual clinical picture. Make notes of instances where they correlate and where they deviate from the expected presentation. Devise a care plan based on the data collected.

Answers to Neurologic Exercises

A. Physiologic Anatomy

1. 1500 (*page 315*)
2. Falx cerebri, tentorium cerebelli (*page 316*)
3. Dura mater (*page 316*)
4. Pia, arachnoid (*page 316*)
5. Arachnoid (*page 316*)
6. Pia (*page 318*)
7. Pyramidal or corticospinal, frontal (*page 318*)
8. Frontal, temporal, parietal, occipital (*page 318*)
9. Any two of the following functions (*page 318*):
   a. For the right hemisphere
      1. geometrical
      2. spatial
      3. visual
      4. musical
   b. For the left hemisphere
      1. verbal
      2. linguistic
      3. arithmetical
      4. calculating
      5. analytical
10. Basal ganglia (*page 318*)
11. Thalamus (*page 318*)
12. Hypothalamus (*pages 318, 319*)
13. Affective and visceral aspects of emotions, part of memory (*page 321*)
14. Midbrain, pons, medulla, pons and medulla (*page 321*)
15. Arousal, alertness, or focusing (*page 322*)
16. Cerebellum (*page 323*)
17. Internal carotid, vertebral or basilar (*page 323*)
18. Middle (*page 323*)
19. Vertebral (*page 324*)
20. Circle of Willis (*page 324*)
21. External carotid, dura mater (*page 324*)
22. Mean arterial pressure, intracranial pressure, 60 (*page 324*)
23. a. Perfusion pressure
    b. $paCO_2$
    c. paO_2 (*page 324*)
24. 80–180 mm water or 5–15 mm Hg, 60% of the serum glucose (*page 327*)
25. Lateral ventricles, 500 cc/day (*page 327*)
26. Lateral ventricles, foramen of Monro, third ventricle, aqueduct of Sylvius, fourth ventricle, foramina of Luschka and Magendie, subarachnoid space, arachnoid villi (*pages 327, 328*)
27. Axons (*page 328*)
28. Ranvier (*page 328*)
29. Neuroglial cells (*page 328*)
30. Glucose (*page 330*)
31. 20 (*page 330*)
32. Water, gases, glucose (*page 330*)
33. Acetylcholine (*page 331*)
34. Dopamine or gamma-aminobutyric acid (*page 331*)
35. Facilitated (*page 332*)
36. Decreased or suppressed (*page 333*)
37. Cervical (especially the first two), thoracic, lumbar (*page 333*)
38. 1st cervical, 2nd lumbar (*page 334*)
39. Anterior, posterior (*page 334*)
40. White, funiculi, fasciculi (*pages 335, 336*)
41. Cortex, spinal cord, descending (*page 336*)
42. Spinal cord, thalamus, ascending (*page 336*)
43. Posterior, opposite, thalamus (*page 336*)
44. Peripheral nerve, posterior horn, posterior or ascending white columns, contralateral brainstem, thalamus, and parietal lobe (*page 337*)
45. Upper (*page 338*)
46. Frontal lobe, basal ganglia, brainstem, contralateral anterior and lateral white columns in spinal cord, anterior horn, peripheral motor nerve, skeletal muscle (*pages 339, 340*)
47. Thoracic, lumbar; cranial, sacral (*page 341*)
48. Dermatomes (*page 341*)
49. Cauda equina (*page 391*)
50. Acetylcholinesterase (*page 342*)
51. II or optic, VIII or acoustic (*pages 343, 344*)
52. III or oculomotor, IV or trochlear, VI or abducens (*pages 343, 344*)
53. V or trigeminal, VII or facial (*page 344*)
54. IX or glossopharnygeal, X or vagus (*page 345*)
55. XI or spinal accessory, XII or hypoglossal (*page 345*)
56. This is an exercise in individual creativity. There are many right images that can result (*pages 343, 344*)
57. Parasympathetic (*page 348*)
58. Norepinephrine (*page 348*)

B. Nursing Assessment Data Base

1. Dysarthria (*page 349*)
2. Anosmia (*page 349*)
3. Optic chiasm, optic tract (between the optic chiasm and the occipital lobe) (*page 350*)
4. III or oculomotor, IV or trochlear, VI or abducens (*page 351*)
5. V or trigeminal, VII or facial (*page 351*)
6. IX or glossopharnygeal, X or vagus (*page 352*)
7. Extension or dorsiflexion, upper (*page 353*)
8. Any two of these (*pages 353, 354*):
   a. Dystaxia
   b. Hypotonia
   c. Nystagmus
   d. Dysarthria
9. 3rd and 4th cervical, 4th thoracic, 10th thoracic, 1st sacral (*pages 354, 355*)
10. Any two of these (*page 355*):
    a. Stereognosis
    b. Topognosis
    c. Graphognosis
    d. Tactile inattention
11. a. Yes
    b. No
    c. No
    d. Yes (*page 355*)
12. a. Eye opening
    b. Best motor response
    c. Best verbal response (*pages 356, 357*)
13. Tentorial herniation or increased intracranial pressure (*page 357*)
14. Dilate, III or oculomotor, constrict (*page 357*)
15. II or optic, III or oculomotor (*page 357*)
16. a. Frontal lobe and increased intracranial pressure
    b. Internal capsule or cerebral hemispheres
    c. Brainstem (*page 358*)
17. Nystagmus, deviation of the eyes toward the irrigated ear (*page 359*)
18. VIII or acoustic, III or oculomotor, VI or abducens (*page 359*)
19. a. **1**
    b. **2**
    c. **3** (*page 360*)
20. Systolic blood pressure or pulse pressure, decrease (*page 360*)
21. Hyperreflexia, hyporeflexia or areflexia (*page 361*)
22. Vascular (*page 363*)
23. Increased (*page 363*)
24. Intracranial pressure (*page 365*)

C. Commonly Encountered Nursing Diagnoses

1. 60 mm Hg, 20 mm Hg (*page 366*)
2. 80 mm Hg, 10 gm (*page 367*)
3. Increased, decreased (*page 370*)
4. Any three of these (*pages 366–375*):
   a. Alteration in cerebral tissue perfusion
   b. Impaired gas exchange
   c. Ineffective breathing pattern
   d. Ineffective airway clearance
   e. Potential for fluid volume deficit
   f. Potential for fluid volume excess
   g. Potential for infection
   h. Impaired verbal communication
   i. Impaired physical mobility
   j. Alteration in thought processes
   k. Ineffective family coping

D. Patient Health Problems

1. Down, increase (*page 375*)
2. Cerebrospinal fluid, cerebral blood volume (*page 375*)
3. Rises (*page 376*)
4. Mean systemic arterial pressure, intracranial pressure (*page 376*)
5. Dilate (*page 376*)
6. Increased CO_2, decreased O_2 (*page 376*)
7. Tentorial or uncal, tonsillor or medullary (*page 377*)
8. Mass lesions, cytotoxic cerebral edema, vasogenic cerebral edema (*pages 377, 378*)
9. Vasogenic, cytotoxic (*pages 377, 378*)
10. a. Increase
    b. Increase
    c. Increase
    d. Increase
    e. Increase
    f. Decrease
    g. Increase
    h. Decrease (*pages 377–385*)
11. Any two of these (*pages 379, 382*):
    a. Level of consciousness
    b. Motor activity
    c. Pupillary size and reflexes
    d. Other cranial nerves
    e. Vital signs
12. Ten (10–20 considered moderate elevation) (*pages 380, 382*)
13. Intraventricular, subarachnoid, epidural, intraparenchymal (*pages 380, 381*)

14. An A wave, plateau wave, or Lundberg wave (*page 383*)
15. Any three of these (*pages 383–385*):
    a. Increase venous return from cranial vault
    b. Limit measures that increase pressure as much as possible
    c. Decrease intracranial volume of cerebrospinal fluid, tissue fluid, or blood
    d. Glucocorticoids
    e. Barbiturate coma
    f. Paralyzing agents
    g. Sedation
16. Communicating or nonobstructive, noncommunicating or obstructive (*page 385*)
17. Any two of these (*page 385*):
    a. Mass lesions
    b. Subarachnoid hemorrhage
    c. Intraventricular hemorrhage
    d. Meningitis
18. Higher (*page 386*)
19. Basilar (*page 388*)
20. Frontal bone, anterior fossa (*page 388*)
21. Anterior (*page 388*)
22. Middle (*page 388*)
23. Cerebellum, medulla or brainstem (*page 389*)
24. Infection, abscess formation (*page 389*)
25. Concussion (*page 391*)
26. One and two, three and four (*page 391*)
27. Resolve, increase in severity (*page 392*)
28. Increased intracranial pressure (*pages 392, 393*)
29. Venous (*page 393*)
30. Epidural (*page 394*)
31. Chronic subdural (*page 394*)
32. Epidural (*page 394*)
33. Same or ipsilateral, opposite or contralateral (*page 394*)
34. a. Wiggle or move
    b. Lift off bed (against gravity)
    c. Perform against resistance (abduct, adduct, flex, extend) (*page 396*)
35. Fasciculus gracilis and cuneatus or posterior column's (*page 397*)
36. Spinothalamic (*page 398*)
37. Upper, lower (*page 399*)
38. Brown-Séquard (*page 399*)
39. 4th cervical vertebra (*page 399*)
40. Reflexes, motor tone (*page 399*)
41. Sympathetic, the 5th thoracic vertebra (*page 400*)
42. Temperature (*page 400*)
43. Any two of these (*page 400*):
    a. Anticoagulation
    b. Antiembolic stockings
    c. Alternating pressure devices
    d. Passive motion (exercises, chairs, moving beds)
44. Gastric dilation or ileus, Cushing's ulcer or stress ulcer (*page 403*)
45. Occlusion or thrombosis, hemorrhage or bleeding (*page 407*)
46. Transient ischemic attacks, reversible ischemic neurologic deficits (*page 408*)
47. a. Left
    b. Right
    c. Right
    d. Left
    e. Left (*pages 409, 410*)
48. Hyperactive (*page 410*)
49. Circle of Willis (*page 412*)
50. IV (*page 414*)
51. Rebleeding, vasospasm (*pages 414, 415*)
52. Any two of these (*page 415*):
    a. Hypervolemia
    b. Hemodilution
    c. Hypertension
    d. Calcium channel blockers
53. Intracranial hemorrhage, seizures (*page 417*)
54. Any two of these (*page 418*):
    a. Cerebral edema
    b. Intracranial hypertension
    c. Seizures
    d. Focal neurologic deficits
    e. Hydrocephalus
    f. Hormonal changes
55. Gliomas (*pages 418, 420*)
56. Headache (*page 420*)
57. a. Left frontal lobe
    b. Right parietal lobe
    c. Temporal lobe
    d. Parietal lobe
    e. Occipital lobe
    f. Cerebellum
    g. Left temporal lobe
    h. Frontal lobe
    i. Frontal lobe (*pages 420, 421*)
58. Any three of these (*page 424*):
    a. Headache
    b. Neck or back pain
    c. Nausea and vomiting
    d. Irritability, confusion
    e. Photophobia

f. Brudzinski's sign
g. Kernig's sign
59. Meningococcal (*page 424*)
60. Cranial nerves (*page 425*)
61. Waterhouse-Friderichsen (*page 425*)
62. Increased, decreased, increased (*page 425*)
63. Younger, older (*pages 427, 428*)
64. Any two of these (*pages 428, 429*):
   a. Tonic-clonic (grand mal)
   b. Absence (petit mal)
   c. Myoclonic
   d. Akinetic
65. Jacksonian seizures (*page 429*)
66. Automatisms or temporal lobe attacks or psychomotor seizures (*page 429*)
67. Up, up (*page 432*)
68. Anticonvulsant medications, alcohol, central nervous system depressants (*page 433*)
69. Decreased, decreased, increased, decreased, increased (*pages 433, 434*)
70. Renal (*page 434*)
71. Less (*page 436*)
72. Demyelination, decrease, distal, up (*pages 437, 438*)
73. Impaired motor function (*page 438*)
74. Increased protein without increased white cells or albuminocytologic dissociation (*page 439*)
75. Blood pressure, heart rate (*pages 439, 440*)
76. Acetylcholine receptor sites on muscle (*page 442*)
77. Upper (*page 443*)
78. Repetitive (*page 443*)
79. Edrophonium chloride or tensilon (*page 443*)
80. Myasthenic, cholinergic (*pages 444–446*)
81. Any two of these (*pages 444–446*):
   a. Anticholinesterase agents
   b. Corticosteroids
   c. Thymectomy
   d. Plasmapheresis
82. Miosis (*pages 448, 449*)
83. Decreased, decreased, decreased, decreased (*page 448*)
84. Up, nervous, gastrointestinal (*page 449*)
85. Dilate, decrease, prolonged (*pages 450, 451*)
86. Liver (*page 450*)
87. Any two of these (*pages 454, 455*):
   a. Gastric lavage
   b. Induction of vomiting
   c. Absorption of toxin
88. a. 3rd
   b. 1st
   c. 2nd (*page 458*)
89. Neostigmine or pyridostigmine, naloxone (*page 460*)
90. Any two of these (*pages 455, 456*):
   a. Dialysis
   b. Hemoperfusion
   c. Forced osmotic diuresis
   d. Forced acid or alkaline diuresis
91. Increased, increased, decreased, rigidity (*pages 461, 462*)
92. Dantrolene (*page 462*)

E. Summary of Patient Health Problems

Refer to the following pages in the Core Curriculum

1. Increased Intracranial Pressure (*pages 375–385*)
2. Hydrocephalus (*pages 385, 386*)
3. Scalp Lacerations (*pages 386, 387*)
4. Skull Fractures (*pages 387–391*)
5. Closed-Head Injuries (*pages 391–393*)
6. Intracranial Hematomas (*pages 393–395*)
7. Acute Spinal Cord Injuries (*pages 395–407*)
8. Stroke (*pages 407–412*)
9. Intracranial Aneurysms (*pages 412–416*)
10. Arteriovenous Malformations (*pages 416–418*)
11. Brain Tumors (*pages 418–423*)
12. Meningitis (*pages 423–427*)
13. Seizures (*pages 427–432*)
14. Status Epilepticus (*pages 432–437*)
15. Guillain-Barré Syndrome (*pages 437–442*)
16. Myasthenia Gravis (*pages 442–447*)
17. Drug Intoxication (*pages 447–457*)
18. Recovery from Anesthesia (*pages 457–462*)

THE NEUROLOGIC SYSTEM

Post Quiz

The following questions are designed to test understanding of some of the key points in the section. Select the letter that best completes the following. The answers are at the end of the test.

1. The subarachnoid space lies between the
   a. dura and pia mater
   b. arachnoid and pia mater
   c. arachnoid and dura mater
   d. dural layers
2. The spinal cord ends at
   a. T-10
   b. L-2
   c. L-5
   d. S-1
3. Cerebrospinal fluid enters the subarachnoid space via
   a. aqueduct of Sylvius
   b. foramina of Magendie and Luschka
   c. dural sinuses
   d. foramen ovale
4. The cerebral lobe primarily responsible for sensation is the
   a. frontal
   b. parietal
   c. temporal
   d. occipital
5. The CNS structure responsible for coordination and refinement of voluntary muscle movement is the
   a. hypothalamus
   b. temporal lobe
   c. thalamus
   d. cerebellum
6. The diencephalon structure involved in the relay of sensory impulses to the cerebral cortex is the
   a. hypothalamus
   b. thalamus
   c. basal ganglia
   d. pons
7. The cranial nerve responsible for hearing and equilibrium is the
   a. III
   b. V
   c. VIII
   d. X
8. Afferent vessels of the Circle of Willis include the
   a. basilar artery
   b. anterior communicating artery
   c. anterior cerebral artery
   d. inferior cerebellar artery
9. In the adult, the extension of the great toe toward the head on plantar stimulation is
   a. normal
   b. absence of the Babinski sign

c. presence of the Babinski sign
d. a lower motor neuron problem

10. A breathing pattern that changes irregularly in both depth and rate is called
a. apneustic
b. Cheyne-Stokes
c. ataxic
d. cluster

11. Which of the following would be a likely clinical feature of a cerebrovascular accident involving the right cerebral hemisphere?
a. speech disturbances
b. right-sided weakness
c. deviation of the head and eyes to the left
d. blindness in the left half of the visual field

12. A subdural hematoma
a. involves bleeding into the space under the dura
b. is usually arterial
c. can only occur immediately after head trauma
d. usually causes contralateral pupil dilation

13. A concussion is a head injury associated with
a. transient loss of cerebral function
b. residual focal neurologic deficits
c. skull fractures
d. progressive deterioration

14. The third and fourth cranial nerves' nuclei are found in the
a. diencephalon
b. midbrain
c. pons
d. medulla

15. Which of the following would be most likely to be contraindicated in a patient with increased intracranial pressure?
a. osmotic diuretics
b. steroids
c. fluid limitation
d. flat position

16. Which of the following is *not* a sign of meningitis?
a. hyperthermia
b. severe headache
c. convulsions
d. negative Kernig's and Brudzinski's signs

17. Examination of the CSF in bacterial meningitis will reveal *all but* which of the following?
a. increased cloudiness
b. increased white blood cells
c. decreased protein
d. increased pressure

18. Guillain-Barré syndrome results from
a. decreased acetylcholine formation
b. demyelination of the nerves
c. inflammation of the Guillain cells
d. meningismus

19. Myasthenia gravis
a. is a result of too much acetylcholine
b. can be temporarily improved by Tensilon
c. produces symmetrical ascending weakness
d. can result in respiratory alkalosis

20. Seizures typified by short lapses of consciousness that may or may not be associated with focal myoclonus are
    a. petit mal
    b. akinetic
    c. Jacksonian
    d. psychomotor
21. Major complications of status epilepticus include
    a. alkalosis
    b. hyperglycemia
    c. respiratory distress
    d. hypothermia
22. In a typical neuron
    a. there are several axons and one dendrite
    b. the impulse is transmitted from the dendrites to the cell body to the axon
    c. the dendrites are myelinated
    d. the neurotransmitters are stored in the nodes of Ranvier
23. The middle meningeal artery
    a. is often the source of a subarachnoid bleed
    b. is a branch of the internal carotid arteries
    c. supplies the pia and arachnoid maters
    d. may cause an epidural hematoma when damaged by head injury
24. The cranial nerve responsible for facial sensation is
    a. III
    b. V
    c. VII
    d. IX
25. The anterior horns
    a. consist of white matter
    b. contain the nerve roots for sensory impulses
    c. primarily contain the nuclei for fibers of the autonomic nervous system
    d. are the outlet for efferent impulses
26. The lateral spinothalamic tract
    a. consists primarily of gray matter
    b. is a descending column
    c. crosses to the contralateral side at the base of the brainstem
    d. conveys impulses for sensations of pain and temperature
27. The parasympathetic division of the autonomic nervous system
    a. originates in the thoracolumbar areas of the spinal cord
    b. has short preganglionic fibers that end in a ganglion chain very near the spinal cord
    c. causes a generalized rather than a local response
    d. has short postganglionic fibers that secrete acetylcholine
28. Cerebral blood flow
    a. normally varies greatly with changes in the blood pressure
    b. increases when the intracranial pressure is close to the mean arterial pressure
    c. increases in response to a high $paCO_2$ due to vasodilation
    d. decreases in response to a low paO_2 due to vasoconstriction
29. The blood-brain barrier is least permeable to
    a. glucose
    b. water
    c. gas molecules
    d. electrolytes
30. Signs of cerebellar dysfunction would *not* include
    a. dystaxia

b. hypotonia
c. nystagmus
d. dysphasia

31. In decerebrate rigidity, the upper extremities
a. extend and adduct
b. extend and abduct
c. flex and adduct
d. flex and abduct

32. The rare postoperative complication treated by dantrolene is
a. sepsis
b. vasodilator shock
c. cerebral ischemia
d. malignant hyperthermia

33. Classic signs of increased intracranial pressure would *not* include
a. headache
b. a decreased level of consciousness
c. decreasing motor function
d. narrowing pulse pressure

34. A spinal cord disorder typified by motor losses more pronounced in the upper than lower extremities is
a. central cord syndrome
b. Brown-Séquard syndrome
c. anterior cord syndrome
d. Guillain-Barré syndrome

35. What level of spinal cord injury causes total loss of respiratory function?
a. above C-4
b. C-4 to C-8
c. T-1 to T-5
d. T-5 to L-2

36. Spastic paralysis may be related to
a. upper motor neuron dysfunction
b. lower motor neuron dysfunction
c. cerebellar dysfunction
d. spinal shock

37. Waterhouse-Friderichsen syndrome is a complication of
a. viral meningitis
b. meningococcal meningitis
c. Guillain-Barré syndrome
d. Myasthenia gravis

38. Myoglobinuria is a possible complication of
a. status epilepticus
b. spinal cord injury
c. myasthenia gravis
d. Guillain-Barré syndrome

39. A respiratory pattern that gradually increases and then decreases in depth until a period apnea ends the cycle and allows another to begin is called
a. Cheyne-Stokes
b. central neurogenic hyperventilation
c. apneustic
d. ataxic

40. The most frequent manifestations of autonomic dysfunction are alterations in
a. temperature
b. blood pressure and heart rate
c. level of consciousness
d. cranial nerve function

41. Which would be one of the more advanced symptoms in a patient with a supratentorial lesion?
    a. dilated pupil
    b. disorientation
    c. flexor posturing
    d. hemiparesis
42. Which of the following is most likely to result in an increase in intracranial pressure?
    a. increased intrathoracic pressure
    b. hyperventilation
    c. mild hypovolemia
    d. increased intracranial compliance
43. Patients with hydrocephalus who require intracranial pressure monitoring would be *least* benefited by
    a. an intraventricular cannula in the anterior horn
    b. an intraventricular cannula in the posterior horn
    c. a subarachnoid screw
    d. an epidural transducer
44. Spinal cord injured patients who cannot make a fist but can flex and extend the arms are most likely to have a lesion at the level of
    a. C-4 or above
    b. C-7 to C-8
    c. T-4 to T-6
    d. L-1 to L-2
45. A sign that spinal shock is subsiding in acute spinal cord injury patients is
    a. flaccid paralysis
    b. presence of response to plantar stimulation
    c. lack of sacral nerve reflexes
    d. decreased deep tendon reflexes
46. When a patient is admitted with possible meningitis and a skin rash or petechiae, precautions should be taken against the transmission of this
    a. bacterial infection
    b. viral infection
    c. fungal infection
    d. gram negative infection
47. When a patient with myasthenia gravis presents with respiratory failure, the cause can be
    a. myasthenic crisis
    b. cholinergic crisis
    c. either myasthenic or cholinergic crisis
    d. meningismus
48. Apomorphine or ipecac may be used in patients who ingested overdoses of certain drugs and
    a. have maintained consciousness
    b. have received activated charcoal
    c. are in shock
    d. have been lavaged to clear
49. Indications that the patient recovering from anesthesia has returned to level of function capable of supporting spontaneous respiration include
    a. presence of cough reflex
    b. presence of gag reflex
    c. response to verbal stimuli
    d. presence of head and neck motor strength
50. A patient who presents with disequilibrium, dystaxia, and dysarthria without impaired consciousness is most likely to have a
    a. frontal lobe lesion

b. parietal lobe lesion
c. temporal lobe lesion
d. posterior fossa lesion

Answers to Neurologic System Post Quiz

1. **b** (*page 316*)
2. **b** (*page 334*)
3. **b** (*page 328*)
4. **b** (*page 318*)
5. **d** (*pages 322–323*)
6. **b** (*page 318*)
7. **c** (*page 344*)
8. **a** (*pages 323–324*)
9. **c** (*pages 353, 358*)
10. **c** (*pages 359–360*)
11. **d** (*pages 409–410*)
12. **a** (*pages 393–394*)
13. **a** (*page 391*)
14. **b** (*page 321*)
15. **d** (*pages 383–385*)
16. **d** (*pages 424–425*)
17. **c** (*page 425*)
18. **b** (*pages 437–438*)
19. **b** (*pages 442–443*)
20. **a** (*page 429*)
21. **c** (*pages 433–435*)
22. **b** (*pages 328–329*)
23. **d** (*pages 324, 394*)
24. **b** (*page 344*)
25. **d** (*pages 334–336*)
26. **d** (*pages 334–336*)
27. **d** (*pages 347–348*)
28. **c** (*pages 324, 376–377*)
29. **d** (*pages 330–331*)
30. **d** (*pages 353–354*)
31. **a** (*page 358*)
32. **d** (*pages 461–462*)
33. **d** (*pages 377, 379–380*)
34. **a** (*page 399*)
35. **a** (*page 399*)
36. **a** (*page 338*)
37. **b** (*page 425*)
38. **a** (*page 434*)
39. **a** (*page 360*)
40. **b** (*pages 439–440*)
41. **c** (*pages 377, 379–380*)
42. **a** (*pages 375–379, 383–385*)
43. **d** (*pages 380–381, 385–386*)
44. **b** (*pages 397–399*)
45. **b** (*pages 399–400*)
46. **a** (*pages 423–424*)
47. **c** (*pages 445–447*)
48. **a** (*pages 454–455*)
49. **d** (*pages 458–461*)
50. **d** (*pages 322, 353–354*)

These are primarily the comprehend or recall, and apply or analyze levels of questions. Examples of synthesis or evaluative questions can be found in the comprehensive examination at the end of the book on pages 278 to 293.

4

The Renal System

SECTION-RELATED TIPS FOR THOSE STUDYING TO TAKE THE CERTIFICATION EXAMINATION

For many nurses the most difficult aspect of renal function is the chemistry involved. The author of this chapter of the *Core Curriculum* effectively presents renal physiology without using an overwhelming amount of chemistry. This approach is consistent with the certification examination, as emphasis is not placed on this aspect on the examination either.

The one additional area that is appropriate to review is fluid physiology, which is helpful in understanding fluid and electrolyte imbalances commonly encountered in the critically ill and on the examination blueprint. It is also helpful in understanding the rationale behind the selection of intravenous therapies for various disorders. The certification examination often has several questions involving alterations in fluid status, alterations in electrolyte balance, and appropriate intravenous fluids.

This aspect of critical care nursing also requires an understanding of osmolality. All four major causes of alterations in serum osmolality are on the examination blueprint (hypernatremia, hyponatremia, hyperglycemia, and uremia). The following material addresses all of these issues.

FLUID PHYSIOLOGY

The laws that govern the behavior of fluids separated by semipermeable membranes are fairly well defined.

Behavior of Solutes

The vast majority of solutes found in the body's fluids are electrolytes. Only a small fraction are noncharged particles. The movement of solutes small enough to cross the membrane is affected by three general phenomena:

1. Each solute passively diffuses from the area of higher to lower concentration (see Figure 4–5).
2. Electrolytes move as necessary to maintain electrical neutrality, an equal number of cations and anions.
3. Convection or bulk flow tends to draw all solutes across the membrane.

Behavior of Solvents

The body's solvent is water. The behavior of water is determined primarily by concentration gradients. Concentration can be expressed as osmolality, i.e., a measurement of particles per unit volume (milliosmols per liter). Differences in osmolality cause osmosis, i.e., the movement of water from the more dilute to the more concentrated side (see Figure 4–6).

The majority of extracellular osmolality is due to sodium and chloride ions. Urea and glucose are noncharged components that do not contribute significantly to osmolality at normal levels but can when elevated. Serum osmolality can be estimated by the formula:

$$S\ .\ osm = (Na \times 2) + \frac{BS}{18} + \frac{BUN}{3} = 285\text{–}295\ mosm/L$$

where S = serum, BS = blood sugar, and BUN = blood urea nitrogen.

Using this formula, it can be seen that the major causes of hyperosmolar states are hypernatremia, hyperglycemia, and uremia. Sodium and glucose are confined to the extracellular space, creating osmotic gradients between intracellular and extracellular compartments. This event can cause fluid to shift from the cell to the plasma. Urea, however, tends to build up inside cells as well as outside and does not usually cause fluid to shift. The exception is when the BUN is lowered rapidly during dialysis, faster than the urea is cleared from cells. This leads to a risk of cerebral edema or dysequilibrium syndrome.

The only cause of hypo-osmolar states is hyponatremia. It is instructive to apply this formula to several of your patients to appreciate the relative magnitude of changes.

The most abundant intracellular electrolytes are phosphate and potassium. Amino acids and magnesium are the other important contributors to the osmolality of cells (see Figure 4–9).

Fluid Compartments of the Body

About 60% of the adult lean body weight is fluid, which is distributed between two major compartments. Two thirds are found in the intracellular space. One third is extracellular. The extracellular is further divided into three-fourths interstitial and one-fourth plasma. The "third space" volume is the fluid abnormally sequestered in any other space.

The barriers between the compartments are important factors in fluid physiology. The cell membrane separates the intracellular from the extracellular spaces. The capillary membrane further subdivides the extracellular into vascular and interstitial compartments.

The cell membrane is a complex structure designed to counter passive diffusion with active transport mechanisms, which we are only beginning to fully understand. Much of the energy the body expends is used by these membrane pumps. The gradients created are a key trigger for many chemical reactions requisite to life.

Fluid flux across the capillary membrane is normally the product of the balance of two forces (see Figure 4–6). The hydrostatic pressure gradient pushes fluid from the plasma into the interstitium. The osmotic pressure gradient created by colloids confined to the bloodstream is called the colloid osmotic pressure. It attracts fluid back to the plasma.

Fluid Status Changes

Compartmental volume changes occur commonly in the critically ill. By remembering the principles governing fluid physiology, the secondary effects of every primary change can be predicted. Here are some examples:

1. Acute hemorrhage decreases capillary hydrostatic forces and results in a secondary decrease in interstitial volume as it moves into the bloodstream.
2. Dehydration, or water loss, tends to affect all compartments proportionately owing to changes in osmolality.
3. Overhydration, or water gain, similarly is distributed about one-third extracellular, two-thirds intracellular.
4. Sodium and water retention, on the other hand, is largely confined to the extracellular compartment. Since the sodium is kept from entering the cells, the water is also kept out.
5. Similarly, sodium and water loss is largely confined to the extracellular compartment.

Another way of looking at potential changes is to consider the primary mechanisms responsible for compartmental shifts.

1. Fluid shifts from the plasma to the interstitial spaces whenever the plasma hydrostatic pressure is high, the plasma colloid osmotic pressure (COP) is low, or the capillary membrane is more permeable.
2. Fluid shifts from the interstitial space to the plasma whenever the plasma hydrostatic pressure drops, or the plasma COP is high.
3. Fluid may shift from the intracellular to extracellular space whenever there is an osmolality gradient in that direction. The usual causes of high extracellular osmolality ar hypernatremia and hyperglycemia.
4. Fluid may shift from the extracellular to intracellular space when the cells become more concentrated. A common cause is inadequate energy available to keep the sodium pumps functioning. Sodium and water are allowed to enter the cell.

Clinical Assessment

Assessing the fluid status of patients involves evaluation of the overall volume status, as well as the volume of each compartment.

1. The overall volume status is reflected in the intake and output and in the weight. Third-space changes can make either misleading.
2. The easiest compartment volume to assess is the blood volume. It is reflected first by changes in venous distention or atrial pressures, and later by changes in arterial pressure. It can be measured by radionuclide techniques.
3. Interstitial space volume changes are reflected by changes in skin turgor or edema.
4. Intracellular volumes are difficult to assess directly. One of the clinical clues is weight change *without* edema. If a patient has a significant weight gain due to fluid retention and does not look edematous, it could be water retention in which two thirds have disappeared from clinical view into cells. The reverse is also true.

Comparison of Types of Replacement Solutions

The ultimate distribution of intravenous fluids administered can be predicted by knowing where its solutes are found and how they are metabolized.

The crystalloids contain electrolytes and/or glucose in various combinations. Commonly used examples are 5% dextrose in water (D_5W), normal saline, and Ringer's lactate. The time it takes one half of these solutions to distribute themselves to the appropriate compartments after administration is approximately 10 to 30 minutes. Glucose is metabolized so D_5W is distributed as free water (one-third extracellular, two-thirds intracellular). Normal saline and Ringer's lactate contain extracellular electrolytes and are distributed one-fourth plasma, three-fourths interstitial.

The colloids contain larger molecules that are confined to the bloodstream until metabolized. Examples include dextran solutions, albumin solutions, and hetastarch solutions. It takes approximately 12 to 24 hours for one half of these solutions to be metabolized. Meanwhile, the presence of colloids increases the plasma COP and draws fluid from the interstitial to the vascular space.

Please see the instructions at the beginning of the book for important general suggestions that are relevant to the bulk of the *Core Curriculum* content. They apply to this section as well as to all of the others.

FIGURES AND TABLES

Refer to these figures and tables while reading the renal section of the Core Curriculum.

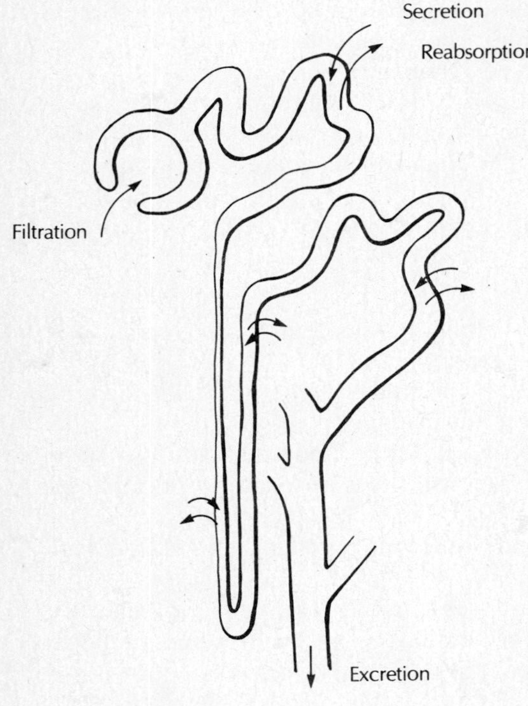

Figure 4–1. The four processes of urine formation. Filtration refers to the passage of fluid and substrates from the glomerulus into Bowman's capsule, reabsorption to those substances taken back from the tubular luminal fluid into the peritubular capillary, secretion to those going from tubular cells into the tubular luminal fluid, and excretion to those passed to the bladder for elimination (*page 472*).

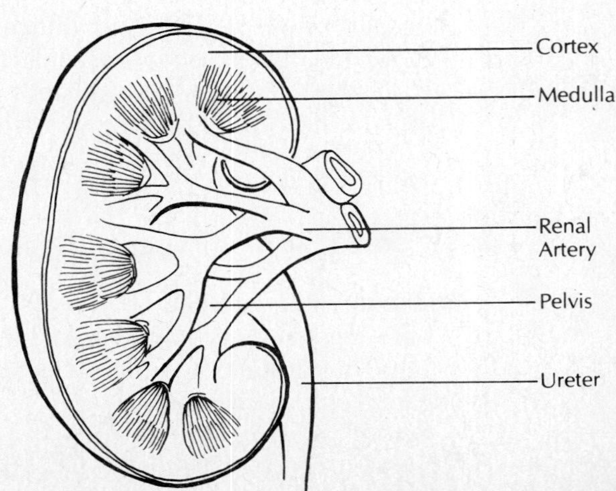

Figure 4–2. Cross-sectional anatomy of the kidney (*pages 472–473*).

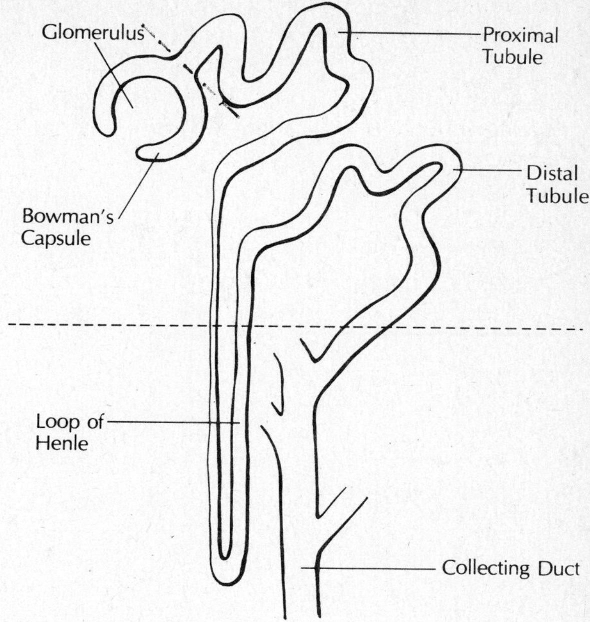

Figure 4–3. Anatomy of the nephron. The dashed line on the upper left indicates the division between the two functional parts of the nephron; the horizontal dashed line indicates the division between the cortex above and the medulla below (*pages 472–475*).

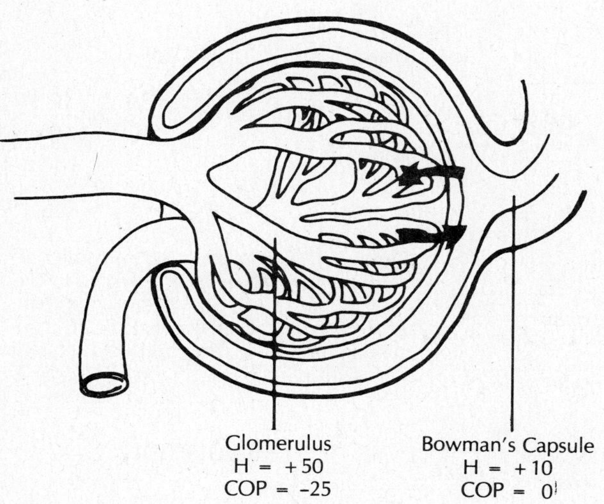

Figure 4–4. Factors involved in glomerular ultrafiltration. The normal hydrostatic pressures (H) and colloid osmotic pressure (COP) in both the glomerulus (*left*) and Bowman's capsule (*middle*) are indicated. The net pressure differences between the two compartments are listed (*right*). All pressures are in mm Hg (*page 475*).

Table 4–1. CALCULATION OF GFR USING CREATININE CLEARANCE (*page 476*)

$$GFR = \frac{U_{Cr}\ V}{P_{Cr}}$$

Example: If $U_{Cr} = 50$ mg/100 cc
$V = 2$ L/day or 1.38 cc/min
$P_{Cr} = 2$ mg/100 cc

$$\text{Then GFR} = \frac{50 \times 1.38}{2} = 34.5 \text{ cc/min}$$

Normal = 125 cc/min

GFR = glomerular filtration rate; U_{Cr} = urine creatinine; V = urine volume; P_{Cr} = plasma creatinine.

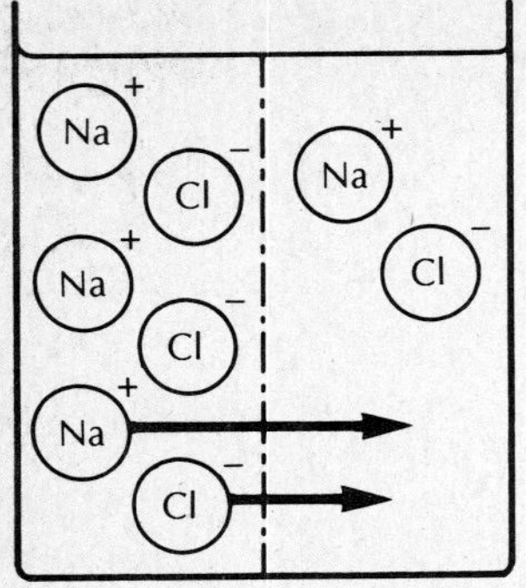

Figure 4–5. Solutes diffuse from the area of higher to lower concentration (*page 476*).

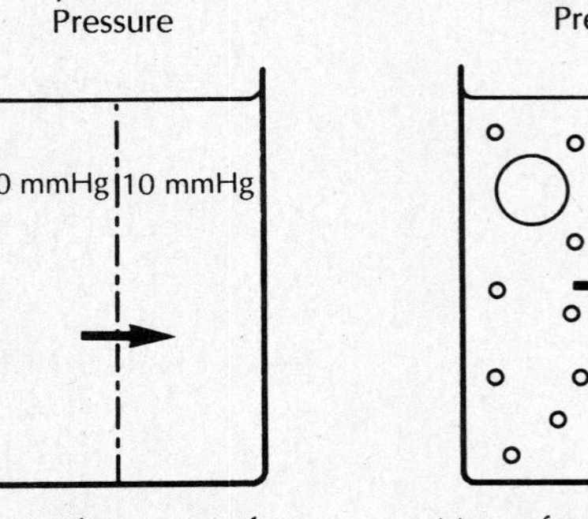

Figure 4–6. Behavior of solvent (water) (*pages 476–477*).

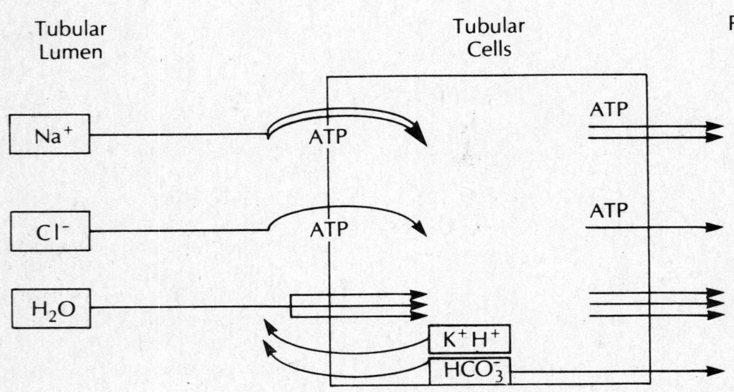

Figure 4–7. Examples of reabsorption (*arrows pointing to right*) and secretion (*arrows pointing to left*) in tubular system. Active adenosine triphosphate (ATP) consuming processes are indicated (*pages 476, 477*).

Table 4–2. COMPARISON OF PRIMARY FUNCTIONS OF THE PARTS OF THE TUBULAR SYSTEM (*pages 477–478*)

Area	Function	Type of Fluid Leaving
Proximal Tubule	60%–80% sodium, chloride, and water reabsorbed Acid-base balanced (bicarbonate absorbed, hydrogen secreted) Organic acids and foreign substances secreted	Isotonic
Loop of Henle		
Descending	Water reabsorbed	Hypertonic
Ascending	Sodium and chloride reabsorbed (impermeable to water)	Hypotonic
Distal Tubule and Collecting Duct	Water, sodium, and chloride reabsorbed Potassium and ammonia secreted Acid-base balanced (bicarbonate absorbed, hydrogen secreted)	Adjusted to meet needs by hormones

Table 4–3. COMPARISON OF SUBSTRATE REABSORPTION IN THE PROXIMAL TUBULE (PT), DESCENDING LOOP OF HENLE (↓ LH), ASCENDING LOOP OF HENLE (↑ LH), DISTAL TUBULE (DT), AND COLLECTING DUCT (CD). PRIMARY SITES FOR EACH ARE UNDERLINED (*pages 477–478*)

Components of Glomerular Filtrate	Tubular Reabsorption	Urine
125 cc of water	Most reabsorbed in <u>PT</u>, ↓ LH, DT, CD	Some left
Electrolytes	Most reabsorbed in <u>PT</u>, ↑ LH, DT, CD	Some left
Glucose	All reabsorbed in <u>PT</u>	None left
Waste Products	Few reabsorbed	Most left

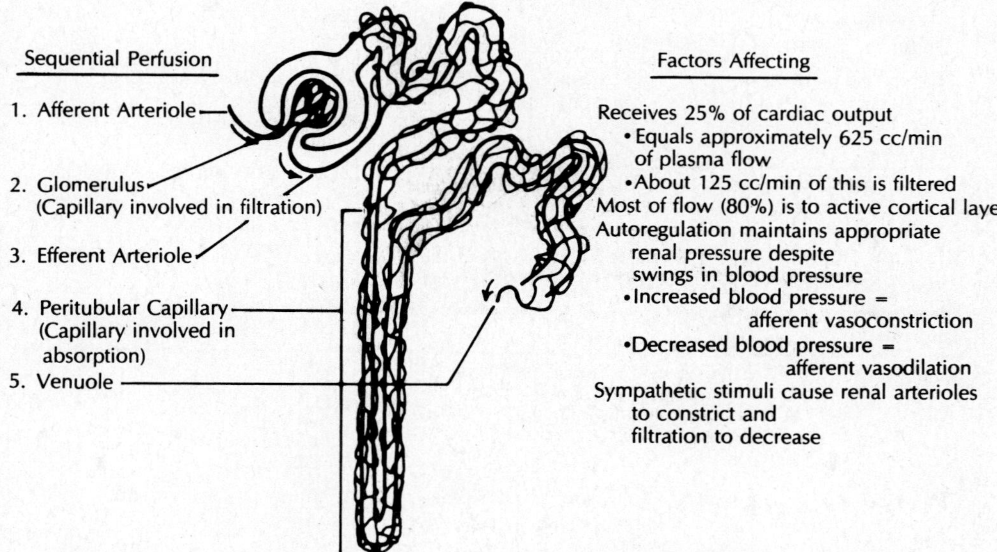

Figure 4–8. Microcirculation of the nephron and factors that affect it (*pages 478–480*).

Figure 4–9. The major intracellular and extracellular electrolytes. Normal levels in milliequivalents per liter are indicated (*pages 482–486*).

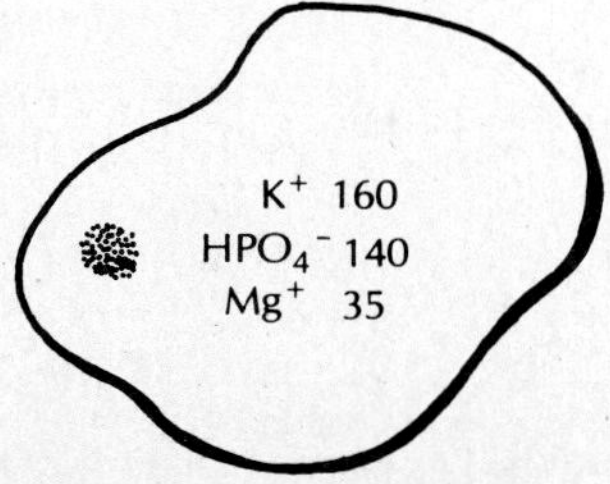

Table 4–4. SUMMARY OF ORIGIN, STIMULI, AND EFFECTS OF THE MAJOR HORMONES AFFECTING URINE FORMATION (*pages 480–485*)

Hormone	Origin	Stimuli	Effects
Aldosterone	Adrenal cortex	Low renal blood flow (1) *Renin* released from JG cells in kidney (2) Becomes *angiotensin I* in bloodstream (3) Converted to *angiotensin II* in lungs (4) Stimulates *aldosterone* release from adrenal cortex Stress Hyperkalemia Hyponatremia	Retention of Na Retention of H_2O Secretion of K
Antidiuretic Hormone	Made and controlled by hypothalamus Stored in and released from the posterior pituitary	High serum osmolality* Hypernatremia* Hypotension, stress	↑ Retention of H_2O Serum osmolality falls and urine osmolality rises
Parathormone	Parathyroid gland	Hypocalcemia Hyperphosphatemia	↑ Calcium into serum from bones Increased phosphate excretion

* These also cause hypothalamus to stimulate thirst to help decrease serum osmolality.

Table 4–5. SUMMARY OF THE ROLE AND FACTORS AFFECTING RENAL PROCESSING OF THE MAJOR ELECTROLYTES (*pages 482–486*)

Electrolyte	Role	Factors Affecting
Sodium	Controls extracellular osmolality and therefore volume Involved in neuromuscular transmission	GFR Aldosterone "Third factor" Increased ADH Diuretics
Potassium	Involved in intracellular physiology Involved in neuromuscular transmission	Intracellular potassium Acid-base balance GFR Diuretics Aldosterone
Calcium	Involved in neuromuscular transmission Needed for clotting Needed for structure of bone and teeth Involved in cellular membrane permeability	Parathormone Vitamin D Corticosteroids Diuretics
Phosphate	Needed for bone structure Involved in intracellular physiology (ATP; 2,3-DPG; DNA; RNA)	Parathormone GFR
Magnesium	Involved in intracellular physiology primarily through enzymes	Sodium availability Parathormone
Chloride	Involved in acid-base balance (goes with sodium, goes opposite bicarbonate)	↓ pH = ↑ HCO_3^- reabsorption = ↓ Cl reabsorption ↑ pH = ↓ HCO_3^- reabsorption = ↑ Cl reabsorption

GFR = glomerular infiltration rate; ADH = antidiuretic hormone; ATP = adenosine triphosphate; 2,3-DPG = 2,3-diphosphoglycerate; HCO_3^- = bicarbonate.

Table 4–6. SUMMARY OF RENAL ROLE IN REGULATION OF BLOOD PRESSURE (*pages 488, 489*)

Factor	Effect	Comments
Extracellular Fluid Volume Maintenance	Volume changes can cause pressure changes	
Renin-Angiotensin Aldosterone System		Renin released from the juxtaglomerular apparatus is triggered by:
Renin	Becomes angiotensin I in bloodstream	Low renal arteriolar pressure
Angiotensin I	Converted to angiotensin II when blood flows through the lungs	Low sodium in distal tubule
Angiotensin II	Causes aldosterone release from adrenal cortex Causes vasoconstriction	Sympathetic stimulation
Aldosterone	Causes increased reabsorption of sodium in distal tubule and, therefore, can increase water reabsorption	
Renal Prostaglandins	Most cause vasodilation Modulate effects of other agents that vasoconstrict Cause decreased renal pressure and increased renal blood flow Inhibit ADH effects in distal tubule and, therefore, more water is excreted	Prostaglandin inhibitors reverse these effects Examples include: Salicylic acid Ibuprofen Indomethacin Naproxen

Table 4–7. SUMMARY OF MAJOR TYPES OF DIURETIC AGENTS (*pages 506–508*)

Agent (Examples)	Mechanism of Action
Volume Expansion (oral and intravenous fluids)	Increased glomerular filtration rate
Osmotic Diuretics (mannitol)	Plasma volume expansion Increased glomerular filtration Decreased absorption of water in renal tubules
Loop Diuretics (furosemide and ethacrynic acid)	Decreased absorption of sodium chloride in ascending loop of Henle and, therefore, decreased water reabsorption later Renal vasodilation and increased glomerular filtration rate
Thiazide Diuretics (hydrochlorothiazide)	Decreased absorption of sodium in ascending loop of Henle and distal tubule and, therefore, decreased water reabsorption
Potassium-Sparing Diuretics (spironolactone)	Inhibition of aldosterone leading to loss of sodium and water with retention of potassium
Carbonic Anhydrase Inhibitors (acetazolamide)	Decreased bicarbonate and sodium absorption leading to increased water loss and a drop in the serum pH

Table 4–8. SUMMARY OF FACTORS COVERED IN THE PHYSIOLOGIC AND ASSESSMENT SECTIONS THAT HAVE IMPORTANT CLINICAL APPLICATIONS WORTH EMPHASIZING (*pages 472–521*)

Item	Application	Page
Four Processes of Urine Formation	These terms have specific definitions that are key to understanding renal physiology: (1) Filtration refers to the movement of fluid and substrates into the nephron from the glomerulus due to pressure gradients (2) Reabsorption refers to fluid and substrates that are retrieved from the glomerular filtrate by the tubular cells (3) Secretion refers to the substrates that are added to the filtrate by the tubular cells (4) Excretion refers to the fluid, present after the first 3 steps, that leaves the collecting duct and that will be eliminated	472
Nephron's Ability to Compensate	There is a tremendous amount of renal reserve due to the numbers of nephrons (one million per kidney) and their ability to compensate. End-stage renal failure does not occur until 90% of nephron function is lost.	474, 544
Net Filtration Pressure	Visualizing the hydrostatic and colloid osmotic pressures involved helps in understanding some causes of altered glomerular filtration. Other causes are those that affect glomerular membrane permeability.	475, 476
Glomerular Filtration Rate (GFR)	Creatinine clearance may be used to calculate the GFR, a sensitive monitor of current renal function.	475–476
Diffusion and Osmosis	These principles of fluid physiology are key in the understanding of not only nephron function but also fluid and electrolyte balance, intravenous therapy, and dialysis techniques.	476–477
Renal Blood Flow	The fact that 80% of the renal blood flow goes to the cortex partly explains why cortical renal failure is often associated with factors that reach the kidney via the bloodstream. The fact that the medulla only gets 20% partly explains why ischemic injury (shock) can cause medullary renal failure.	479
Antidiuretic Hormone and Aldosterone	When studying these hormones, be careful to differentiate their effect on the serum from their effect on the urine. The effects are opposite to each other.	481–484
The "Third Factor"	A third factor or hormone that affects renal function is atrial natriuretic hormone. It is released from the heart when the atria are distended and appears to cause both vasodilation and loss of sodium followed by the loss of water in the nephron.	482–483
Prostaglandin Inhibitors	One of many potential complications of high dose or overdoses of these drugs is renal failure by vasoconstriction. Many such drugs are available over the counter.	489
Erythropoietin	Increased levels in response to renal hypoxia are thought to be the mechanism behind polycythemia often seen in patients with such entities as chronic heart and lung disease.	489
Urinalysis	There are several values with a wide range of normals reflecting the normal kidney's ability to alter output depending on need. One helpful hint in trying to assess if renal response is appropriate is to use the principle "the urine should be worse than the serum" when abnormalities in blood tests also exist. Examples include: (1) An acidotic patient should have more acidotic urine. (2) An alkalotic patient should have more alkalotic urine. (3) A hyperphosphatenic patient should have higher urine phosphate levels. (4) A hypokalemic patient should have lower urine potassium levels. (5) A hyperosmolar patient should have more hyperosmolar urine. When these normal and corrective responses do not exist, look for problems in the kidney or the hormones involved.	496–498

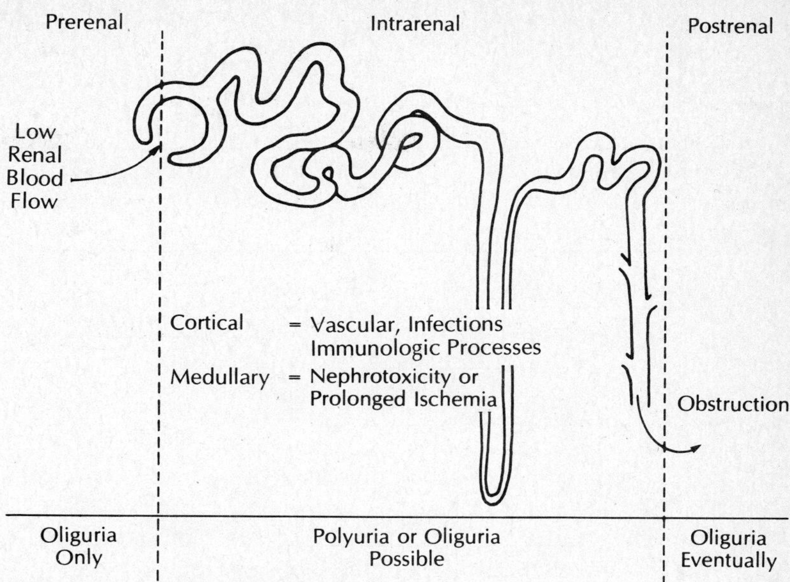

Figure 4–10. Comparison of causes of acute pre-, intra-, and postacute renal failure above line and effect on urinary output below line (*pages 521–524*).

Table 4–9. COMPARISON OF LABORATORY FINDINGS IN PRERENAL AND INTRARENAL FAILURE (*page 527*)

Test	Prerenal	Intrarenal	
		Cortical	*Medullary*
Urine Na^+	Low	Low	High
Urine Specific Gravity	High	Varies	Low to normal
BUN/Creatinine	↑ ↑ ↑/↑	↑ ↑/↑ ↑	↑ ↑/↑ ↑
Proteinuria	Little or none	Moderate to high	Little to moderate
Urine Sediment	None	Presence of cells, casts Numerous erythrocytes	Heavy presence of cells, casts Rare erythrocytes

Table 4–10. COMPARISON OF STAGES OF CHRONIC RENAL FAILURE (*pages 544–549*)

Stage	Nephron Loss	Common Lab Findings	Creatinine Clearance	Symptoms
Diminished Renal Reserve	50%	Serum creatinine doubles	Decreases to ½ normal	Free of symptoms
Renal Insufficiency	75%	Serum creatinine mildly elevated (quadrupled); urine slightly dilute; anemia	10–50 mL/min	Symptoms begin to develop
End-Stage Renal Disease	90%	Serum electrolyte and acid-base status altered Serum creatinine high (10 mg/dL or more) until treated	10–15 mL/min <5 mL/min to require dialysis	Symptoms require artificial support (dialysis) or transplant
Uremic Syndrome	90% or less	Findings reflect multiorgan system involvement Creatinine level depends on therapy	10–15 mL/min or below Usually <5 mL/min	Symptoms of multiorgan system involvement

THE RENAL SYSTEM

Exercises

After reading the renal section of the Core Curriculum, *fill in the blanks in the following statements. It can be done one topic at a time or all at once. The answers are at the end of the exercises.*

A. Physiologic Anatomy (*pages 472–490*)

1. The four processes involved in urine formation are as follows:
   a. ____________________
   b. ____________________
   c. ____________________
   d. ____________________
2. The most highly metabolic layer of the renal cross-sectional anatomy is the ____________________.
3. The ____________________ layer of the kidney contains the collecting ducts and tips of the loops of Henle.
4. The number of nephrons per kidney is normally about ____________________.
5. The type of nephron that has a greater concentrating ability is the ____________________.
6. The two functional segments of the nephron are the ____________________ and the ____________________.
7. The glomerular membrane is relatively impermeable to ____________________ and ____________________.
8. The normal glomerular capillary hydrostatic pressure is ____________________ mm Hg and its colloid osmotic pressure is ____________________ mm Hg.
9. The normal glomerular filtration rate is ____________________ cc per minute.
10. How will the following factors affect the glomerular filtration rate (increase or decrease)?
    a. Decreased renal blood flow ____________________
    b. Afferent arterial dilation ____________________
    c. Hypoproteinemia ____________________
    d. Urinary tract obstruction ____________________
11. The passive movement of a solute through a semipermeable membrane from an area of higher to lower concentration is called ____________________.
12. The passive movement of water through a semipermeable membrane from an area of lower to higher concentration is called ____________________.
13. When absorption requires energy expenditure to move against a concentration gradient, it is called ____________________ transport.
14. In the proximal tubules, 60%–80% of the ____________________ are reabsorbed actively, and an equal amount of ____________________ is reabsorbed passively.
15. Organic acids and foreign substances go directly into the tubular lumen from the cells lining them, a process referred to as ____________________.
16. Water is reabsorbed in the ____________________ loop of Henle

and electrolytes are reabsorbed in the ____________ loop of Henle.

17. The ____________ limb of the loop of Henle is impermeable to water.
18. The ____________ and ____________ segments of the nephron are the two parts most directly affected by aldosterone and antidiuretic hormones.
19. The vessels immediately before and after the glomerulus are the ____________ and the ____________, respectively.
20. Renin is secreted by the ____________ apparatus, which consists of the ____________ and the ____________.
21. The kidneys receive ____________% of the cardiac output.
22. The majority of blood flow is received by the aerobic but highly metabolic ____________ layer of the kidney.
23. In order to regulate renal perfusion to appropriate levels, the afferent arteriole constricts in response to ____________ blood pressure.
24. In response to sympathetic stimuli, the renal afferent and efferent arteries ____________ and the glomerular filtration rate may ____________.
25. Indicate whether the following can increase or decrease the glomerular filtration rate.
    a. Increase sympathetic tone ____________
    b. Angiotensin II ____________
    c. Low-dose dopamine ____________
26. The thirst center is located in the ____________ and is stimulated by a rise in intracellular ____________.
27. Antidiuretic hormone is made by the ____________ and is stimulated by a rise in the serum ____________.
28. When antidiuretic hormone is secreted, the urine osmolality goes ____________ and the serum osmolality goes ____________.
29. At the beginning of the loop of Henle, the osmolality of the filtrate is ____________, and by the end of the loop of Henle, it is ____________.
30. Sodium is the major ion of the ____________ space and therefore affects its volume.
31. Most of the sodium is reabsorbed in the ____________ of the nephron.
32. The three major factors that affect sodium absorption in the nephron are as follows:
    a. ____________
    b. ____________
    c. ____________
33. Aldosterone is produced by the ____________ and causes the nephron to reabsorb more ____________ and ____________, and reabsorb less ____________.
34. Three major factors affecting potassium absorption in the nephron are as follows:
    a. ____________
    b. ____________
    c. ____________

35. The four major factors affecting calcium absorption are as follows:
    a. ______
    b. ______
    c. ______
    d. ______
36. Phosphate is found primarily in ______ fluid, and its renal absorption is affected primarily by ______ and ______.
37. Magnesium is a major cation in the ______ space and its renal reabsorption is affected by the presence of ______ and ______.
38. Acidosis causes the normal kidney to ______ the amount of bicarbonate reabsorbed and ______ the amount of chloride excreted.
39. Alkalosis causes the normal kidney to ______ the amount of bicarbonate reabsorbed and ______ the amount of chloride excreted.
40. When urine flow rates decrease, the BUN goes ______ owing to ______.
41. Indicate whether the following result in an increase in BUN, an increase in creatinine, or an increase in both:
    a. Decreased nephron function ______
    b. Catabolic states ______
    c. Hypovolemia ______
42. A high serum creatinine level can be attributed to ______.
43. The kidney can directly affect acid base concentration by altering the amount of the two electrolytes, ______ and ______ in the urine.
44. When the patient has alkalemia, the normal kidney responds by ______ the amount of hydrogen secreted and ______ the amount of bicarbonate reabsorbed.
45. Two examples of ways in which the kidney affects the blood pressure are through ______ and ______.
46. The factors leading to the release of renin are ______, ______, and ______.
47. Angiotensin II causes the vessels to ______, and the adrenal gland to release ______.
48. Generally, renal prostaglandins cause the renal perfusion pressure to ______ and renal blood flow to ______ via vasodilation, and the ______ of antidiuretic hormone.
49. The hormone produced or catalyzed by the kidney that increases red blood cell production is ______.

B. Nursing Assessment Data Base (*pages 490–500*)

1. In the presence of biliuria the urine appears ______.
2. The urine will be hematest positive by dipstick when either ______ or ______ is present.
3. Two possible causes of edema in patients with renal failure are increased ______ and decreased ______.
4. When the patient's hand begins flapping uncontrollably after sustained voluntary hyperextension of the wrist and spreading of the fingers, it is referred to as ______.

5. Two examples of sites of pain that may be due to renal disorders are ______________________ and ______________________.
6. When the BUN to creatinine ratio exceeds ______________ ______ to ______________________, extrarenal causes of the excessive BUN elevation are suspected.
7. The serum osmolality normally is kept between ____________ __________ and ____________________ mosm, whereas the urine varies between ____________________ and ______________ ______ mosm.
8. Specific gravity tests the ______________________ of urine, not the actual concentration or osmolality.
9. Creatinine clearance is used to quantify the function of the ___________ ___________.
10. The average pH of urine is about ______________________.
11. Renal tubular acidosis may be present if the patient's serum pH is ______________________ and the urine pH is ______________________.
12. List three causes of acetone excretion in the urine:
    a. ______________________
    b. ______________________
    c. ______________________
13. Two examples of contraindications for intravenous pyelography are ______________________ and ______________________.

C. **Commonly Encountered Nursing Diagnoses** (*pages 500–521*)

1. Physical signs of fluid volume excess include ____________ __________ and ______________________.
2. Normal insensible losses in the adult are about ____________ ____________ cc per day, and oxidative losses are about ____________ ____________ cc per day.
3. Physical signs of fluid volume deficits include ______________ _______ and ______________________.
4. In renal failure the electrolytes found abundantly in intracellular fluid are more likely to go ______________________.
5. Signs that a renal patient's nutritional requirements are not being met include ______________________ and ______________________.
6. Complications of diuretic therapy include ______________ _____ and ______________________.
7. Three of the seven types of diuretic agents are ____________ ___________, ______________________, and ______________ _______.
8. Indicate the action by which the following drugs increase the urinary output:
    a. Furosemide ______________________
    b. Mannitol ______________________
    c. Spironolactone ______________________
    d. Acetazolamide ______________________
9. Indicate the action by which the following drugs decrease the blood pressure:
    a. Methyldopa ______________________
    b. Propranolol ______________________
    c. Nitroprusside ______________________
    d. Hydralazine ______________________
    e. Captopril ______________________

10. The most common acid-base imbalance in patients with renal failure is ________________________.
11. Electrolyte imbalances that may occur with metabolic acidosis include ________________________ potassium, ________________________ calcium, and ________________________ chloride.
12. Two causes of anemia in patients with chronic renal failure include ________________________ and ________________________.
13. Uremic syndrome occurs when the GRF has decreased to ________________________ cc/min.
14. The most common complication leading to death in patients with acute renal failure is ________________________.
15. Renal patients with secondary hyperparathyroidism have ________________________ serum calcium and ________________________ serum phosphate along with skeletal system deterioration.
16. Secondary hyperparathyroidism may be treated by the administration of ________________________, ________________________, and ________________________.
17. Two factors that alter the response of renal patients to drugs are ________________________ and ________________________.
18. Suicide rates in patients with chronic renal failure are about ________________________ times higher than that of the general population.

D. Patient Health Problems (*pages 521–606*)

1. Oliguric acute renal failure has a ________________________ mortality rate than the nonoliguric type.
2. Prerenal failure is caused by ________________________ and results in ________________________ urine production.
3. Intrarenal failure caused by vascular or immunologic insults are more likely to affect the ________________________ layer.
4. The two primary causes of medullary intrarenal failure or acute tubular necrosis are ________________________ and ________________________.
5. Oliguric medullary intrarenal failure may progress through the following four stages:
   a. ________________________
   b. ________________________
   c. ________________________
   d. ________________________
6. Indicate which type of renal failure is associated with each of the following conditions:
   a. Malignant hypertension ________________________
   b. Hypovolemia ________________________
   c. Acute glomerulonephritis ________________________
   d. Aminoglycoside toxicity ________________________
   e. Severe sustained ischemia ________________________
   f. Prostatic hypertrophy ________________________
7. Nephron injury is more likely to occur when the ischemic insult lasts over ________________________ minutes.
8. When renal failure leads to metabolic acidosis, the respiratory rate and/or depth may go ________________________.
9. Oliguria can be defined as a 24-hour urine volume under ________________________ cc.

10. When prerenal failure is present, the BUN rises ______________________ than the creatinine, the urine concentration goes ______________________, and the urine sodium goes ______________________.
11. The category of renal failure most likely to result in increased urinary sodium levels is ______________________.
12. The major types of dialysis are ______________________, ______________________, and ______________________.
13. Relative contraindications for hemodialysis include ______________________ and ______________________.
14. Relative contraindications for peritoneal dialysis include ______________________ and ______________________.
15. External shunts used for hemodialysis may be assessed for patency by ______________________ and ______________________.
16. In dialysis, when patients have shunts or fistulas in the left arm, blood pressures and venipunctures should be done in the ______________________ arm.
17. The three primary physiologic principles that operate in simple dialysis membranes are as follows:
    a. ______________________
    b. ______________________
    c. ______________________
18. The movement of fluid from the area of lower to higher concentration is ______________________, whereas the movement of molecules from higher to lower concentration is ______________________.
19. Peritoneal dialysis with 4.25% dialysate solutions will result in ______________________ fluid removal from the patient than 1.5% solutions.
20. Peritoneal dialysis may cause ______________________ serum glucose.
21. Continuous arterial-venous hemofiltration procedures remove small molecules like ______________________ and ______________________ in addition to water.
22. Continuous arterial-venous hemodialysis usually removes ______________________ urea than hemofiltration.
23. Indicate which electrolyte imbalance a renal failure patient is most likely to be developing when the following changes occur:
    a. Peaked T waves ______________________
    b. Hyperactive bowel sounds ______________________
    c. Tetany or seizures ______________________
    d. Paralytic ileus ______________________
24. Bricker's "intact nephron" hypothesis states that when some nephrons decrease function slowly over time, the remaining nephrons ______________________.
25. List the four stages of chronic renal failure and indicate the percentage of nephron function loss for the first three phases:
    a. ______________________
    b. ______________________
    c. ______________________
    d. ______________________
26. The most common cause of interstitial nephritis is ______________________.
27. Two types of chronic renal failure that commonly cause proteinuria are ______________________ and ______________________.
28. The most common cause of the presence of white cell casts in the urine

without accompanying red cells or protein is ______________________.

29. Indicate the creatinine clearance and serum creatinine levels associated with these stages of renal failure:
    a. Renal insufficiency:
       Creatinine clearance ______________________ cc/min
       Creatinine ______________________ mg/dL
    b. End-stage renal disease:
       Creatinine clearance ______________________ cc/min
       Creatinine ______________________ mg/dL
30. Indicate whether the following are more likely to increase or decrease in patients with chronic renal failure:
    a. Blood pressure ______________________
    b. Hemoglobin ______________________
    c. Serum bicarbonate ______________________
    d. Serum potassium ______________________
    e. Respiratory rate ______________________
    f. Serum phosphate ______________________
    g. Muscle mass ______________________
31. A substance found in dialysate solution that can be converted into bicarbonate by the patient is ______________________.
32. Patients with anemia resulting from chronic renal failure usually tolerate a hematocrit as low as ______________________%.
33. For each of the following groups of manifestations, indicate which complication of chronic renal failure is most likely to be present.
    a. Chest pain that is relieved by sitting up and forward and widespread ST segment elevation on the ECG ______________________.
    b. Pulsus paradoxus, distant heart sounds, distended jugular veins, and hypotension ______________________.
    c. "Restless leg syndrome" and diminished leg strength and paresthesia ______________________.
    d. Hypocalcemia, bone pain, and pathologic fractures ______________________.
34. Chronic ambulatory peritoneal dialysis techniques can replace approximately ______________________% of renal function.
35. Indicate whether the following are usually considered contraindications for renal transplant:
    a. Age of 50 years ______________________
    b. Irreversible end-stage renal disease ______________________
    c. Presence of preexisting antibodies ______________________
    d. Tendency to frequent chronic infections ______________________
    e. Functioning urinary tract ______________________
36. The four types of tests done in tissue typing to determine the compatibility between donor and recipient of a renal transplant are as follows:
    a. ______________________
    b. ______________________
    c. ______________________
    d. ______________________
37. List the primary immunologic factor involved in each of the following types of rejection in patients undergoing renal transplantation:
    a. Hyperacute rejection ______________________
    b. Acute rejection ______________________
    c. Chronic rejection ______________________
38. Patients with uremic bowel syndrome have alternating episodes of ______________________ and ______________________.

39. Complications of immunosuppressant therapy include ____________ __________ and ______________________.
40. Signs of rejection of a transplanted kidney include ______________ ______ blood pressure, ______________________ weight, and ______________________ urinary output.
41. Drugs used to control rejection of a transplanted kidney may include ______________________ and ______________________.
42. Two examples of common causes of hyperkalemia are ___________ ___________ and ______________________.
43. In hyperkalemia, the motility of the gastrointestinal tract may go ______________________.
44. The early ECG change associated with hyperkalemia is __________ ___________.
45. Muscle weakness associated with hyperkalemia usually begins in the ______________________.
46. In severe hyperkalemia, potassium may be driven from the serum to the cells by the administration of ______________________, __________ ______________, and ______________________.
47. Kayexalate has two effects on specific electrolytes: the serum _____ __________________ goes up and the serum __________________ _____ goes down.
48. Causes of hypokalemia include ______________________ and _____ __________________.
49. Indicate whether hypokalemia is more likely to increase or decrease the following:
    a. Muscle strength ______________________
    b. Cardiac irritability ______________________
    c. Gastrointestinal motility ______________________
    d. Blood pressure ______________________
    e. Urinary output ______________________
50. Two electrolyte imbalances, ______________________ and ______ ________________, can increase the tendency to develop digitalis toxicity.
51. Hypernatremia may result when sodium retention goes __________ ___________ or total body water goes ______________________.
52. Two electrolyte imbalances that can lead to excess water loss are ______________________ potassium and __________________ _____ calcium.
53. Patients with high serum sodium levels from sodium retention tend to have signs of ______________________ hydration.
54. In patients with high serum sodium levels from loss of water, the heart rate usually goes ______________________, the hematocrit goes _____ __________________, and the serum osmolality goes ____________ _________.
55. Hyponatremia may develop when sodium retention goes ________ ______________ or water retention goes ______________ _______.
56. Causes of excessive sodium loss include ______________________ and ______________________.
57. Water intoxication can cause the hematocrit to ___________ ___________, the central venous pressure to ____________ _________, the serum osmolality to ______________________, and body weight to ______________________.

58. Intravenous therapy for patients with hyponatremia and signs of dehydration would be ______________________ solutions.
59. In hypercalcemia related to bedrest, severe hyperthyroidism and hyperparathyroidism, the calcium has gone from the ______________________ to the serum.
60. The electrolytes, calcium and ______________________ are often inversely related.
61. In patients with hypercalcemia, muscle tone may go ______________________ and urinary output may go ______________________.
62. Two of the possible interventions for hypercalcemia are ______________________ and ______________________.
63. Patients with chronic renal failure may develop hypocalcemia from two mechanisms: ______________________ and ______________________.
64. The two hormones that play an important role in calcium regulation are ______________________ and ______________________.
65. Hypocalcemia can cause the bronchi to ______________________ and cardiac contractility to ______________________.
66. The two classic early signs of the neuromuscular irritability associated with hypocalcemia are ______________________ and ______________________.
67. Hyperphosphatemia occurs in the ______________________ stage of the course of renal disease.
68. The agents commonly used to bind phosphate in the gastrointestinal tract are the ______________________.
69. Phosphates may be taken from the serum into the cell when ventilation goes ______________________ or the serum glucose has been ______________________.
70. Hypophosphatemia may result in muscle ______________________, ______________________ anemia, and hypoxia primarily due to lack of the red blood cell enzyme ______________________.
71. Indicate whether the following are more likely to cause the serum phosphate to increase or decrease:
    a. Cytotoxic drugs ______________________
    b. Hyperparathyroidism ______________________
    c. Acetazolamide ______________________
    d. Chronic alcoholism ______________________
    e. Hypercalcemia ______________________
72. Hypermagnesemia can cause neuromuscular activity to ______________________, respiratory rate to ______________________, heart rate to ______________________, and the T wave to ______________________.
73. In conjunction with treating the cause, severe hypermagnesemia can be treated by ______________________ or ______________________.
74. Indicate whether the following are more likely to cause the serum magnesium to increase or decrease:
    a. Acidosis ______________________
    b. Renal failure ______________________
    c. Pancreatitis ______________________
    d. Prolonged parenteral nutrition ______________________
    e. Hypoparathyroidism ______________________
    f. Excessive gastrointestinal losses ______________________
75. Hypomagnesemia can cause neuromuscular irritability to ______________________

_____________, cardiac irritability to _____________________, and the T wave to ____________________.

76. Renal trauma is ____________________ common in blunt injuries than in penetrating injuries.
77. The majority of renal injuries are ____________________ which lead to hematuria and spare the urine collection system.
78. Patients with renal trauma also have incurred damage to other organs ____________________% of the time.
79. Tomography is ____________________ useful than ultrasound in diagnosing nonpenetrating renal trauma.
80. In minor renal trauma, healing will occur in ____________________ weeks.

E. Summary of Patient Health Problems (*pages 521–606*)

After reading each disease, summarize the pathophysiology, nursing assessment data base, and nursing diagnoses. The certification examination holds you responsible for knowing the etiology and risk factors, the signs and symptoms, the collaborative diagnosis, the complications,and the management and treatment goals. Those preparing to take it should also summarize these areas. If they are not clearly covered in the Core, *a second resource may be necessary. The space allotted is purposefully limited to encourage concise descriptions of concepts and careful selection of key points. It is not as helpful to write the things you already know as it is to write those you need to study.*

1. Acute Renal Failure

Pathophysiology	*Etiology/Risk Factors*	*Signs/Symptoms*

Collaborative Diagnosis	*Complications*	*Management/Goals*

2. Chronic Renal Failure

Pathophysiology	*Etiology/Risk Factors*	*Signs/Symptoms*

Collaborative Diagnosis	*Complications*	*Management/Goals*

3. Hyperkalemia

Pathophysiology	*Etiology/Risk Factors*	*Signs/Symptoms*

Collaborative Diagnosis	*Complications*	*Management/Goals*

4. Hypokalemia

Pathophysiology	*Etiology/Risk Factors*	*Signs/Symptoms*

Collaborative Diagnosis	*Complications*	*Management/Goals*

5. Hypernatremia

Pathophysiology	*Etiology/Risk Factors*	*Signs/Symptoms*

Collaborative Diagnosis	*Complications*	*Management/Goals*

6. Hyponatremia

Pathophysiology	*Etiology/Risk Factors*	*Signs/Symptoms*

Collaborative Diagnosis	*Complications*	*Management/Goals*

7. Hypercalcemia

Pathophysiology	*Etiology/Risk Factors*	*Signs/Symptoms*

Collaborative Diagnosis	*Complications*	*Management/Goals*

8. Hypocalcemia

Pathophysiology	*Etiology/Risk Factors*	*Signs/Symptoms*

Collaborative Diagnosis	*Complications*	*Management/Goals*

9. Hyperphosphatemia

Pathophysiology	*Etiology/Risk Factors*	*Signs/Symptoms*

Collaborative Diagnosis	*Complications*	*Management/Goals*

10. Hypophosphatemia

Pathophysiology	*Etiology/Risk Factors*	*Signs/Symptoms*

Collaborative Diagnosis	*Complications*	*Management/Goals*

11. Hypermagnesemia

Pathophysiology	*Etiology/Risk Factors*	*Signs/Symptoms*

Collaborative Diagnosis	*Complications*	*Management/Goals*

12. Hypomagnesemia

Pathophysiology	*Etiology/Risk Factors*	*Signs/Symptoms*

Collaborative Diagnosis	*Complications*	*Management/Goals*

13. Renal Trauma

Pathophysiology	*Etiology/Risk Factors*	*Signs/Symptoms*

Collaborative Diagnosis	*Complications*	*Management/Goals*

F. Application to Clinical Practice

Care for patients with renal disorders. Relate the anatomy and physiology, assessment and pathophysiology found in this section to their individual clinical pictures. Make note of instances where they correlate and those where they deviate from the expected presentation. Devise a care plan based on the data collected.

Answers to Renal System Exercises

A. Physiologic Anatomy

1. a. Filtration
   b. Absorption
   c. Secretion
   d. Excretion (*page 472*)
2. Cortex (*page 472*)
3. Medullary (*page 472*)
4. One million (*page 472*)
5. Juxtamedullary or long looped (*page 474*)
6. Glomerulus or corpuscle, tubule (*page 474*)
7. Large proteins, red blood cells (*page 474*)
8. 50, 25 (*page 474*)
9. 125 (*page 475*)
10. a. Decrease
    b. Increase
    c. Increase
    d. Decrease (*pages 476–480*)
11. Diffusion (*page 476*)
12. Osmosis (*pages 476–477*)
13. Active (*page 477*)
14. Electrolytes, water (*page 477*)
15. Secretion (*page 478*)
16. Descending, ascending (*page 478*)
17. Ascending (*page 478*)
18. Distal tubule, collecting duct (*page 478*)
19. Afferent arteriole, efferent arteriole (*page 479*)
20. Juxtaglomerular, juxtaglomerular cells, macula densa (*page 479*)
21. 20%–25% (*page 479*)
22. Cortical (*page 479*)
23. Increased (*page 479*)
24. Constrict, decrease (*page 480*)
25. a. Decrease
    b. Decrease
    c. Increase (*page 480*)
26. Hypothalamus, concentration or osmolality (*pages 480–481*)
27. Hypothalamus, concentration or osmolality (*page 481*)
28. Up, down (*page 481*)
29. Near isotonic or about 300 mosm, hypotonic or dilute (*pages 481–482*)
30. Extracellular (*page 482*)
31. Proximal tubule (*page 482*)
32. a. Glomerular filtration rate
    b. Aldosterone
    c. Third factor (*pages 482–483*)
33. Adrenal cortex, sodium, water, potassium (*pages 482–483*)
34. a. Cellular potassium level
    b. High flow rate through distal portion of the nephron
    c. Aldosterone (*pages 483–484*)
35. a. Parathormone
    b. Vitamin D
    c. Corticosteroids
    d. Diuresis (*pages 484–485*)
36. Intracellular, parathormone, glomerular filtration rate (*page 485*)
37. Intracellular, sodium, parathormone (*page 485*)
38. Increase, increase (*page 485*)
39. Decrease, decrease (*page 485*)
40. Up, decreased filtration or backleak or increased reabsorption (*page 486*)
41. a. Increased BUN and creatinine
    b. Increased BUN
    c. Increased BUN (*page 486*)
42. Decreased kidney function (*page 486*)
43. Hydrogen, bicarbonate (*pages 486–487*)
44. Decreasing, decreasing (*page 488*)
45. Any two of these (*pages 488, 489*):
    a. Maintenance of fluid volume
    b. Aldosterone
    c. Renin-angiotensin aldosterone system
    d. Prostaglandins
46. Decreased glomerular filtration rate, decreased sodium in distal tubule, increased sympathetic tone (*page 488*)
47. Constrict, aldosterone (*page 488*)
48. Decrease, increase, inhibition (*page 489*)
49. Erythropoietin (*page 489*)

B. Nursing Assessment Data Base

1. Orange (*page 490*)
2. Hemoglobin, myoglobin (*page 490*)
3. Water and sodium retention, albumin (*page 494*)
4. Asterixis (*page 495*)
5. Any two of these (*pages 490–496*):
   a. Costovertebral angle
   b. Flank
   c. Groin
6. 20, 1 (*page 496*)
7. 285, 295, 50, 1200 (*page 497*)
8. Density (*page 497*)
9. Nephron (*page 497*)
10. 6.0 (4.5–8.0) (*page 497*)
11. Low or acidotic, high or alkalotic (*page 497*)
12. a. Diabetic ketoacidosis

b. Starvation
c. Salicylate administration (*page 497*)

13. Any two of these (*pages 498, 499*):
a. Poor renal function
b. Multiple myeloma
c. Pregnancy
d. Congestive heart failure
e. Diabetes mellitus
f. Sickle cell anemia

C. Commonly Encountered Nursing Diagnoses

1. Any two of these (*pages 500, 501*):
a. Intake in excess of output
b. Weight gain
c. Decreased urinary output
d. Hypertension
e. Edema or anasarca
f. Distended neck veins or elevated central venous pressure
g. Bounding pulses
h. Dyspnea, orthopnea
i. Crackles
j. Diminished heart sounds
k. Anxiety, restlessness
l. Decreased level of consciousness
2. 600–800, 300–350 (*page 501*)
3. Any two of these (*page 502*):
a. Weight loss
b. Output in excess of intake
c. Hypotension
d. Tachycardia
e. Poor skin turgor
f. Dry skin and mucous membranes
g. Thirst
h. Flattened neck veins
i. Weakness
j. Altered level of consciousness
k. Altered urinary output
4. Up (*page 503*)
5. Any two of these (*page 505*):
a. Muscle wasting
b. Weight loss
c. Frequent infections
d. Decreased serum protein and albumin
e. Decreased anthropometric measurements
6. Any two of these (*page 507*):
a. Hypovolemia
b. Hypokalemia or hyperkalemia
c. Hyperuricemia
d. Hyponatremia
e. Metabolic alkalosis
f. Hypochloremia
g. Azotemia
7. Any three of these (*pages 507, 508*):
a. Increased fluid intake
b. Osmotic diuretics
c. Loop diuretics
d. Thiazide diuretics
e. Potassium-sparing diuretics
f. Carbonic anhydrase inhibitors
g. Cardiotonic agents
8. a. Loop diuretic
b. Osmotic diuretic
c. Aldosterone-inhibiting (potassium-sparing)
d. Carbonic anhydrase inhibitor (*pages 507–508*)
9. a. Central nervous system-sympathetic blockade
b. Beta-sympathetic blockade
c. Direct vasodilation
d. Direct vasodilation
e. Angiotensin-converting enzyme inhibition (*pages 509–510*)
10. Metabolic acidosis (*page 511*)
11. Increased, increased, increased (*page 512*)
12. Any two of these (*page 512*):
a. Lack of erythropoietin
b. Blood loss
c. Uremia
d. Vitamin deficiency
13. 10–15 (*page 513*)
14. Infection (*page 514*)
15. Increased, increased (*pages 515–516*)
16. Aluminum hydroxide gels, activated vitamin D, calcium (*page 516*)
17. Any two of these (*page 518*):
a. Decreased fat stores for lipid-soluble drugs
b. Decreased cardiac output for renal perfusion and elimination
c. Dilution by water retention
d. Decreased cell uptake with acidemia
e. Decreased serum protein for binding and deactivating some agents
f. Altered drug absorption
g. Decreased excretion by drug or metabolics
18. 100 (*page 520*)

D. Patient Health Problems

1. Higher (*page 521*)
2. Decreased renal perfusion, decreased (*page 521*)
3. Cortical (*page 521*)
4. Nephrotoxicity and ischemic injury (*page 521*)
5. a. Initial phase of poor perfusion or toxic insult

b. Oliguric phase
c. Diuretic phase
d. Recovery phase (*pages 522–523*)

6. a. Cortical intrarenal
b. Prerenal
c. Cortical intrarenal
d. Medullary intrarenal
e. Medullary intrarenal
f. Postrenal (*pages 523–524*)
7. 40 (*page 524*)
8. Up (*page 526*)
9. 400 (*page 526*)
10. Faster, up, down (*page 527*)
11. Medullary intrarenal (*page 527*)
12. Hemodialysis, peritoneal dialysis, continuous arterial-venous hemofiltration or hemodialysis (*pages 531–532*)
13. Intolerance of systemic heparinization, cardiovascular instability (*page 531*)
14. Any two of these (*page 531*):
a. Bleeding disorder
b. Abdominal adhesions
c. Recent abdominal surgery
15. Palpating for a thrill, inspecting the character of blood in the tubing (*page 533*)
16. Right (*page 534*)
17. a. Osmosis
b. Diffusion
c. Filtration (*page 534*)
18. Osmosis, diffusion (*page 534*)
19. More (*pages 535–536*)
20. Increased (*page 536*)
21. Any two of these (*page 536*):
a. Potassium
b. BUN
c. Creatinine
22. More (*pages 536–537*)
23. a. Hyperkalemia
b. Hyperkalemia
c. Hypocalcemia
d. Hypokalemia (*pages 537, 538*)
24. Hypertrophy or compensate (*page 543*)
25. a. Diminished reserve, 50%
b. Renal insufficiency, 75%
c. End-stage renal disease, 90%
d. Uremic syndrome (*page 544*)
26. Pyelonephritis (*page 544*)
27. Glomerulonephropathy, nephrotic syndrome (*page 548*)
28. Urinary tract infection (*page 548*)
29. a. 10–50, four times baseline value
b. 10–15, 10 or greater (*page 549*)
30. a. Increase
b. Decrease
c. Decrease
d. Increase
e. Increase
f. Increase
g. Decrease (*pages 547–559*)
31. Acetate or lactate (*page 551*)
32. 20–24 (*page 551*)
33. a. Pericarditis
b. Cardiac tamponade
c. Peripheral neuropathy
d. Osteomalacia or renal rickets (*pages 552–558*)
34. 10 (*page 560*)
35. a. No
b. No
c. Yes
d. Yes
e. No (*page 562*)
36. a. ABO typing
b. Human leukocyte antigen (HLA) typing
c. Mixed leukocyte culture (MLC) typing
d. Crossmatch for preformed antibodies (*page 563*)
37. a. Preexisting antibodies
b. B-cell lymphocytes
c. T-cell lymphocytes (*pages 563–565*)
38. Diarrhea, constipation (*page 566*)
39. Any two of these (*page 568*):
a. Increased risk of infection
b. Increased risk of malignancy
c. Esophagitis
d. Peptic ulcer
e. Pancreatitis
40. Increased, increased, decreased (*page 569*)
41. Any two of these (*page 570*):
a. Corticosteroid
b. Cyclosporin A
c. Antilymphocyte globulin
d. Monoclonal antibodies
e. Cyclophosphamide
42. Any two of these (*pages 572–573*):
a. Renal disease
b. Cellular destruction
c. Excessive potassium intake
d. Adrenal cortical insufficiency
e. Decreased cardiac output
f. Sodium deficit
g. Acidosis
43. Up (*page 573*)
44. Peaked T waves (*page 574*)
45. Lower extremities (*page 574*)
46. Glucose, insulin, bicarbonate (*pages 574–575*)
47. Sodium, potassium (*page 575*)

48. Any two of these (*pages 575, 576*):
    a. Alkalosis
    b. Gastrointestinal losses
    c. Liver disease
    d. Diuretic therapy
    e. Renal tubular acidosis
    f. Increased adrenal cortical function
    g. Diarrhea
    h. Starvation
49. a. Decrease
    b. Increase
    c. Decrease
    d. Decrease
    e. Increase (*page 576*)
50. Hypokalemia, hypercalcemia (*pages 578, 586*)
51. Up, down (*page 578*)
52. Decreased, increased (*page 578*)
53. Over (*pages 579–582*)
54. Up, up, up (*pages 580–582*)
55. Down, up (*page 582*)
56. Any two of these (*page 582*):
    a. Diuretics, diuresis
    b. Diarrhea
    c. Nasogastric suction
    d. Diaphoresis
    e. Some renal diseases
    f. Hyperglycemia
57. Decrease, increase, decrease, increase (*page 584*)
58. Saline or hypertonic saline (*page 585*)
59. Bone (*page 585*)
60. Phosphorus (*page 585*)
61. Down, up (*pages 586, 587*)
62. Any two of these (*page 588*):
    a. Saline with diuretic therapy
    b. Corticosteroids
    c. Drugs to increase bone uptake of calcium such as mithramycin
    d. Phosphate
63. Hyperphosphatemia, vitamin D resistance (*page 588*)
64. Parathormone, thyrocalcitonin (*pages 588–589*)
65. Constrict or spasm, decrease (*pages 590–591*)
66. Chvostek's, Trousseau's (*page 590*)
67. Late (*page 592*)
68. Aluminum hydroxide gels (*page 592*)
69. Up, up (*page 593*)
70. Weakness; hemolytic; 2,3 diphosphoglycerate (*pages 593–594*)
71. a. Increase
    b. Decrease
    c. Decrease
    d. Decrease
    e. Decrease (*pages 591–595*)
72. Decrease, decrease, decrease, peak (*page 596*)
73. Any two of these (*page 597*):
    a. Dialysis
    b. Diuretics
    c. Saline-induced diuresis
    d. Calcium gluconate
74. a. Increase
    b. Increase
    c. Decrease
    d. Decrease
    e. Decrease
    f. Decrease (*pages 596–598*)
75. Increase, increase, flatten or invert (*pages 598–599*)
76. More (*page 600*)
77. Contusions (*page 600*)
78. 60–80 (*page 602*)
79. More (*page 603*)
80. 4–6 (*page 604*)

E. Summary of Patient Health Problems

Refer to the following pages in the Core Curriculum

1. Acute Renal Failure (*pages 521–543*)
2. Chronic Renal Failure (*pages 543–572*)
3. Hyperkalemia (*pages 572–575*)
4. Hypokalemia (*pages 575–578*)
5. Hypernatremia (*pages 578–582*)
6. Hyponatremia (*pages 582–585*)
7. Hypercalcemia (*pages 585–588*)
8. Hypocalcemia (*pages 588–591*)
9. Hyperphosphatemia (*pages 591–593*)
10. Hypophosphatemia (*pages 593–595*)
11. Hypermagnesemia (*pages 595–597*)
12. Hypomagnesemia (*pages 597–600*)
13. Renal Trauma (*pages 600–606*)

THE RENAL SYSTEM

Post Quiz

The following questions are designed to test understanding of some of the key points in the section. Select the best answer for each of the following. The answers are at the end of the test.

1. The glomeruli, proximal tubules, and distal tubules are located in the
   a. renal cortex
   b. renal medulla
   c. adrenal gland
   d. pyramid
2. The peritubular capillaries
   a. form the glomerulus
   b. come before the efferent arteriole
   c. come before the afferent arteriole
   d. are in the area of the tubules and loop of Henle
3. Which of the following statements concerning glomerular filtrate is *false?*
   a. It is a protein-free, plasma-like fluid.
   b. It is filtered at the rate of approximately 125 cc/min.
   c. It is directly related to renal blood flow.
   d. It occurs in the renal medulla.
4. Which of the following statements concerning normal tubular function is *false?*
   a. All but approximately 1% is reabsorbed.
   b. All of the waste products are reabsorbed.
   c. All of the glucose is reabsorbed in patients with normal blood sugars.
   d. Reabsorption becomes more selective as the filtrate travels through the nephron.
5. Aldosterone
   a. causes sodium and water excretion
   b. causes potassium retention
   c. comes from the posterior pituitary
   d. increases in response to angiotensin II
6. Antidiuretic hormone (ADH)
   a. causes sodium and water excretion
   b. causes potassium retention
   c. is released from the posterior pituitary
   d. increases in response to renin secretion
7. Conditions that might cause prerenal failure include
   a. high doses of nephrotoxins
   b. beta-hemalytic infections
   c. nephron degeneration
   d. decreased cardiac output
8. Causes of an elevated BUN include
   a. low protein intake
   b. overhydration
   c. anabolic metabolism
   d. gastrointestinal bleeding
9. Oliguria is a 24-hour urine output of
   a. nothing
   b. less than 400 cc
   c. 400–700 cc
   d. less than 700 cc

10. Most electrolytes are absorbed in the
    a. proximal tubule
    b. loop of Henle
    c. distal tubule
    d. collecting duct
11. Aldosterone and antidiuretic hormones act primarily in the
    a. proximal tubule
    b. glomerulus and proximal tubule
    c. distal tubule and collecting duct
    d. loop of Henle
12. Osmosis is
    a. a type of active reabsorption
    b. the equilibration of solutes across a concentration gradient
    c. the movement of water from the area of lower to higher concentration
    d. another name for hydrostatic pressure
13. Active transport
    a. includes osmosis and diffusion
    b. involves mechanisms that require energy
    c. does not occur in the kidney
    d. is the result of natural principles governing the behavior of solutes and solvents
14. One stimulus for aldosterone secretion is
    a. low serum sodium
    b. low serum potassium
    c. hypervolemia
    d. hyperosmolality
15. Parathyroid hormone
    a. increases phosphate reabsorption
    b. increases calcium reabsorption
    c. increases sodium and water retention
    d. decrease phosphate excretion
16. Stimuli for ADH include
    a. decreased atrial stretch
    b. hypertension
    c. hyponatremia
    d. hypo-osmolality
17. Chloride
    a. is a cation
    b. usually moves opposite bicarbonate
    c. is usually increased in metabolic alkalosis
    d. is absorbed primarily with potassium
18. When the patient has a low pH, the kidneys will try to compensate by
    a. increasing H^+ retention
    b. increasing bicarbonate secretion
    c. increasing H^+ secretion
    d. decreasing bicarbonate reabsorption
19. Laboratory signs of intrarenal failure usually include
    a. polycythemia
    b. elevated BUN with a normal creatinine
    c. concentrated urine
    d. abnormal casts or cells in the urine
20. The diet for a patient with chronic renal failure
    a. should provide for a negative nitrogen balance
    b. is relatively high in protein
    c. should maintain an anabolic state
    d. includes sodium and potassium supplements

21. The net filtration pressure across the glomerular membrane will increase when
    a. renal blood flow decreases
    b. there is an obstruction in the ureter
    c. interstitial edema is present
    d. the serum albumin level is low
22. One of the factors involved in the countercurrent mechanism is
    a. a hypotonic medullary interstitium causing urine concentration
    b. the descending loop of Henle being permeable only to NaCl
    c. the ascending loop of Henle being permeable only to water
    d. the existence of a healthy and functioning loop of Henle and vasa recta
23. Intrarenal failure is more likely to involve the cortex when it is triggered by
    a. prolonged prerenal failure (ischemia)
    b. abruptio placentae
    c. nephrotoxicity
    d. ureteral obstruction
24. A patient with severe hyperkalemia
    a. will exhibit a shortened ST segment
    b. can be treated by insulin, glucose, and sodium bicarbonate
    c. may have hyperparathyroidism
    d. is likely to have resultant alkalemia
25. A patient with hypophosphatemia
    a. will exhibit a depressed ST segment and the development of a u wave
    b. can be treated with aluminum hydroxide gels
    c. may develop hemolytic anemia
    d. often has an associated hypocalcemia
26. The term used to refer to the movement of substances from the renal tubular cells into the tubular lumen is
    a. filtration
    b. absorption
    c. secretion
    d. excretion
27. Hemodialysis is preferred over peritoneal dialysis when the patient
    a. has had recent abdominal surgery
    b. is less than 2 years old
    c. is hemodynamically unstable
    d. is actively bleeding
28. Trousseau's and Chovstek's signs are indicative of
    a. hyperkalemia
    b. hypernatremia
    c. hypermagnesemia
    d. hypocalcemia
29. A major intracellular cation involved in enzyme systems is
    a. phosphate
    b. magnesium
    c. sodium
    d. chloride
30. An intravenous pyelogram
    a. is indicated when patients have poor renal function
    b. can cause nephrotoxicity and dehydration
    c. is used to measure glomerular filtration
    d. is the test of choice for patients with diabetes mellitus
31. Increased glomerular filtration rates can lead to excess
    a. retention of phosphorus
    b. retention of potassium
    c. retention of calcium
    d. loss of sodium

32. Patients on prostaglandin-inhibiting agents may develop
    a. increased renal perfusion
    b. increased glomerular filtration rate
    c. increased water excretion
    d. renal arterial vasoconstriction
33. Patients with renal failure accompanied by increasing BUN and serum glucose can be expected to have
    a. an elevated serum osmolality
    b. a decreased serum osmolality
    c. increased urine osmolality
    d. decreased urine osmolality
34. When a patient's serum creatinine rises from 0.6 mg/dL to 1.2 mg/dL, renal function
    a. is normal
    b. is 50% of normal
    c. is 25% of normal
    d. is 10% of normal
35. Mechanisms that result in increased urinary output include
    a. increasing sodium reabsorption
    b. increasing the effect of aldosterone
    c. inhibiting carbonic anhydrase
    d. increasing renal vascular resistance
36. Which diuretic would be more appropriate for a patient with hyperkalemia, heart failure, and metabolic acidosis?
    a. mannitol
    b. furosemide
    c. acetazolamide
    d. spironolactone
37. Which of the following is part of the current understanding of the pathophysiology of chronic renal failure?
    a. the kidney has very limited reserves
    b. clinical manifestations occur early in the disease progression
    c. loss of nephron function causes remaining nephrons to hypertrophy
    d. decreased creatinine clearance occurs late in the course of disease
38. Laboratory manifestations of chronic renal failure are more likely to include
    a. hypocalcemia
    b. hypophosphatemia
    c. hypokalemia
    d. concentrated urine
39. Which of the following is more likely to cause water intoxication?
    a. inhibition of antidiuretic hormone
    b. excessive diuretic therapy
    c. congestive heart failure
    d. hypercalcemia
40. Which of the following is more likely to cause hypomagnesemia?
    a. excessive gastrointestinal fluid loss
    b. hyperparathyroidism
    c. hypothyroidism
    d. renal failure

Answers to the Renal System Post Quiz

1. **a** (*page 572*)
2. **d** (*page 479*)
3. **d** (*page 475*)
4. **b** (*pages 476–477*)
5. **d** (*pages 482–483*)
6. **c** (*page 481*)
7. **d** (*pages 521–524*)
8. **d** (*page 486*)
9. **b** (*page 526*)

10. **a** (*page 577*)
11. **c** (*page 478*)
12. **c** (*page 476*)
13. **b** (*pages 476–477*)
14. **a** (*pages 482–483*)
15. **b** (*pages 484–485*)
16. **a** (*page 481*)
17. **b** (*page 485*)
18. **c** (*pages 486–488*)
19. **d** (*page 527*)
20. **c** (*pages 504–505, 565–566*)
21. **d** (*page 475*)
22. **d** (*pages 481–482*)
23. **b** (*pages 521–524*)
24. **b** (*pages 572–575*)
25. **c** (*pages 597–599*)
26. **c** (*pages 476–478*)
27. **a** (*page 531*)
28. **d** (*pages 590–591*)
29. **b** (*page 485*)
30. **b** (*pages 498–499*)
31. **d** (*pages 482–485*)
32. **d** (*page 489*)
33. **a** (*page 476*)
34. **b** (*page 549*)
35. **c** (*pages 506–508*)
36. **b** (*pages 506–508*)
37. **c** (*pages 543–544*)
38. **a** (*pages 548–550*)
39. **c** (*page 582*)
40. **a** (*pages 597–598*)

These are primarily the comprehend or recall, and apply or analyze levels of questions. Examples of synthesis or evaluate questions can be found in the comprehensive examination at the end of the book on pages 278 to 293.

5

The Endocrine System

SECTION-RELATED TIPS FOR THOSE STUDYING TO TAKE THE CERTIFICATION EXAMINATION

This section is like the pulmonary section in that it uses a lot of abbreviations and like the neurologic section in that you gain more in studying if you start by memorizing the functions of the major glands and hormones. Although the abbreviations are not used on the examination, the list below is fairly short and reviewing them will help when reading through this section. Figure 5–2 and Table 5–3 may be helpful in memorizing the important glands, their significant hormones, and their major functions.

Keep in mind that only a small percentage of the examination questions are on the endocrine system and that the lower the percentage devoted to a system on the examination, the less difficult the questions asked.

Abbreviation	*Hormone*
ACTH	Adrenocorticotropic hormone or adrenocorticotropin
ADH	Antidiuretic hormone or vasopressin
CRH*	Cortisol-releasing hormone
CT	Calcitonin
GH	Growth hormone or somatotropin
GRH*	Growth-releasing hormone
PTH	Parathormone
T_3, T_4	Active thyroid hormones
TRH*	Thyroid-releasing hormone
TSH	Thyroid-stimulating hormone

* CRH, GRH, and TRH are factors the hypothalamus releases to stimulate the anterior pituitary to release ACTH, GH, and TSH, respectively.

Please see the instructions at the beginning of the book for important general suggestions that are relevant to the bulk of the *Core Curriculum* content. They apply to this section as well as the others.

FIGURES AND TABLES

Refer to these figures and tables while reading the endocrine section of the Core Curriculum.

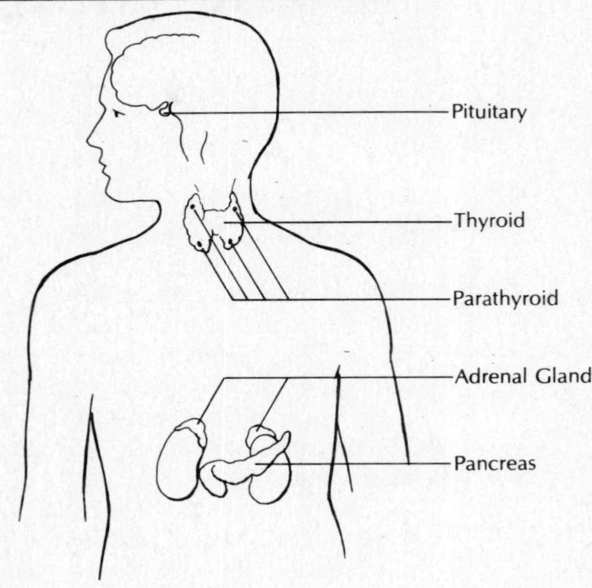

Figure 5–1. Locations of the major glands of the endocrine system (*pages 609–623*).

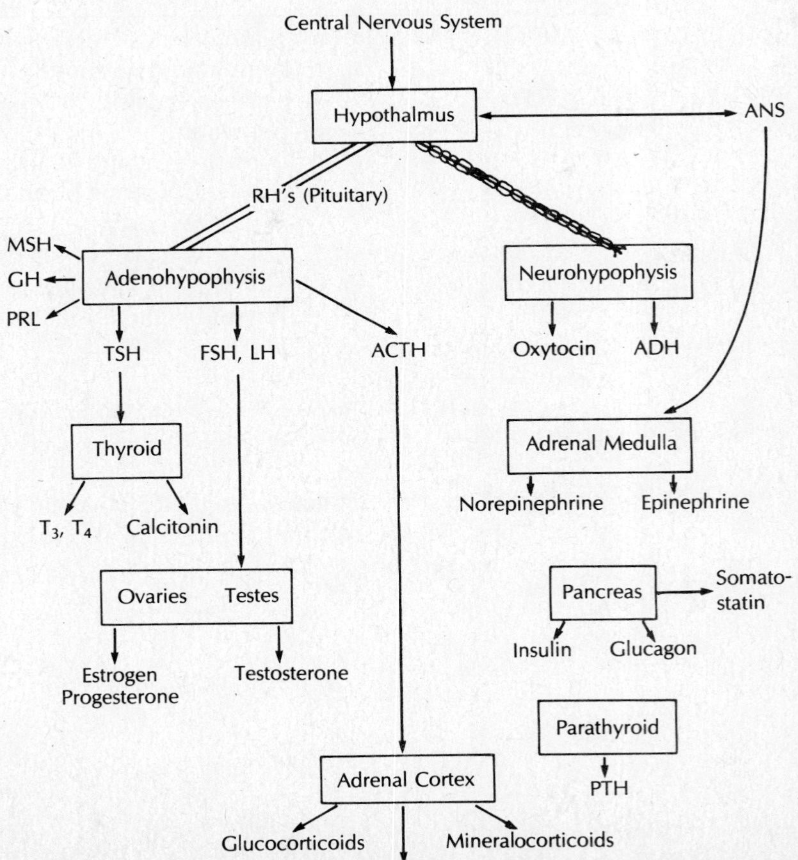

Figure 5–2. Interrelationships between glands of the endocrine system. The hypothalamus stimulates the adenohypophysis via releasing factors secreted into small veins linking them. It stimulates the neurohypophysis via nerve fibers (*pages 612–623*).

Table 5–1. SUMMARY OF THE HORMONES—ORIGINS, STIMULI, AND EFFECTS (*pages 614–623*)

Hormones	Releasing Stimuli	Target/Effect
Anterior Pituitary Hormones	***Stimulus for Releasing Factors from Hypothalamus***	
Growth Hormone (Somatotropin)	Genetic cycles, daily cycles Hypoglycemia, starvation Exercise, stress Inhibited by hyperglycemia and elevated corticosteroids	Growth of cells capable of it Increases blood sugar (by antagonism of insulin) Mobilizes fatty acids Growth aspect synergistic with insulin and thyroxin
Adrenocorticotropic Hormone (Corticotropin)	Diurnal variations Stress Hypoglycemia Inadequate levels of adrenocortical hormone (cortisol)	Stimulates production and release of adrenal cortical hormones
Thyroid-Stimulating Hormone (Thyrotropin)	Inadequate levels of thyroid hormones Inhibited by somatostatin	Stimulates growth production and output of thyroid gland
Posterior Pituitary Hormones	***Stimulus for Releasing Impulse from Hypothalamus***	
Antidiuretic Hormone (Vasopressin)	Increased serum osmolality Hypoxia Hypotension, hypovolema Stress Various drugs	Physiologic levels: Water retention in kidney High levels: Arteriolar vasoconstriction Also potentiates coagulation
Oxytocin	Childbirth Suckling	Uterine contraction Breast lactation
Thyroid Hormones	***Releasing Stimuli***	
T_4 = 90% T_3 = 10% (most potent)	Thyroid-stimulating hormone from pituitary (T_4 to T_3 conversion in periphery is blocked by stress, drugs, liver, and kidney failure, and malnutrition)	Increases metabolic rate in almost all tissues Increased fat, carbohydrate and protein metabolism Stimulates growth Increased temperature
Calcitonin (Thyrocalcitonin)	Hypercalcemia	Slightly decreases serum calcium (and phosphate)
Parathyroid Hormones		
Parathyroid (Parathormone)	Hypocalcemia Catecholamines, cortisol Inhibited by abnormal serum magnesium or high vitamin D metabolites Diurnal variations	Increased absorption of calcium from kidney, bone, and GI tract Increased excretion of phosphate and HCO_3^- in urine Increased absorption of magnesium in kidney
Adrenal Cortical Hormones		
Glucocorticoids (Cortisol)	ACTH from pituitary Diurnal variations	Increases blood sugar by increased glucose synthesis and decreased glucose uptake by cells Stimulates breakdown of protein and fat for glucose synthesis Anti-inflammatory Facilitates other hormones
Mineralocorticoids (Aldosterone)	Low renal blood flow (renin) ACTH from pituitary Hyperkalemia Hyponatremia	Increased sodium retention, Increased water retention, Decreased potassium retention } Does this in kidneys, skin, and GI tract

Continued on the following page

Table 5–1. SUMMARY OF THE HORMONES—ORIGINS, STIMULI, AND EFFECTS (*pages 614–623*) *Continued*

Hormones	Releasing Stimuli	Target/Effect
Androgens	ACTH from pituitary	Small amounts so minimal effects
Adrenal Medullary Hormones		
Epinephrine (Adrenalin) 80% Norepinephrine 20%	Sympathetic nerve stimulus Hypoglycemia Hypoxia Hypotension	Antagonize insulin Hyperglycemia Generalized adrenergic response
Pancreatic Hormones		
Insulin	Hyperglycemia GI hormones Inhibited by catecholamines and many other substrates	Transport glucose into cells (especially muscle and fat cells) Increased liver glycogen stores Stimulates synthesis and inhibits breakdown of both fat and protein
Glucagon	Hypoglycemia High protein die Catecholamines and GI hormones Inhibited by somatostatin	Stimulates carbohydrate, protein, fat breakdown into glucose Antagonizes insulin activity
Somatostatin	Negative feedback systems	Decreases insulin, glucagon, growth hormone, TSH and GI hormones

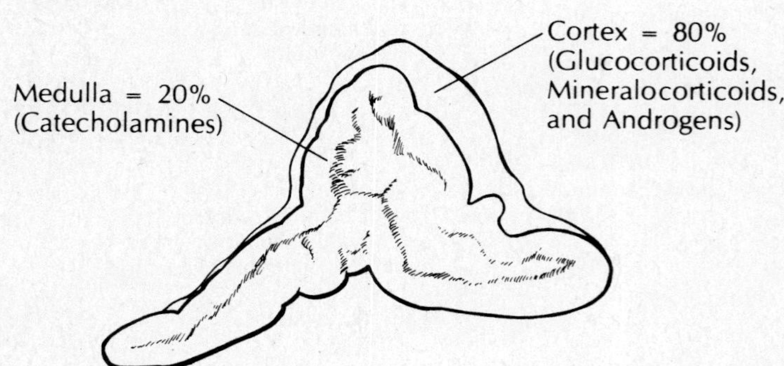

Figure 5–3. Cross-sectional anatomy of the adrenal gland. Cortex and medulla are indicated, with the hormones they secrete (in parenthesis) (*pages 618–620*).

Exocrine Function
Acinar Cells
(Digestive Juices)

Endocrine Function
Islets of Langerhans (2% of cells)
- Alpha Cells (glucagon)
- Beta Cells (insulin)
- Delta Cells (somatostatin, gastrin)

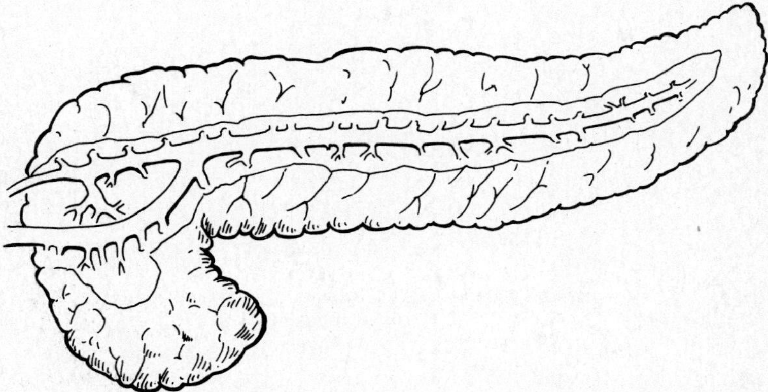

Figure 5–4. Pancreatic cell types, with the substances they secrete (in parenthesis) (*pages 618–623*).

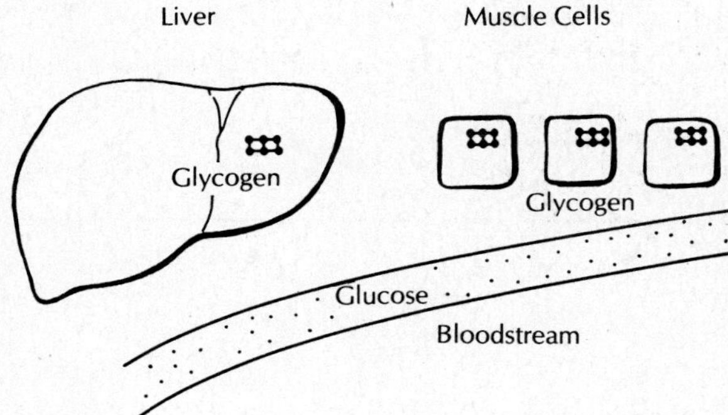

Figure 5–5. Sites of two forms of carbohydrate. Glucose is a simple sugar found in the bloodstream; glycogen is a complex sugar stored in the liver and in muscle cells (*pages 618–623*).

Table 5–2. TERMS USED TO DESCRIBE CARBOHYDRATE METABOLISM AND HORMONES THAT STIMULATE THEM (*pages 618–623*)

Term	Definition	Hormones Controlling It
Glucogenesis	Increasing blood sugar (making glucose)	Glucagon, cortisol, catecholamines, growth hormone
Gluconeogenesis	Increasing blood sugar by breaking down fat and protein stores	Glucagon, cortisol, catecholamines, growth hormone
Glycogenolysis	Increasing blood sugar by breaking down glycogen stores	Glucagon, cortisol, catecholamines

Table 5–3. SUMMARY OF THE MAJOR ENDOCRINE GLAND FUNCTIONS AND DISORDERS (*pages 613–623*)

Gland	Hormone	Function	Dysfunction	
			Hyposecretion	Hypersecretion
Adenohypophysis	GH	Stimulates growth	Dwarfism	Giantism Acromegaly
	TSH	Stimulates thyroid	(See thyroid gland)	
	ACTH	Stimulates adrenal cortex	(See adrenal gland)	
Neurohypophysis	ADH	Stimulates water retention, concentrates urine	Diabetes insipidus	Syndrome of inappropriate ADH
Thyroid	T_3, T_4	Stimulates metabolic rate	Hypothyroidism Myxedema coma	Hyperthyroidism Thyroid crisis
	Calcitonin	Decreases serum calcium		
Parathyroid	Parathyroid	Affects calcium and phosphorus balance	Hypocalcemia	Hypercalcemia
Pancreas	Insulin	Decreases blood sugar	Type I diabetes mellitus	Hypoglycemia
	Glucagon	Increases blood sugar		
Adrenal Cortex	Glucocorticoids (cortisol)	Increases blood glucose Affects protein and carbohydrate metabolism Anti-inflammatory	Addison's disease Acute adrenal crisis	Cushing's syndrome
	Mineralocorticoids (aldosterone)	Sodium and water retention Potassium loss		Hyperaldosteronism
Adrenal Medulla	Epinephrine Norepinephrine	Stress response		Pheochromocytoma

Table 5–4. SUMMARY OF FACTORS COVERED IN THE PHYSIOLOGIC ANATOMY SECTION THAT HAVE IMPORTANT CLINICAL APPLICATIONS WORTH MENTIONING (*pages 609–623*)

Factor	Clinical Application	Page
Hormone Receptors	Down regulation of receptor sites by high level of hormones partly explains not only the etiology of some endocrine disorders, but also the altered patient response to endogenous and exogenous catecholamines. High levels over a period of time tend to decrease receptor sites and drug effects.	610
Foundational Concepts	Endocrine disorders can occur from dysfunction in any step of a typical sequence: (1) Inability to monitor the need for hormone release (2) Inability to make or release a hormone (3) Altered transport in the bloodstream (4) Altered responsiveness of target cells (5) Inability to monitor the need has been met (6) Inability to inhibit further hormone release	609–612
Growth Hormone	Growth hormone released from the anterior pituitary at first primarily increases the blood sugar. Growth of bone and cartilage occurs only after a second step, release of somatomedins from the liver. Under stress this step is inhibited by steroids and therefore does not result in growth. Children with liver failure or who chronically receive steroids may not grow and develop properly.	614
ACTH	Critically ill patients often have ACTH and cortisol levels sustained at a high level, which interferes with their ability to rest and sleep. The ability to increase circulating levels of ACTH and cortisol, however, is a critical component of the stress response. Patients with unidentified adrenal insufficiency have a high mortality rate from acute illness.	615
ADH	Many factors that stimulate ADH release from the posterior pituitary may coexist in a critically ill patient (hypoxia, hypovolemia, hypotension, stress, pain, and drugs like narcotics, tranquilizers, and general anesthesia). For this reason, syndrome of inappropriate ADH or high ADH activity is one of the most common endocrine disorders in critical care.	616
T_3, T_4	Hypothyroid function is fairly common in women and in the older patient population. It may be unmasked by admission to critical care by further blocking of the conversion of T_4 to T_3, the more active form, and other effects of stress on thyroxine activity. Factors that contribute are severe illness, mechanical ventilation, malnutrition, steroids, propranolol, and the development of liver or renal failure.	617
Calcitonin	Although endogenous calcitonin does not play a major role in normal calcium metabolism, pharmacologically it can be very useful in the treatment of hypercalcemia and bone pain (Calcimar is the trade name of the drug).	618
PTH	Calcium imbalances are common in critical care. So are alterations in PTH levels. The relationship between them in various patient subsets is under current investigation.	618
Cortisol	The presence of high endogenous secretion of cortisol and the frequency with which patients receive or have received steroids prior to admission place critically ill patients at risk for the consequences. They include hyperglycemia, catabolic metabolism, and anti-inflammatory effects. The latter place the patient at higher risk of infection.	619
Aldosterone	Aldosterone levels are often altered in the critically ill and knowledge of its effects is an important aspect of practice. This is addressed in detail in the Renal Section.	619–620
Insulin	Insulin has two important types of effects. High levels are required to lower the blood sugar by increasing glucose transport into cells. At lower levels, it also prevents catabolism of protein, fat, and glycogen into glucose. Type I diabetics who often have very low insulin levels have problems lowering their blood sugars and are chronically catabolic.	622
Growth-Promoting Hormones	The three hormones that promote growth synergistically are growth hormone, insulin, and thyroid. Low levels may result in altered growth and development or may be unmasked during a later growth phase, pregnancy (gestational thyroid and insulin abnormalities). These three may also be important in healing and in growth of new tissue and are under investigation in their effect on wound healing and anabolism in critically ill patients.	622

THE ENDOCRINE SYSTEM

Exercises

After reading the endocrine section of the Core Curriculum, *fill in the blanks in the following statements. It can be done one topic at a time or all at once. The answers are at the end of the exercises.*

A. Physiologic Anatomy (*pages 609–623*)

1. Hormones are substances made by one type of cell and released into the ______________ where they travel to target cells, which are determined by the presence of ______________ for that hormone.
2. The presence of a high concentration of a hormone may ______________ the number of available receptor sites.
3. Three mechanisms of hormone action are
   a. ______________
   b. ______________
   c. ______________
4. Negative feedback is the mechanism by which the amount of hormone release is ______________.
5. The pituitary is embedded in the ______________ bone at the base of the brain.
6. The hypothalamus is linked to the anterior pituitary via ______________, and to the posterior pituitary via ______________.
7. Name three major hormones secreted by the adenohypophysis.
   a. ______________
   b. ______________
   c. ______________
8. Indicate whether the following will increase or decrease the activity of growth hormone:
   a. Hyperglycemia ______________
   b. Stress ______________
   c. Corticosteroid administration ______________
9. The effects of growth hormone include ______________ of protein synthesis, ______________ of fatty acid mobilization, and ______________ of insulin activity.
10. Indicate whether the following will increase or decrease the release of adrenocorticotropin:
    a. Stress ______________
    b. Increased cortisol levels ______________
    c. Hypoglycemia ______________
11. Adrenocorticotropin has a diurnal pattern that reaches its highest levels each day in the ______________ hours and its lowest levels in the ______________ hours.
12. Indicate whether the following will increase or decrease the release of antidiuretic hormone:
    a. Hypoxia ______________
    b. Hypo-osmolality ______________
    c. Ethanol ______________
    d. Hypotension ______________
    e. Morphine ______________

13. Of the two thyroid hormones produced, ________________ is the most abundant and ________________ is the most potent.
14. Three drugs that suppress the conversion of T_4 to T_3 are ________________, ________________, and ________________.
15. The term sick euthyroid syndrome is used to describe the adaptive ________________ in T_3 and T_4 levels during times of critical illness.
16. Name the four hormones involved in growth.
    a. ________________
    b. ________________
    c. ________________
    d. ________________
17. Thyrocalcitonin causes the serum calcium to go ________________, whereas parathormone causes it to go ________________.
18. Indicate whether the following will increase or decrease the release of parathormone:
    a. Hypocalcemia ________________
    b. Sleep ________________
    c. Magnesium imbalances ________________
19. The effects of cortisol include ________________ serum glucose levels, ________________ insulin activity, ________________ fat and protein breakdown, and ________________ inflammatory response.
20. Indicate whether the following will increase or decrease the release of aldosterone:
    a. Hypokalemia ________________
    b. Hypervolemia ________________
    c. Renin release ________________
    d. Hyponatremia ________________
21. The effects of aldosterone on the renal tubules include ________________ sodium absorption, ________________ fluid absorption, and ________________ potassium absorption.
22. Adrenal medullary hormones are the primary first line of defense during ________________ and the major hormone released is ________________.
23. Under stress, the release of catecholamines from the adrenal medulla causes the blood sugar to ________________, gastrointestinal activity to ________________, insulin activity to ________________, cardiac output to ________________, and bronchi to ________________.
24. The islet cells of the pancreas include the ________________ cells, which produce insulin; the ________________ cells, which produce glucagon; and the ________________ cells, which produce somatostatin.
25. The effects of insulin include ________________ glucose uptake by muscle and fat cells, ________________ glycogen synthesis, and ________________ fat and protein synthesis.
26. The effects of glucagon include ________________ glycogenolysis, ________________ gluconeogenesis, and ________________ insulin activity.
27. Because somatostatin ________________ several hormones, it

may be of therapeutic value in some cancer patients with endocrine complications.

28. Two examples of hormones that raise the blood sugar are ______ ______ and ______.
29. Indicate which gland secretes each of the following hormones:
    a. Growth hormone ______
    b. Cortisol ______
    c. Calcitonin ______
    d. Glucagon ______
    e. Catecholamines ______
30. Indicate which hormone imbalances can lead to each of the following disorders:
    a. Acromegaly ______
    b. Addison's disease ______
    c. Cushing's syndrome ______
    d. Hypocalcemia ______

B. Nursing Assessment Data Base (*pages 623–627*)

1. List three pathologic mechanisms that can cause endocrine disorders.
    a. ______
    b. ______
    c. ______
2. List three types of pharmacologic agents that may alter hormone activity.
    a. ______
    b. ______
    c. ______

C. Patient Health Problems (*pages 629–672*)

1. Diabetes insipidus is a(n) ______ in antidiuretic hormone activity resulting in ______ excretion of water.
2. The four mechanisms that can lead to diabetes insipidus are
    a. ______
    b. ______
    c. ______
    d. ______
3. Signs of diabetes insipidus include ______ sensation of thirst, ______ mucous membranes, ______ serum osmolality, ______ urine osmolality, and ______ serum sodium.
4. Goals of therapy in patients with diabetes insipidus include ______ serum osmolality and ______ urine volume.
5. Patients with acute transient forms of diabetes insipidus may be treated with ______ and ______.
6. The syndrome of inappropriate antidiuretic hormone is ______ antidiuretic hormone activity, resulting in ______ water excretion.
7. Indicate whether the following agents can increase or decrease antidiuretic hormone activity:
    a. Vincristine ______
    b. Pentamidine ______
    c. Chlorpropamide ______
    d. Acetaminophen ______
    e. Thiazide diuretics ______

f. ETOH ______________________
g. Phenytoin ______________________
h. Chlordiazepoxide ______________________

8. Indicate how the following conditions can affect antidiuretic hormone activity (increase, decrease, or both):
a. Head trauma ______________________
b. Brain tumor ______________________
c. Meningitis ______________________
d. Pyelonephritis ______________________
e. Pneumonia ______________________
f. Positive pressure ventilation ______________________
g. Hypoxia ______________________

9. Signs of the syndrome of inappropriate antidiuretic hormone include ______________________ serum sodium, ______________________ serum osmolality, ______________________ urine osmolality, and ______________________ water retention.

10. Therapy for severe acute syndrome of inappropriate antidiuretic hormone may include ______________________ intravenous solutions.

11. The concern over the above therapy is the potential for ______________________ damage if the sodium concentration goes ______________________ too fast.

12. The pathophysiology of thyroid crisis is related to both thyroid hormone and the response to ______________________, which is altered owing to ______________________ number of receptor sites.

13. Signs of hyperthyroid crisis may include ______________________ temperature, ______________________ heart rate, ______________________ skin, ______________________ pulse pressure, and ______________________ reflexes.

14. Laboratory findings associated with hyperthyroid crisis include ______________________ T_3 and T_4, ______________________ TSH, ______________________ serum calcium, and ______________________ blood sugar.

15. Three agents used to treat hyperthyroid crisis that seem to act, at least in part, by decreasing the conversion of T_4 to T_3 are ______________________, ______________________, and ______________________.

16. A substrate that can be part of the cause of hyperthyroid crisis but paradoxically can be part of its treatment is ______________________.

17. Myxedema coma may be accompanied by ______________________ edema, ______________________ temperature, ______________________ deep-tendon reflexes, ______________________ weight, ______________________ ventilation, and fluid ______________________.

18. Laboratory findings associated with myxedema coma may include ______________________ T_3 and T_4 levels, ______________________ serum sodium, ______________________ hemoglobin, ______________________ CPK, and ______________________ cholesterol.

19. In primary hypothyroidism, the thyroid-stimulating hormone level goes ______________________.

20. Indicate whether the following are more likely to cause increased or decreased parathormone activity:
a. Hyperplasia of the gland ______________________

b. Chronic renal failure ____________
c. Malignancies ____________
d. Thyroidectomy ____________
e. Hypomagnesemia ____________

21. The most common cause of primary adrenal insufficiency is ____________, but it can also be associated with suppression or caused by the administration of exogenous ____________.
22. Patients with adrenal insufficiency may have ____________ appetite, ____________ bowel sounds, ____________ blood pressure, and ____________ temperature.
23. Indicate the type of adrenal insufficiency (primary or secondary) most likely to be associated with the following.
    a. Aldosterone deficiency ____________
    b. Hyperpigmentation ____________
    c. Increased adrenocorticotropic hormone ____________
    d. Increased cortisol after adrenocorticotropic hormone ____________
    e. Hypothyroidism ____________
24. Laboratory findings associated with adrenal insufficiency may include ____________ blood glucose, ____________ serum potassium, and ____________ serum sodium.
25. Adrenal insufficiency can be treated with intravenous solutions containing ____________ and ____________, and with ____________, which can reverse the symptoms of both cortisol and aldosterone deficiency.
26. Insulin-inhibiting hormones include ____________ and ____________.
27. The pathophysiology of diabetic ketoacidosis related to insulin deficiency includes ____________ gluconeogenesis, ____________ lipolysis, ____________ serum osmolality, ____________ serum bicarbonate, and ____________ serum pH.
28. Drugs that can inhibit insulin include ____________ and ____________.
29. Early in diabetic ketoacidosis the total body potassium level goes ____________ while the serum potassium level goes ____________.
30. Signs of diabetic ketoacidosis include ____________ thirst, ____________ skin, ____________ level of consciousness, ____________ respirations, and ____________ blood pressure.
31. Interventions for patients with diabetic ketoacidosis include replacement of the electrolytes ____________ and ____________.
32. The goals of therapy in patients include volume resuscitation and lowering the blood sugar by ____________ mg/hour until a level of ____________ mg is eventually reached.
33. In hyperglycemic hyperosmolar nonketotic coma, ketosis does not occur because ____________.
34. The kidney can contribute to rising serum glucose levels in patients with hyperglycemic hyperosmolar nonketotic coma when ____________.

35. Hyperglycemic hyperosmolar nonketotic coma is associated with Type ____________ diabetes mellitus.
36. Compared with those with diabetic ketoacidosis, patients with hyperglycemic crisis have ____________ osmolality, ____________ serum pH, ____________ blood sugar, ____________ serum acetone, and ____________ fluid deficits.
37. Hypoglycemia stimulates the release of the hormones ____________ and ____________.
38. Two endocrine disorders that can lead to hypoglycemia are ____________ and ____________.
39. Signs of hypoglycemia include ____________ skin, neuromuscular ____________, and ____________ heart rate.

D. Summary of Patient Health Problems (*pages 629–672*)

After reading each disease, summarize the pathophysiology, nursing assessment data base, and nursing diagnoses. The certification examination holds you responsible for knowing the etiology and risk factors, the signs and symptoms, the collaborative diagnosis, and the management and treatment goals. Those preparing to take it should also summarize these areas. If they are not clearly covered in the Core, *a second resource may be necessary. The space allotted is purposefully limited to encourage concise descriptions of concepts and careful selection of key points. It is not as helpful to write the things you already know as it is to write those you need to study.*

1. Diabetes Insipidus

Pathophysiology	*Etiology/Risk Factors*	*Signs/Symptoms*

Collaborative Diagnosis	*Complications*	*Management/Goals*

2. Syndrome of Inappropriate Antidiuretic Hormone

Pathophysiology	*Etiology/Risk Factors*	*Signs/Symptoms*

Collaborative Diagnosis	*Complications*	*Management/Goals*

3. Hyperthyroid Crisis

Pathophysiology	*Etiology/Risk Factors*	*Signs/Symptoms*

Collaborative Diagnosis	*Complications*	*Management/Goals*

4. Myxedema Coma

Pathophysiology	*Etiology/Risk Factors*	*Signs/Symptoms*

Collaborative Diagnosis	*Complications*	*Management/Goals*

5. Acute Adrenal Insufficiency

Pathophysiology	*Etiology/Risk Factors*	*Signs/Symptoms*

Collaborative Diagnosis	*Complications*	*Management/Goals*

6. Diabetic Ketoacidosis

Pathophysiology	*Etiology/Risk Factors*	*Signs/Symptoms*

Collaborative Diagnosis	*Complications*	*Management/Goals*

7. Hyperglycemic Hyperosmolar Nonketotic Coma

Pathophysiology	*Etiology/Risk Factors*	*Signs/Symptoms*

Collaborative Diagnosis	*Complications*	*Management/Goals*

8. Hypoglycemic Episodes

Pathophysiology	*Etiology/Risk Factors*	*Signs/Symptoms*

Collaborative Diagnosis	*Complications*	*Management/Goals*

E. Application to Clinical Practice

Care for patients with endocrine disease. Relate the anatomy, physiology, assessment, and pathophysiology found in this section to their individual clinical pictures. Make note of those instances where they correlate and those where they deviate. Devise a care plan based on the data collected.

Answers to Endocrine System Exercises

A. Physiologic Anatomy

1. Bloodstream, receptor sites or substrates (*pages 609–610*)
2. Decrease (*page 610*)
3. a. Activation of cyclic AMP
   b. Activation of genes
   c. Activation of calcium channels or release of intracellular substrates (*pages 610–611*)
4. Decreased (*page 612*)
5. Sphenoid or sella turcica (*page 612*)
6. Vessels, nerves (*pages 612–614*)
7. Any three of these (*pages 614–615*):
   a. Growth hormone
   b. Adrenocorticotropic hormone
   c. Thyroid-stimulating hormone
   d. Gonadotropins
   e. Prolactin
8. a. Decrease
   b. Increase
   c. Decrease (*page 614*)
9. Stimulation, stimulation, inhibition (*page 614*)
10. a. Increase
    b. Decrease
    c. Increase (*page 615*)
11. Early morning (5 a.m. to 8 a.m.), late night (10 p.m. to 2 a.m.) (*page 615*)
12. a. Increase
    b. Decrease
    c. Decrease
    d. Increase
    e. Increase (*page 616*)
13. T_4, T_3 (*page 617*)
14. Glucocorticoids, propranolol, propylthiouracil (*page 617*)
15. Decrease (*page 617*)
16. a. Insulin
    b. Growth hormone
    c. Sex steroids
    d. Thyroid hormones (*page 617*)
17. Down, up (*pages 617–618*)
18. a. Increase
    b. Increase
    c. Decrease (*page 618*)
19. Increased, decreased, increased, decreased (*page 619*)
20. a. Decrease
    b. Decrease
    c. Increase
    d. Increase (*page 620*)
21. a. Increased
    b. Increased
    c. Decreased (*page 620*)
22. Stress, epinephrine (*page 620*)
23. Increase, decrease, decrease, increase, dilate (*pages 620–621*)
24. Beta, alpha, delta (*page 622*)
25. Increased, increased, increased (*page 622*)
26. Increased, increased, decreased (*page 622*)
27. Inhibits (*page 623*)
28. Any two of these (*pages 613–623*):
    a. Glucagon
    b. Epinephrine
    c. Cortisol
    d. Growth hormone
29. a. Anterior pituitary
    b. Adrenal cortex
    c. Thyroid
    d. Pancreas
    e. Adrenal medulla (*pages 613–623*)
30. a. Increased growth hormone
    b. Decreased adrenal corticoids or corticotropin
    c. Increased adrenal corticoids or corticotropin
    d. Decreased parathormone (*pages 613–623*)

B. Nursing Assessment Data Base

1. Any three of these (*page 623*):
   a. Trauma
   b. Necrosis
   c. Surgical interventions
   d. Infection
   e. Inflammation
   f. Autoimmune disorders
   g. Irradiation
   h. Neoplasm
   i. Chemotherapy
   j. Infiltrative disorders
   k. AIDS
2. Any three of these (*page 625*):
   a. Central nervous system depressants
   b. Chemotherapy
   c. Anti-inflammatory agents
   d. Ethanol
   e. Antidepressants
   f. Calcium channel blockers
   g. Thiazide diuretics
   h. Antibiotics
   i. Iodine-containing agents

C. Patient Health Problems

1. Decrease, increased (*pages 629–630*)
2. a. Central or neurogenic (decreased production)

   b. Nephrogenic (lack of renal response)
   c. Pharmacologic (inhibition of secretion or action)
   d. Undertreatment of known diabetes insipidus (*page 630*)
3. Increased, dry, increased, decreased, increased (*page 631*)
4. Decreased, decreased (*page 631*)
5. Intravenous fluids, vasopressin (*page 632*)
6. Increased, decreased (*page 634*)
7. a. Increase
   b. Increase
   c. Increase
   d. Increase
   e. Increase
   f. Decrease
   g. Decrease
   h. Decrease (*pages 630–634*)
8. a. Both
   b. Both
   c. Both
   d. Decrease
   e. Increase
   f. Increase
   g. Increase (*pages 630–634*)
9. Decreased, decreased, increased, increased (*pages 634–635*)
10. Hypertonic saline (*page 636*)
11. Brain, up (*page 636*)
12. Catecholamines, increased (*page 636*)
13. Increased, increased, moist or flushed, increased, increased (*pages 637–639*)
14. Increased, decreased, increased, increased (*pages 639–640*)
15. Propylthiouracil or methimazole, propranolol, glucocorticoids (*page 640*)
16. Iodine (*pages 637–640*)
17. Nonpitting, decreased, decreased, increased, decreased, retention (*pages 644–648*)
18. Decreased, decreased, decreased, increased, increased (*page 646*)
19. Up (*page 646*)
20. a. Increased
    b. Increased
    c. Increased
    d. Decreased
    e. Decreased (*pages 649–650*)
21. Autoimmune destruction or Addison's disease, corticosteroids (*page 651*)
22. Decreased, increased, decreased, increased (*pages 651–652*)
23. a. Primary
    b. Primary
    c. Primary
    d. Secondary
    e. Secondary (*pages 650–652*)
24. Decreased, increased, decreased (*page 652*)
25. Glucose, saline, hydrocortisone (*page 653*)
26. Any two of these (*pages 655–657*):
    a. Glucagon
    b. Cortisol
    c. Catecholamines
    d. Growth hormone
27. Increased, increased, increased, decreased, decreased (*pages 655–657*)
28. Any two of these (*page 656*):
    a. Thiazide diuretics
    b. Glucocorticoid
    c. Phenytoin
    d. Sympathomimetic agents
    e. Diazoxide
29. Down, up (*pages 655–657*)
30. Increased, dry or flushed, decreased, increased or Kussmaul, decreased (*pages 656–657*)
31. Any two of these (*page 657*):
    a. Sodium
    b. Potassium
    c. Phosphate
32. 75–100, 150–200 (*page 659*)
33. There is enough insulin to prevent it (*page 663*)
34. Dehydration or decreased glomerular filtration rates lead to decreased glucose excretion (*page 664*)
35. II (*page 664*)
36. Higher, higher, higher, lower, higher (*pages 663–666*)
37. Any two of these (*page 667*)
    a. Glucagon
    b. Epinephrine
    c. Cortisol
    d. Growth hormone
38. Adrenal insufficiency, panhypopituitarism (*page 668*)
39. Diaphoretic, weakness, increased (*page 669*)

D. Summary of Health Care Problems

Refer to the following pages in the Core Curriculum

1. Diabetes Insipidus (*pages 629–634*)
2. Syndrome of Inappropriate ADH (*pages 634–637*)
3. Hyperthyroid Crisis (*pages 637–644*)
4. Myxedema Coma (*pages 644–650*)
5. Acute Adrenal Insufficiency (*pages 650–654*)
6. Diabetic Ketoacidosis (*pages 655–662*)
7. Hyperglycemic Hyperosmolar Nonketotic Coma (*pages 662–667*)
8. Hypoglycemic Episodes (*pages 667–672*)

THE ENDOCRINE SYSTEM

Post Quiz

The following questions are designed to test understanding of some of the key points in the section. Select the one best answer for each. The correct answers are at the end of the test.

1. The pituitary gland is controlled by the
   a. thalamus
   b. hypothalamus
   c. adenohypophysis
   d. neurohypophysis
2. Inappropriately high antidiuretic hormone secretion would cause
   a. decreased urine formation
   b. increased urine formation
   c. hyperkalemia
   d. hypokalemia
3. A hormone that causes protein anabolism is
   a. cortisol
   b. growth hormone
   c. glucagon
   d. adrenocorticotropic hormone
4. Thyroxine
   a. stimulates the thyroid gland
   b. comes from the anterior pituitary
   c. increases metabolic activity
   d. causes hypocalcemia
5. Parathyroid hormone release
   a. increases calcium and decreases phosphorus
   b. increases phosphorus and decreases calcium
   c. is controlled by the hypothalamus
   d. is controlled by the anterior pituitary
6. Cortisol release results in
   a. increased sodium and water excretion
   b. inflammatory response
   c. decreased blood sugar
   d. protein catabolism
7. Stimulation of the adrenal medulla results in *all but* which of the following?
   a. pupillary constriction

b. peripheral vasoconstriction
c. decreased peristalsis
d. increased blood sugar

8. Which of the following is *least* likely to inhibit insulin?
a. epinephrine
b. antidiuretic hormone
c. somatostatin
d. glucagon

9. Glucagon
a. increases in response to hyperglycemia
b. is produced by the beta cells of the pancreas
c. causes glucogenolysis and gluconeogenesis
d. is the stored form of glucose

10. Insulin release causes
a. increased cellular glucose metabolism
b. increased blood sugar
c. decreased glycogen stores
d. increased serum osmolality

11. Consequences of severe hypothyroidism include
a. decreased cholesterol
b. pericardial effusions
c. dehydration
d. gastrointestinal hypermotility

12. Diabetes insipidus
a. may be a complication of head trauma
b. causes the urine specific gravity to increase
c. causes water retention
d. is the result of inappropriate antidiuretic syndrome

13. Signs of hyperthyroid crisis may include *all but* which of the following?
a. hyporeflexia
b. flushed diaphoretic skin
c. psychosis
d. exophthalmos

14. Acute adrenal insufficiency
a. is another name for Cushing's disease
b. causes hypotension, hyperkalemia, and fever
c. causes sodium and water retention
d. causes hyperglycemia

15. Which of the following statements about hyperglycemic nonketotic coma is true?
a. Acidosis is more severe than in diabetic ketoacidosis.
b. Hyperglycemia is less severe than in diabetic ketoacidosis.
c. Complications include shock, thrombosis, and electrolyte imbalance.
d. Hypo-osmolality is the key pathologic factor.

16. Typical signs of hypoglycemia include
a. warm dry skin
b. tremors and restlessness
c. bradycardia
d. anorexia

17. Which endocrine gland is located in the sella turcica?
a. hypothalamus
b. pituitary
c. parathyroid
d. thyroid gland

18. If a patient with adrenal insufficiency has an elevated plasma adrenocorticotropic hormone level,
    a. primary adrenal failure is present
    b. treatment should include adrenocorticotropic hormone
    c. hypopituitary function is the cause of the disease
    d. the skin will appear less pigmented than usual
19. The neurohypophysis secretes
    a. thyroid-stimulating hormone
    b. follicle-stimulating hormone
    c. luteinizing hormone
    d. antidiuretic hormone
20. Signs of diabetic ketoacidosis include
    a. Kussmaul respirations and abdominal pain
    b. metabolic alkalosis
    c. hyperphosphatemia
    d. hypercapnea
21. Drugs that can precipitate hypoglycemia include
    a. sulfonamides
    b. catecholamines
    c. propranolol
    d. corticosteroids
22. Signs of myxedema coma may include
    a. weight loss
    b. tachycardia and hypertension
    c. periorbital edema
    d. increased blood pressure
23. Cortisol levels are monitored and controlled by the
    a. anterior pituitary
    b. adrenal medulla
    c. hypothalamus
    d. adrenal cortex
24. One agent that may precipitate the symptoms of thyrotoxic crisis is
    a. propranolol
    b. iodine
    c. diazepam
    d. methimazole
25. Diabetes insipidus may be treated with
    a. concentrated saline solutions given intravenously
    b. mannitol or furosemide
    c. lithium and demeclocycline
    d. desmopressin or vasopressin
26. Patients with diabetes mellitus may require increased doses of insulin when they
    a. exercise more strenuously
    b. develop renal or liver failure
    c. lose weight
    d. are under stress
27. The pathophysiology of hyperthyroid crisis may include
    a. decreased catecholamine bonding sites
    b. catecholamines potentiating peripheral response to thyroid hormones
    c. decreased oxygen demand and consumption
    d. generalized decrease in intracellular chemical activities
28. The pathophysiology of diabetic ketoacidosis includes
    a. increased cellular glucose utilization

b. decreased gluconeogenesis
c. increased lipolysis
d. production of ketones from protein breakdown

29. In severe untreated diabetic ketoacidosis
    a. potassium shifts from the serum to the cells
    b. the total body potassium is depleted
    c. serum potassium does not rise unless the patient is in prerenal failure
    d. acidemia induces hypokalemia
30. Patients with syndrome of inappropriate antidiuretic hormone
    a. may benefit from acetaminophen administration
    b. may develop signs of hypervolemia
    c. are treated with hypotonic intravenous solutions
    d. have very low urine osmolalities

Answers to Endocrine Post Quiz

1. **b** (*page 614*)
2. **a** (*page 634*)
3. **b** (*page 614*)
4. **c** (*pages 616–617*)
5. **a** (*page 618*)
6. **d** (*page 619*)
7. **a** (*pages 620–621*)
8. **b** (*pages 615–622*)
9. **c** (*page 622*)
10. **a** (*pages 621–622*)
11. **b** (*pages 644–646*)
12. **a** (*pages 629–631*)
13. **a** (*pages 637–639*)
14. **b** (*pages 650–652*)
15. **c** (*pages 662–667*)
16. **b** (*pages 669–670*)
17. **b** (*page 612*)
18. **a** (*pages 650–653*)
19. **d** (*pages 615–616*)
20. **a** (*page 657*)
21. **a** (*pages 663, 668*)
22. **c** (*pages 644–645*)
23. **c** (*pages 614–615*)
24. **b** (*pages 637–639*)
25. **d** (*pages 631, 632*)
26. **d** (*pages 656, 668*)
27. **b** (*page 637*)
28. **c** (*pages 655–656*)
29. **b** (*page 655*)
30. **b** (*pages 634–635*)

These are primarily the comprehend or recall, and apply or analyze levels of questions. Examples of synthesis or evaluate questions can be found in the comprehensive examination at the end of the book on pages 278 to 293.

6

Hematology

SECTION-RELATED TIPS FOR THOSE STUDYING TO TAKE THE CERTIFICATION EXAMINATION

Like endocrinology, hematology represents only a small percentage of the examination questions and the questions asked tend to be easier than those on systems representing a higher proportion of the examination. Similarly, many basic nursing curricula do not emphasize content on immunology and hematology. Consequently, our knowledge of related physiologic principles is relatively weak. However, as you study this section, you will be impressed by how relevant these topics are to critical care nursing today. Patients often have local or systemic injury processes, undergo immunosuppression, risk nosocomial infections and septic syndromes, and may have both abnormal bleeding and clotting tendencies.

As with previous systems, reviewing a few terms, synonyms, and definitions is a helpful place to start. One way to do so is to study Figure 6–1 and Tables 6–1 and 6–2 in the *Study Guide* before reading this section of the *Core Curriculum*.

In addition, the following discussion will pull together factors covered in this and other sections of the *Core Curriculum* that highlight the need for monitoring critically ill patients for the common and important complications of immunosuppression, septic syndrome, bleeding tendencies, and thrombotic events. Both immunosuppression and sepsis are on the 1992 examination blueprint and are not addressed directly in the *Core Curriculum*. It would be best to come back and read this part after studying the hematology section.

Immunosuppression

The longer a patient remains critically ill, the more likely he is to become significantly immunosuppressed. Common contributing factors, with examples, are listed below.

Factors	*Examples*
Bypassed skin and irritated mucous membranes	Endotracheal tubes Vascular catheters Foley catheters Nasogastric tubes Surgical procedures Endoscopy
Altered protective mechanisms	Endotracheal tubes that bypass nares, prevent epiglottis function, and inhibit cough Drugs that raise gastric pH above bactericidal levels

Factors	*Examples*
Altered nutrition	Metabolic demands may be hard to estimate or meet Stressed patients tend to use nutrients given in catabolic or acute phase reactions rather than for anabolic needs. They may particularly have difficulty metabolizing glucose calories Poor gastrointestinal (GI) motility may preclude using the tract to feed, thereby potentially further insulting its mucosal integrity
Sequential infections	In response to the first infection, the patient's bone marrow is capable of dramatically increasing the white count using fully mature cells. It takes time to build to that point to respond to a second infection as effectively.
Drugs that can cause immunosuppression	Bone marrow depressing agents Steroids Antibiotics Anesthesia Analgesics
Aspects of history associated with higher risk	Very old or very young age Chronic disease or stress Splenectomy Infection with human immunodeficiency virus (HIV) Diabetes mellitus Renal failure Hepatic failure Malnutrition Prosthetic heart valves Small-bowel resection

Septic Syndrome

Local response to injury may become a generalized response, a septic syndrome. This is often triggered by a nidus of infection, but it may also be triggered by other sources of local injury such as trauma, burns, pancreatitis with peritoneal inflammation, areas of ischemic injury or necrosis, and breakdown products of hematomas and red blood cells, which inflame surrounding tissues.

The substrates released by activated white blood cells in these areas cause a systemic reaction seen clinically as fluctuations in blood pressure, temperature, heart rate, respiratory rate, and level of consciousness. The patient may have chills and/or warm dry skin and later may develop shock.

The activated substrates also cause other systemic reactions that are clinically more subtle. The pathophysiologic reactions and consequences of these septic episodes are as follows.

Reaction	*Consequences*
Inflammation	Systemic vasodilation ($\downarrow$ SvR) Generalized increased permeability (edema) White cells enter normal tissues Potential platelet aggregation and sequestration
Phagocytosis	Engulfing and degrading of normal tissues Release of killing by-products (H_2O_2, free radicals, acids, bleach), causing further tissue injury Increased oxygen metabolism by widespread phagocyte activity
Cardiovascular consequences	Cardiac output increases with high stroke volumes and low ejection fractions Flow is maldistributed with areas of hyperemia and of hypoperfusion
Endocrine consequences	Stress hormones increase the rate of glycogenolysis, gluconeogenesis, and insulin inhibition, all of which can raise the blood sugar and keep the patient catabolic
Multiple-organ failure	The end result of the above reactions may be sequential organ system failure, including Adult respiratory distress syndrome (ARDS) Renal failure Hepatic failure Disseminated intravascular coagulation (DIC) Decreased GI function Encephalopathy Septic shock

The most common cause of death in intensive care today is septic syndrome with multiple-organ failure. There were only 50,000 cases in 1980 and 400,000 cases in 1990. The management of septic syndrome includes:

Treating the cause
Supportive care of oxygenation, ventilation, perfusion, and nutrition
Prevention of secondary infections
Early recognition
Early interventions for the potential sequential organ failure

Pharmacologic interventions are directed at the substrates activated by injury. The local response to injury that becomes generalized and DIC are described in the hematology section of the *Core Curriculum*. Individual organ system failures are each addressed in their respective sections.

Bleeding Tendencies

The critically ill patient is also at high risk for bleeding diathesis. Several of the risk factors and related causes may be present in a single patient.

Risk Factors	*Causes*
Disrupted vessels	Surgery Trauma Invasive procedures

Risk Factors	*Causes*
Thrombocytopenia	Massive transfusion therapy (washout phenomenon)
	Massive fluid resuscitation (dilution phenomenon)
	Trauma, sepsis, DIC, and ARDS (sequestering phenomenon)
	Drug induced via:
	Heparin
	Antibiotics, sulfonamides
	Antiarrhythmics
	Digoxin
	Phenytoin
	Bone marrow depression
	Prosthetic devices (valves, intra-aortic balloon pump, extracorporeal circuits)
	Splenomegaly
Platelet inhibition	Drug induced via fairly strong inhibitors such as ASA, quinidine, or ETOH
	Drug induced via more moderate inhibitors such as β-blockers, calcium channel blockers, anesthesia, antibiotics, tricyclic antidepressants, and colloids (especially dextran)
	Disorders such as renal failure, liver failure, viral infections, and hypothermia
Interference with thrombin formation	Massive transfusion therapy (washout phenomenon)
	Diseases such as liver failure, DIC, and congenital factor deficits such as hemophilia and von Willebrand's disease
	Vitamin K deficiencies caused by malnutrition or antibiotic therapy that decreases the GI flora that produce vitamin K
	Decreased fibrinogen levels due to disease or drugs such as thrombolytic agents
Enhanced clot lysis	Thrombolytic agents such as streptokinase, urokinase, and tissue plasminogen activators

Two conditions appear repetitively on the list above and deserve further emphasis: liver failure and heparin. Liver failure can cause bleeding diatheses by several mechanisms. They include thrombocytopenia via platelet destruction or splenomegaly when portal hypertension is present, platelet inhibition, decreased clotting factor production, and inability to metabolize drugs and other hemostatic factors involved.

Heparin can potentially cause three hemostatic defects. One to two percent of patients develop significant bleeding, 1%–2% of patients develop significant thrombosis, and 30% develop thrombocytopenia. Bleeding and clotting phenomena should be watched for and platelet counts should be monitored. The platelet count may drop gradually over days in patients on therapeutic doses of heparin (pure thrombocytopenia). It can drop suddenly from even minimal doses of heparin in flush solutions in patients developing a risk of thrombotic episodes. This is called heparin-platelet thrombotic—thrombocytopenia—syndrome, or heparin-platelet aggregation syndrome, or white clot syndrome. Patients in whom the latter syndrome is suspected should have a heparin-platelet aggregation study done and all heparin discontinued if the study is positive.

Thrombotic Events

Several aspects of routine nursing care of the critically ill involve the prevention of thrombotic or embolic events. Again, many patients may have multiple risk factors.

Risk Factor	*Contributing Factors*
Stases or reduced blood flow rates	Decreased cardiac output
	Heart failure
	Vasoconstriction
	Vascular obstruction by external compression
	Increased blood viscosity via polycythemia or hyperproteinemia
Vessel damage	Preexisting atherosclerosis
	Trauma or surgery
	Intravascular procedures, studies, or lines
	Irritation by drugs, inflammatory processes, or septic syndrome
Hypercoagulability	Heparin-platelet aggregation syndrome
	Stress
	Catecholamines
	Third trimester pregnancy
	Drugs such as desmopressin or vasopressin
	Red blood cell or platelet disorders
	Smoking
	Immediately postoperative splenectomy due to thrombocytosis

The treatment of thrombotic events depends on the site but may include treatment of the cause, prevention of further clotting by nursing measures and anticoagulation, and lysis of the clot with thrombolytic agents.

Please see the instructions at the beginning of the book for important general suggestions that are relevant to the bulk of the *Core Curriculum* content. They apply to this section as well as all of the others.

FIGURES AND TABLES

Refer to these figures and tables while reading the hematology section of the Core Curriculum.

Figure 6–1. Fully differentiated blood cells. *Synonyms* are indicated in parenthesis (*pages 675–685*).

Red Blood Cells
(Erythrocytes)

Platelets
(Thrombocytes)

Granular Leukocytes
(Granulocytes, Myeloid Series)

Neutrophils
(PMNs, Polys, Segs)

Eosinophils

Basophils
(Mast Cells)

Nongranular Leukocytes

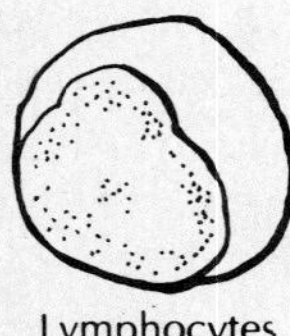

Lymphocytes

B cells — Humoral Immunity
Can become plasma cells

T cells — Cellular Immunity

Null Cells — Natural killer cells

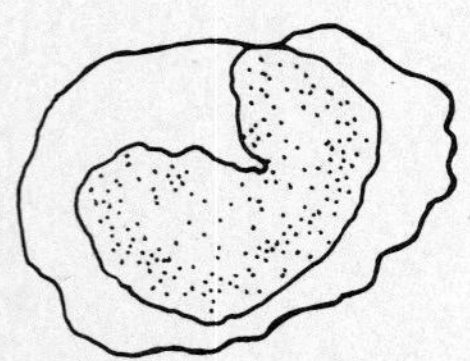

Mononuclear Phagocytes
(Monocytes)

Develop into tissue macrophages

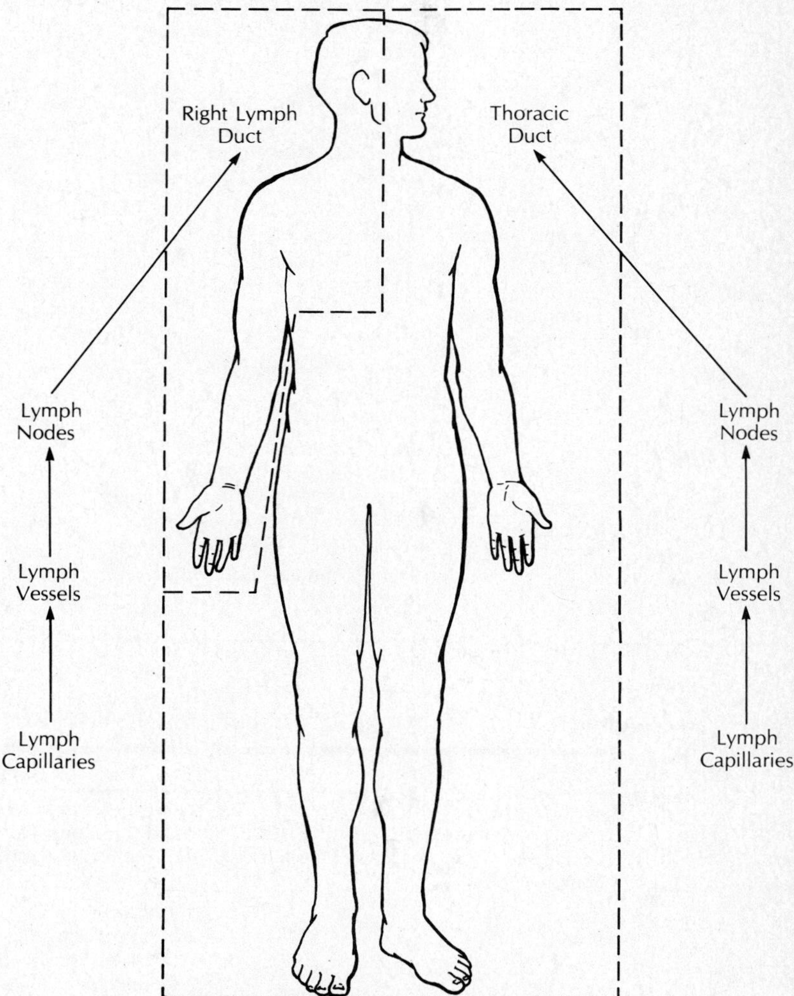

Figure 6–2. Anatomy and circulation of the lymphatic system. Broken line indicates portions of the body drained by the two major lymph ducts—the right lymphatic above and the thoracic duct below. Node Distribution: Head and Neck: Superficial and Deep. Extremities: All Superficial. Mediastinum: All Deep. Abdomen: Superficial and Deep (*pages 677–678*).

Table 6–1. COMPARISON OF THE FORMATION, FUNCTION, AND NUMBERS OF CIRCULATING BLOOD CELLS (*pages 678–684, 696–697*)

Cell	Where Formed (Younger Forms)	Functions	Amount	
Erythrocyte	Bone marrow (reticulocytes)	Transport O_2 Acid-base balance	4.4–5.9 million/μL in men 3.8–5.2 million/μL in women	
Platelet	Bone marrow	Hemostasis	150,000–400,000/μL	
Granulocytes	Bone marrow		60%–70% of WBCs	
1. Neutrophils	(bands, stabs)	Phagocytosis	39%–79% (1500–7500/μL)	Breakdown of granulocytes
2. Eosinophils		Detoxification of allergies Phagocytosis Antiparasites Anaphylaxis	0%–5% (0–500/μL)	
3. Basophils		Increased in allergy, hypersensitivity reactions, chronic inflammation Secrete heparin and histamine	0–2% (0–200/μL)	
Monocytes	Bone marrow, lymph nodes, spleen	Phagocytosis Especially potent if develop into macrophages	3–8% of WBCs (0–1000/μL)	
Lymphocytes	Bone marrow, lymph nodes, spleen		10–40% of WBCs (1000–4500/μL)	
1. T Cells		Produced in response to antigens Cellular immunity	65–85%	Breakdown of lymphocytes
2. B Cells		Produce antibodies (immunoglobulins) Humoral immunity Sensitized, productive B cells are called plasma cells	↓ 35%	
3. Null Cells		Undifferentiated killer cells Important in defense against cancer	↓ 10%	

Table 6–2. HEMATOLOGIC FUNCTION OF ORGANS (*pages 675–693*)

Organ	Functions
Bone Marrow (productive marrow in vertebrae, skull, chest cage, ilium, and proximal long bones)	Only site for production of erythrocytes, granulocytes, and thrombocytes One site for production of lymphocytes and monocytes
Lymphatic System	
Lymph Fluid	High in proteins, fats, enzymes, and antibodies Low in red blood cells, platelets, and fibrinogen Contains granulocytes, macrophages, and lymphocytes
Lymph Nodes	Filter bacteria and foreign material Produce monocytes and lymphocytes
Thymus	Controls cellular immunity and T-cell function
Spleen	
White Pulp	Primarily involved in B-cell function and antibody production
Red Pulp	Red blood cell reservoir (1%–2% red cell mass) Red blood cells culled (hemolyzed) Red blood cells pitted (unwanted parts excised) Platelet reservoir (33% platelet mass) Platelet production and destruction regulated
Liver	Utilizes bilirubin from hemolysis for bile production Phagocytoses toxic substances via fixed macrophages Produces plasma clotting factors and antithrombins

Table 6–3. LIFE CYCLES OF THE BLOOD CELLS (*pages 678–690*)

Erythrocytes	Live about 120 days Destroyed in bone marrow, liver, spleen if too old, damaged, or abnormal By-products of destruction include iron and bilirubin
Granulocytes	Stored in bone marrow (10 × blood level) Circulating half-life is a matter of hours Circulating mass is 50% free, 50% marginated Leave bloodstream into injured or inflamed tissue Lost via use in phagocytosis or in secretions, excretions
Monocytes	Circulating half-life is a matter of hours Most become tissue macrophages: Fixed = bone marrow, Kupffer cells, lung, lymph, spleen Free = inflammation, certain fluids Can live months to years in tissues
Lymphocytes	Circulate continuously between bloodstream and lymph system May live 100–300 days
Platelets	Live about 9–12 days

Table 6–4. FUNCTIONS OF THE T CELL LYMPHOCYTE IN CELLULAR IMMUNITY (*pages 683–684*)

General Role	Trained by thymus to recognize self vs. non-self
Functional Subtypes	Cytotoxic killer T cells Helper and suppressor T cells that mediate immune response Memory T lymphocytes
Processes Involved	Antigen attracts T cells that surround it and become sensitized T cells secrete lymphokines that: (1) Attract macrophages and neutrophils (2) Sensitize more T cells (3) Stimulate B cells (Interleukin-2) (4) Help destroy antigens (lymphotoxin) (5) Inhibit viral growth (Interferon)
Clinical Manifestations	Immunity to intracellular pathogens (viruses, protozoa, fungi) Immune surveillance and tumor immunity Cutaneous delayed hypersensitivity and contact allergy Allograft rejection, graft-versus-host reactions Autoimmune diseases if lack of suppressor T cells

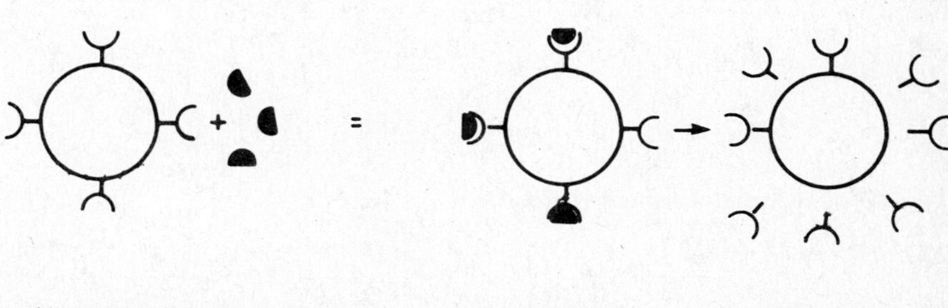

Figure 6–3. The process of activating B cells to produce antibodies (*pages 684–685*).

Table 6–5. CHARACTERISTICS OF THE FIVE TYPES OF IMMUNOGLOBULINS (Ig's) (*page 685*)

Immunoglobulin (% Circulating Antibodies)	Characteristics
IgG (75%)	Primarily antibacterial (some antiviral) Anamestic responses (involve immunologic memory) Neonatal protection
IgA (15%)	Form found in mucous membranes more abundant and more important than form found in serum Protects against antigen adherence and invasion
IgM (10%)	Primarily antibacterial (some antiviral) First response to antigen
IgD (1%)	Activates B cells to plasma cells
IgE (.002%)	Causes symptoms of allergic reaction by attaching to and stimulating cells that secrete the responsible chemicals

Table 6–6. ANTIGENS AND ANTIBODIES PRESENT IN VARIOUS BLOOD GROUPS (*pages 685–686*)

Blood Group	Antigens	Antibodies
OO (universal donor)	None	Both Anti-A and Anti-B
AA, AO	A	Anti-B
BB, BO	B	Anti-A
AB (universal recipient)	A and B	None
RH-D (primary RH-Hr type)	+ = D present − = D absent	No Anti-D Anti-D when sensitized

Table 6–7. THE COMPLEMENT SYSTEM (*pages 687–688*)

Components	Effects
Group of serum proteins (C1 to C9) stimulated most rapidly by antigen-antibody reaction.	Enhance many responses by: facilitating opsonization and phagocytosis Lysing membranes of invaders Agglutinizing organisms Neutralizing viruses Activating basophils Facilitating inflammation

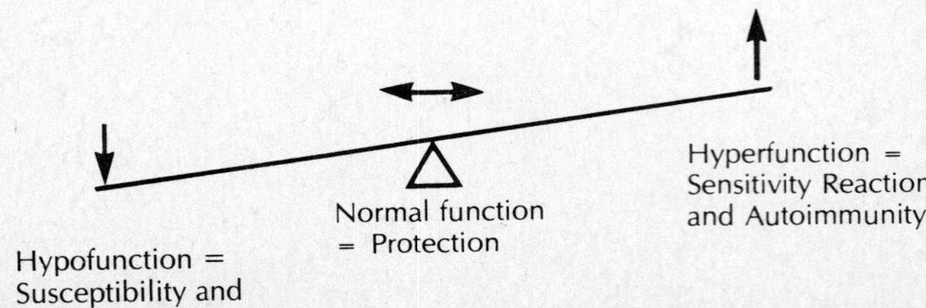

Figure 6–4. Spectrum of immune system function (*pages 685–688*).

Table 6–8. CHARACTERISTICS OF TYPES OF SENSITIVITY REACTIONS (*page 688*)

Type	Characteristics
Immediate (seconds to minutes)	
Cytotoxic	B cells produce antibody and activate complement against foreign or unrecognized cell (transfusion reaction)
Anaphylactic	Antigen-antibody reaction triggers chemicals that primarily affect smooth muscle and vessels
Subacute (minutes to hours)	Antigen-antibody complex, complement, and neutrophils overreact
Arthus	Local skin reaction
Serum Sickness	Systemic reaction
Delayed Hypersensitivity (hours to days)	T-cell mediated reactions such as tuberculin tests and graft rejection

Table 6–9. THE PROCESS OF INFLAMMATION (*pages 688, 689*)

Stage	Reaction	Factors Involved
Vascular Response	Vasodilation Increased vessel permeability Leukocytes enter inflamed area Fluid shifts into extravascular space	Histamine Serotonin Bradykinin
Cellular Response	Local blood flow increases and becomes viscoid	
	Leukocytes marginate and emigrate through vessel toward inflamed tissue	Chemotactic or attracting chemicals
	Phagocytosis occurs by neutrophils and macrophages (includes recognition, engulfment, and killing)	Produce bactericidal chemicals like H_2O_2 and free radicals Process enhanced if local environment is aerobic
	Rest of immune response is triggered (antigen presented to lymphocytes)	
	Inflammation may be isolated into abscess	
Bone Marrow Response	White cells are released into the circulation	
Wound Healing	Normal cells are regenerated to replace damaged cells Scar formation occurs if connective tissue replaces normal cell	

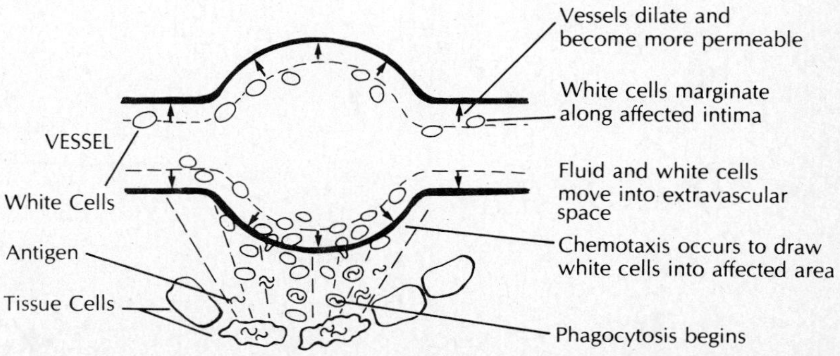

Figure 6–5. Major early stages of inflammation (*pages 688–689*).

Table 6–10. THE NORMAL RESPONSE TO INJURY, IRRITATION OR INFECTION INVOLVES A COMPLEX REACTION OF THE FOLLOWING INTERACTING AND OVERLAPPING 4 COMPONENTS (*pages 680–689*)

Reaction	Description
Phagocytosis	Antigens, injured cells, and pathogens are recognized, engulfed, killed, and degraded by the two main phagocytes: neutrophils and macrophages
Lymphocyte Reaction	T cells regulate the cellular aspects of immunity by helping and then suppressing the aggregation of white cells. B cells regulate the humoral response to immunity, primarily by the synthesis of antibodies or immunoglobulins
Complement Activity	When activated, these proteins initiate enzyme reactions that lead to antigen destruction and enhance the other three components in this table
Inflammation	This local reaction is mediated by the vessel endothelium, which allows the above components to concentrate in injured tissues and phagocytosis to occur

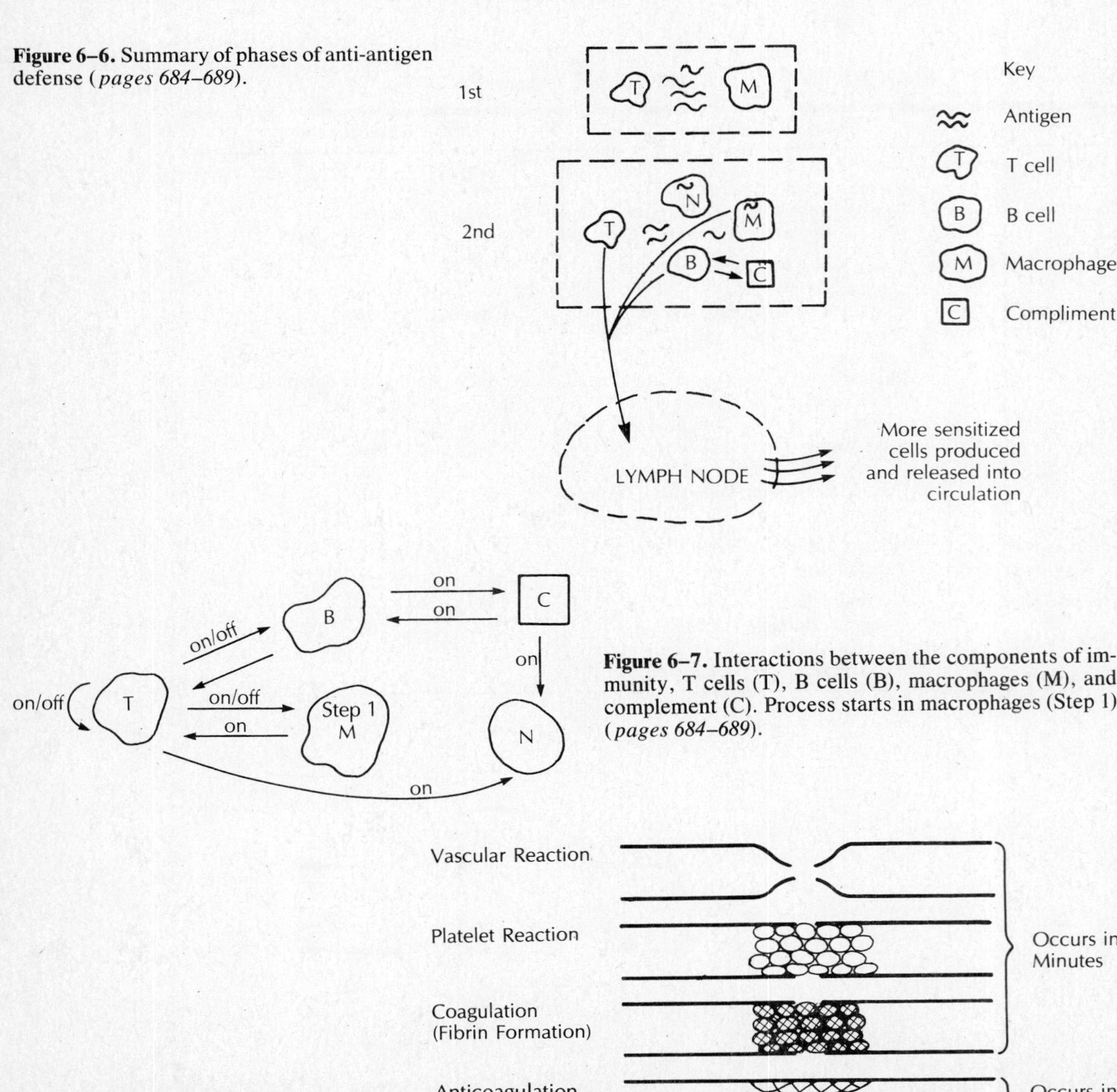

Figure 6–6. Summary of phases of anti-antigen defense (*pages 684–689*).

Figure 6–7. Interactions between the components of immunity, T cells (T), B cells (B), macrophages (M), and complement (C). Process starts in macrophages (Step 1) (*pages 684–689*).

Figure 6–8. Major mechanisms involved in hemostasis (*pages 689–693*).

Figure 6–9. Intrinsic and extrinsic pathways of fibrin formation (*pages 691–692*).

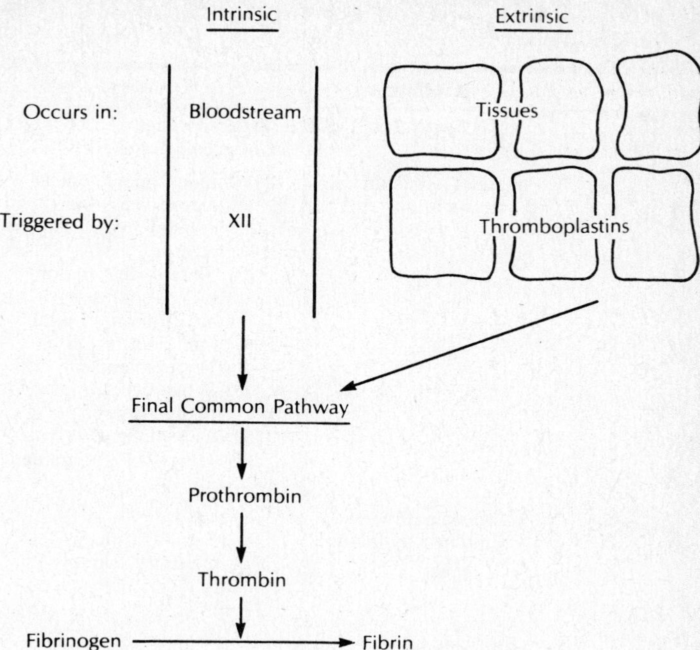

Table 6–11. CHARACTERTISTICS OF MAJOR PHASES OF HEMOSTASIS (*pages 689–693*)

Phase	Mechanism	Disorders	Laboratory Evaluation
Vascular	Vasoconstriction	Vessel damage Collagen defects	
Platelet	Platelet adhesion and aggregation	Thrombocytopenia due to (1) Depressed bone marrow by disease or drugs (2) Platelet destruction by antibodies, autoimmunity, viral infection, or DIC (3) Hypersplenism (4) Sequestering in injured areas	Low platelet count
		Decreased platelet activity (ETOH, ASA, quinidine)	Poor platelet clot retraction or activity tests
Coagulation	Intrinsic pathway Initiated by factor XII	Liver disorders Congenital disorders Multiple transfusions Dietary deficiencies (vitamin K)	PTT—intrinsic and common pathways
	Extrinsic pathway Initiated by thromboplastins		PT—extrinsic and common pathways
	Common pathway Initiated by intrinsic or extrinsic pathway		TT—both pathways
Anticoagulation	Fibrinolysis by plasmin FSPs (or FDPs) and antithrombins help prevent clot from reforming		FSPs (FDPs) titers D-Dimer levels (newer more sensitive test) Antithrombin levels

PTT = partial thromboplastin time; PT = prothrombin time; TT = thrombin time; FSP = fibrin split products; FDP = fibrin-degradation products

Table 6–12. FACTORS COVERED IN THE PHYSIOLOGIC ANATOMY SECTION THAT HAVE CLINICAL APPLICATIONS WORTH EMPHASIZING (*pages 675–693*)

Factor	Clinical Application	Page
Bone Marrow	Because adults have 30–50 cc of bone marrow per kilogram (2100–3500 cc in the 70 kg person), a few hundred cc's of marrow can be donated when necessary with little significant risk to the donor.	675
Lymph Fluid	Although the normal total lymph flow through the lymph system is only 2 cc/min, local obstruction to flow can result in distal edema.	677
Spleen	Because the spleen is an important site of antibody synthesis, patients undergoing a splenectomy have a significantly higher risk of becoming septic or succumbing to even routine infections and need to be instructed on how to reduce the risk postdischarge.	678
RBC Structure	Because the RBC has a relatively simple structure, work is ongoing in manufacturing hemoglobin capable of increasing oxygen-carrying capacity.	679
Hemolysis	The breakdown products of RBCs (iron and bilirubin) are very irritating to surrounding tissue and may trigger inflammation or sepsis. The removal of extravascular hemeffusions or hematomas may reduce this risk.	680
Neutrophils' Role	Gallium is an isotope that is taken up by neutrophils. Since they only concentrate extravascularly in inflamed, injured, or infected tissues, gallium scans can be useful in identifying these areas.	680
Macrophages' Role	Both neutrophils and macrophages are phagocytes. The neutrophils are the abundant circulating mobile pool. The macrophages are part of the primary line of defense in residence in normal body tissue. They are more powerful but less abundant, and they play a regulating role with lymphocytes.	681–682
Lymphocytes	Lymphocytes are the only white blood cells not capable of phagocytosis. Instead, they produce important substances required for immunity and regulate this response. It consists of cellular and humoral components.	683
T-Cell Lymphocytes	The T cell regulates the cells you need on site for immunity. This is the reason it is listed as a component of "cellular" immunity. Helper T cells trigger the immune response. The suppressor T cells inhibit it. Decreased helper T-cell activity is one cause of immunosuppression. Decreased suppressor T-cell activity is one cause of autoimmunity.	684
B-Cell Lymphocytes	B cells produce and release humors or substances that are important for immunity, primarily antibodies. Antigen-specific B cells may produce antibodies on site or in the lymph nodes and spleen. The antibodies then circulate to interact with these antigens wherever they are found. They also activate a second major humor involved in immunity, the complement.	684–685, 687
Acquired Immunity	Since both T cells and B cells develop memory or increased sensitivity to antigens after an initial exposure, subsequent exposures trigger an enhanced response and can be more quickly controlled. This is an important aspect of acquired immunity to commonly encountered antigens.	684–685
ABO Typing	This is one example of tissue typing to determine donor-recipient compatibility. There are about 100 known human tissue antigens found on cell membranes. Each of us is born with 10 of these that mark our cells as "self." The other 90 are "nonself" and are recognized as foreign. The three human tissue antigens most important to blood cell compatibility are A, B, and Rh D.	685–686

Table continued on following page

Table 6–12 FACTORS COVERED IN THE PHYSIOLOGIC ANATOMY SECTION THAT HAVE CLINICAL APPLICATIONS WORTH EMPHASIZING (*pages 675–693*) *Continued*

Factor	Clinical Application	Page
Inflammation	The septic syndrome involves an inappropriate systemic vascular inflammation rather than an appropriate local one. Consequences include: (1) Systemic vasodilation (2) Widespread tissue edema (3) Activation of phagocytosis in normal tissue (4) Depletion of bone marrow stores of white cells (5) Continued activation of inflammation that postpones healing	688–689
Killing and Degradation	The septic syndrome also involves activation of widespread phagocytosis. Consequences include: (1) Increased oxygen combustion and consumption by numerous phagocytes (2) Production and release of noxious oxygen by-products such as lactic acid, hydrogen peroxide, and free radicals into normal tissue	689
Hemostatic Mechanisms	The normal hemostatic mechanism is delicately balanced so that clots form only where risks of extravasation occur and stay until enough healing has occurred. Otherwise, blood is allowed to flow unimpeded. Critically ill patients may have alterations in one or all of the four normal components. The four components are the (1) Vascular reaction—vasoconstriction and platelet attraction (2) Platelet reaction—soft plug formation (3) Plasma clotting factors—fibrin formation (4) Anticoagulation—prevents clot reformation during fibrinolysis and healing, and maintains blood in a fluid state	689–693
Thrombocytopenia	Thrombocytopenia is common in critical care and is often multifactorial. Although the risk of spontaneous bleeding occurs at counts below 30,000, acutely ill patients may also be receiving drugs that decrease activity of the platelets present and may have decreased clotting factors. The combination of factors may contribute to a risk of bleeding at higher platelet counts.	691
Anticoagulants	These drugs are commonly used in critically ill patients to prevent thrombotic or emboli episodes. The agents and mechanisms of action are: (1) Aspirin—inhibits platelet activity (2) Coumadin—inhibits the extrinsic pathway to fibrin formation (3) Heparin—inhibits the intrinsic pathway by potentiating antithrombin	689–692
Fibrinolytic Agents	There are drugs that can be used to lyse clots immediately rather than allowing the normal fibrinolytic mechanisms to progress over days when there is danger of loss of viable tissue and no contraindications to their use. Although they differ in onset, half-life, cost, and subset efficacy, they all act primarily by activating plasminogen into plasmin, a substance that dissolves clots. Extra activated plasmin has a high protein affinity and may bind to fibrinogen and other circulating proteins.	692
Endogenous Anticoagulants	Naturally occurring anticoagulants include antithrombin produced by the liver, heparin produced by mast cells or basophils, and fibrin degradation products that locally prevent clot reformation during fibrinolysis.	692–693

HEMATOLOGY

Exercises

After reading the hematology section of the Core Curriculum, *fill in the blanks in the following statements. It can be done one topic at a time or all at once. The answers are at the end of the exercises.*

A. Physiologic Anatomy (*pages 675–693*)

1. A 50-kg adult has approximately ______________cc of bone marrow, ______________% of which is active in blood cell production.
2. Indicate whether the following sites contain active marrow in adults (yes or no):
   a. Shaft of the femur ______________
   b. Shaft of the humerus ______________
   c. Clavicle ______________
   d. Sternum ______________
   e. Ilium ______________
3. The ______________ is the only organ capable of producing all five types of blood cells.
4. State whether the following are found in relatively low or high amounts in lymph fluid.
   a. Erythrocytes ______________
   b. Granulocytes ______________
   c. Antibodies ______________
   d. Enzymes ______________
5. Of the two lymph ducts, the ______________ is the larger, whereas the ______________ drains primarily the right upper aspects of the body.
6. Indicate whether the lymph nodes are deep, superficial, or both, in each of the following areas:
   a. Head and neck ______________
   b. Mediastinum ______________
   c. Extremities ______________
   d. Abdomen ______________
7. The ______________ controls T-cell function and is relatively ______________ in size in the adult than in the adolescent.
8. The white pulp of the spleen contains white blood cells producing ______________ for humoral immunity.
9. The immediate precursors to erythrocytes are ______________, which normally account for ______________ % of the circulating pool.
10. The production rate of blood cells is controlled by the hormone ______________ and primarily requires energy and the nutrients ______________, ______________, and ______________.
11. Hemolysis occurs primarily in the ______________, ______________, and ______________.
12. Red blood cells are hemolyzed when they are about ______________ days old or earlier if they are ______________.

13. By-products of hemolysis include ______________________ and ______________________.
14. The ______________________ is the most abundant circulating white blood cell and there is about ______________________ times more inside than there is outside the bone marrow.
15. Name the blood cell(s) primarily involved in each of the following:
    a. Oxygen transport ______________________
    b. Acid-base balance ______________________
    c. Phagocytosis ______________________
    d. Heparin and histamine secretion ______________________
    e. Detoxification of allergic responses ______________________
16. The immediate precursor to a mature segmented neutrophil is a ______________________.
17. Most ______________________ become one of two types of macrophages, ______________________ or ______________________.
18. Corticosteroids can suppress the activity of the following white blood cell types:
    a. ______________________
    b. ______________________
    c. ______________________
19. Indicate whether the following are characteristics of B-cell or T-cell lymphocytes:
    a. Synthesize antibodies ______________________
    b. Differentiated by the bone marrow ______________________
    c. Most abundant lymphocytes ______________________
    d. Mediate cellular immunity ______________________
    e. Active in tumor immunity ______________________
    f. Become plasma cells ______________________
    g. Control intracellular pathogens ______________________
    h. Mediate humoral immunity ______________________
20. Two examples of lymphokines produced by T cells include ______________________, which affects other lymphocytes, and ______________________, which limits the growth of viruses.
21. Name the immunoglobulin described by the following phrases:
    a. Most abundant circulating antibody ______________________
    b. Mediates allergic reactions ______________________
    c. Primarily present in secretions ______________________
    d. Develops B cells into plasma cells ______________________
22. Indicate which major antigens are present and which antibodies are produced in patients with the following blood types:

	Antigens	*Antibodies*
a. A	______________________	______________________
b. O	______________________	______________________
c. AB	______________________	______________________

23. When a patient is positive for cold agglutins, transfusion reactions are less likely if the blood is ______________________ prior to administration.
24. Immunity is mediated through various white blood cells and the ______________________ system, a group of serum proteins.
25. The inflammatory response involves vessel ______________________ and ______________________ permeability, leukocyte attraction into the area via a process called ______________________, and antigen engulfment, killing, and degradation or ______________________.

26. The most oxygen- or energy-dependent step of inflammation and phagocytosis is ______________________.
27. The four steps in the normal hemostatic mechanisms are as follows:
    a. ______________________
    b. ______________________
    c. ______________________
    d. ______________________
28. The precursor of the thrombocyte in the bone marrow is the ______________________.
29. Platelets are regulated primarily by the ______________________, which sequesters ______________________ of the total platelet mass.
30. When activated by injured vessels, platelets first aggregate and then release substances that enhance ______________________ and ______________________ formation.
31. Indicate whether or not each of the following is more likely to be associated with thrombocytosis, thrombocytopenia, or inhibition of platelet activity.
    a. Early postsplenectomy ______________________
    b. ETOH ______________________
    c. ASA ______________________
    d. DIC ______________________
    e. Viral disease ______________________
32. Patients are at risk of spontaneous hemorrhage when the platelet count drops below ______________________.
33. Clotting factors that require vitamin K for their synthesis by the ______________________ are factors ______________________, ______________________, ______________________, and ______________________.
34. The ______________________ clotting pathway is activated by factor XII and the ______________________ pathway by tissue thromboplastin.
35. The final step in the hemostasis process is the formation of ______________________, which then converts fibrinogen into ______________________.
36. Anticoagulation factors include ______________________ which lyses fibrin clots, ______________________ which are breakdown products of fibrin, and ______________________ which are synthesized by the liver.

B. Nursing Assessment Data Base and Commonly Encountered Nursing Diagnoses (*pages 692–715*)

1. Indicate whether the following are high, low, or normal.
    a. Erythrocyte count = $3.0 \times 10^6/\mu L$ ______________________
    b. Leukocyte count = $15{,}000/\mu L$ ______________________
    c. Platelet count = $50{,}000/\mu L$ ______________________
    d. Partial thromboplastin time = 40 seconds ______________________
    e. Fibrinogen level = 100 mg/dL ______________________
2. In patients with leukopenia, ______________________ may be the most reliable sign of infection.
3. Indicate whether the following contain coagulation factors and/or platelets.
    a. Packed red blood cells ______________________

b. Plasmanate ____________________
c. Fresh frozen plasma ____________________

4. Indicate the primary expected posttransfusion changes in laboratory values for each of the following.
a. 1 unit whole blood ____________________
b. 1 unit packed red blood cells ____________________
c. 1 unit platelets ____________________

5. List an example of a major blood product that can achieve the following effects.
a. Increased oxygen transport with the smallest increase in blood volume ____________________
b. Increased fibrinogen, factor VIII, and factor XIII ____________________
c. Plasma volume expansion without increased clotting factors ____________________

6. The most common type of tranfusion reaction is a ____________________ reaction.

C. Patient Health Problems (*pages 715–747*)

1. Sickle cell disease is the inheritance from ____________________ of an abnormal type hemoglobin that causes red blood cells to assume a crescent shape whenever they become ____________________.
2. The main pathologic consequences of the sickling of red blood cells are ____________________ and ____________________.
3. Hemoglobin electrophoresis can be used to distinguish sickle cell disease in which ____________________ % is hemoglobin S, and sickle cell trait in which about ____________________ is hemoglobin S.
4. List four compensatory responses to anemia.
a. ____________________
b. ____________________
c. ____________________
d. ____________________
5. The disease associated with a primary increase in red blood cells with associated elevation of platelets and white blood cells is ____________________.
6. Indicate whether neutrophils are more likely to increase or decrease in the following:
a. *Pneumocystis carinii* ____________________
b. Ionizing radiation ____________________
c. Aplastic anemia ____________________
d. Hemodialysis ____________________
7. Neutropenia is defined as an absolute neutrophil count below ____________________ but a count below ____________________ carries a severe threat of infection.
8. Complications of leukemia include ____________________ hemoglobin, and formation of ____________________ in various organs.
9. Indicate which type of leukemia is most commonly associated with each of the following:
a. Increased immature lymphocytes ____________________
b. Increased granulocyte precursors ____________________
c. Abnormal B cells ____________________
d. Presence of Philadelphia chromosome ____________________
10. Multiple myeloma is the production of ____________________ by plasma cells that can lead to the lytic lesions of ____________________

__________, damage to the __________________ and ______ ______________ serum calcium.

11. The laboratory manifestations of multiple myeloma can include __________________ hemoglobin, __________________ serum calcium, and the presence of __________________ protein in the urine.
12. Lymphomas are classified into Hodgkin's or non-Hodgkin's by the presence or absence of __________________, into stage A or B by the presence or absence of __________________, and into level of involvement I through IV by the location of involved __________ __________.
13. Indicate whether or not the following are typical clinical manifestations of lymphomas:
    a. Weight gain __________________
    b. Painful or tender lymph nodes __________________
    c. Cough or dyspnea __________________
    d. Pruritus __________________
    e. Night sweats __________________
14. Anaphylaxis is the result of an __________________-__________________ reaction that stimulates the release of mediating substances like __________________.
15. The shock that results from anaphylaxis is due to __________ __________ and __________________.
16. Human immunodeficiency virus (HIV) is a viral infection of the __________________ cells of the immune system with an incubation period of __________________ to __________________.
17. Describe the states of the Walter-Reed Classifications of HIV (0 through 6)
    a. 0 __________________
    b. 1 __________________
    c. 2 __________________
    d. 3 __________________
    e. 4 __________________
    f. 5 __________________
    g. 6 __________________
18. The condition in which the person harbors the HIV but has not developed AIDS is called __________________.
19. The pathophysiology of disseminated intravascular coagulation involves __________________ production of thrombin, __________ __________ levels of antithrombin, and __________________ availability of clotting factors.
20. The laboratory manifestations of disseminated intravascular coagulation involve __________________ prothrombin time, __________ __________ fibrinogen level, __________________ fibrin split products, and __________________ protamine sulfate test.
21. Indicate which hereditary bleeding disorder(s) is (are) associated with these characteristics:
    a. Transmitted by females to male offspring __________________
    b. Platelet dysfunction and decreased factor VIII __________ __________
    c. Decreased factor VIII alone __________________
    d. Decreased factor IX alone __________________
22. Hemophilia A and B can be followed by specific factor assay or the __________________ time.

D. Summary of Patient Health Problems (*pages 715–742*)

After reading each disease, summarize the pathophysiology, nursing assessment data base, and nursing diagnoses. Since the certification examination holds you responsible for knowing the etiology and risk factors, the signs and symptoms, the collaborative diagnosis, and the management and treatment goals, those preparing to take it should also summarize these areas. If they are not clearly covered in the Core, *a second resource may be necessary. The space allotted is purposefully limited to encourage concise descriptions of concepts and careful selection of key points. It is not as helpful to write the things you already know as it is to write those you need to study.*

1. Sickle Cell Disease

Pathophysiology	*Etiology/Risk Factors*	*Signs/Symptoms*

Collaborative Diagnosis	*Complications*	*Management/Goals*

2. Anemias

Pathophysiology	*Etiology/Risk Factors*	*Signs/Symptoms*

Collaborative Diagnosis	*Complications*	*Management/Goals*

3. Polycythemia

Pathophysiology	*Etiology/Risk Factors*	*Signs/Symptoms*

Collaborative Diagnosis	*Complications*	*Management/Goals*

4. Neutropenia

Pathophysiology	*Etiology/Risk Factors*	*Signs/Symptoms*

Collaborative Diagnosis	*Complications*	*Management/Goals*

5. Leukemia

Pathophysiology	*Etiology/Risk Factors*	*Signs/Symptoms*

Collaborative Diagnosis	*Complications*	*Management/Goals*

6. Acute Lymphoblastic Leukemia

Pathophysiology	*Etiology/Risk Factors*	*Signs/Symptoms*

Collaborative Diagnosis	*Complications*	*Management/Goals*

7. Acute Nonlymphoblastic Leukemia

Pathophysiology	*Etiology/Risk Factors*	*Signs/Symptoms*

Collaborative Diagnosis	*Complications*	*Management/Goals*

8. Chronic Lymphocytic Leukemia

Pathophysiology	*Etiology/Risk Factors*	*Signs/Symptoms*

Collaborative Diagnosis	*Complications*	*Management/Goals*

9. Chronic Myeloid Leukemia

Pathophysiology	*Etiology/Risk Factors*	*Signs/Symptoms*

Collaborative Diagnosis	*Complications*	*Management/Goals*

10. Multiple Myeloma

Pathophysiology	*Etiology/Risk Factors*	*Signs/Symptoms*

Collaborative Diagnosis	*Complications*	*Management/Goals*

11. Lymphomas

Pathophysiology	*Etiology/Risk Factors*	*Signs/Symptoms*

Collaborative Diagnosis	*Complications*	*Management/Goals*

12. Anaphylaxis

Pathophysiology	*Etiology/Risk Factors*	*Signs/Symptoms*

Collaborative Diagnosis	*Complications*	*Management/Goals*

13. Human Immunodeficiency Virus

Pathophysiology	*Etiology/Risk Factors*	*Signs/Symptoms*

Collaborative Diagnosis	*Complications*	*Management/Goals*

14. Disseminated Intravascular Coagulation

Pathophysiology	*Etiology/Risk Factors*	*Signs/Symptoms*

Collaborative Diagnosis	*Complications*	*Management/Goals*

15. Select Hereditary Bleeding States

Pathophysiology	*Etiology/Risk Factors*	*Signs/Symptoms*

Collaborative Diagnosis	*Complications*	*Management/Goals*

E. Application to Clinical Practice

Care for patients with hematologic disorders. Relate the anatomy, physiology, assessment, and pathophysiology found in this section to their individual clinical pictures. Make note of instances where they correlate and those where they deviate. Devise a care plan based on the data collected.

Answers to Hematology Exercises

A. Physiologic Anatomy

1. 1500–2500, 50 (*page 675*)
2. a. No
   b. No
   c. Yes
   d. Yes
   e. Yes (*page 675*)
3. Bone marrow (*page 675*)
4. a. Low
   b. High
   c. High
   d. High (*page 677*)
5. Thoracic, right lymph duct (*page 677*)
6. a. Both
   b. Deep
   c. Superficial
   d. Both (*pages 677, 678*)
7. Thymus, smaller (*page 678*)
8. Antibodies or immunoglobulins (*page 678*)
9. Reticulocytes, 1–2 (*page 678*)
10. Erythropoietin, iron, B_{12}, folic acid (*page 679*)
11. Spleen, liver, bone marrow (*page 679*)
12. 120, abnormal (*pages 678–679*)
13. Iron, bilirubin (*page 680*)
14. Neutrophil, 10 (*page 680*)
15. a. Erythrocytes
    b. Erythrocytes
    c. Neutrophils, monocytes, macrophages
    d. Basophils
    e. Eosinophils (*pages 679–682*)
16. Band (*page 681*)
17. Monocytes, fixed, free (*pages 681, 682*)
18. a. Eosinophils
    b. Monocytes
    c. Lymphocytes (especially B cells) (*pages 681–683*)
19. a. B cell
    b. B cell
    c. T cell
    d. T cell
    e. T cell
    f. B cell
    g. T cell
    h. B cell (*pages 682–685*)
20. Interleukin-2, interferon (*page 684*)
21. a. IgG
    b. IgE
    c. IgA
    d. IgD (*page 685*)
22.

	Antigens	Antibodies
a.	A	Anti B
b.	Neither	Anti A, Anti B
c.	A, B	Neither (*page 686*)

23. Warmed (*page 687*)
24. Complement (*page 687*)
25. Dilation, increased, chemotaxis, phagocytosis (*pages 688–689*)
26. Killing or degradation (*page 689*)
27. a. Vascular reaction
    b. Platelet reaction
    c. Clot formation
    d. Anticoagulation during healing and fibrinolysis (*pages 689–693*)
28. Megakaryocyte (*page 690*)
29. Spleen, one third (*page 690*)
30. Coagulation, platelet plug (*page 690*)
31. a. Thrombocytosis
    b. Inhibited activity
    c. Inhibited activity
    d. Thrombocytopenia
    e. Thrombocytopenia (*pages 690, 691*)
32. 30,000 (*page 691*)
33. Liver, II, VII, IX, X (*page 691*)
34. Intrinsic, extrinsic (*page 691*)
35. Thrombin, fibrin (*page 692*)
36. Plasmin, fibrin split or degradation products, antithrombins (*pages 692–693*)

B. Nursing Assessment Data Base and Commonly Encountered Nursing Diagnoses

1. a. Low
   b. High
   c. Low
   d. Normal
   e. Low (*pages 696–699*)
2. Fever (*page 705*)
3. a. Neither
   b. Neither
   c. Coagulation factors (*pages 710–711*)
4. a. Hemoglobin increased .5 gm%/unit, hematocrit increased 1%–2%/unit
   b. Hemoglobin increased 1 gm%, hematocrit increased 2%–3%/unit
   c. Platelets increased 10,000/unit/sq. meter (*pages 710–711*)
5. a. Packed red blood cells
   b. Cryoprecipitate, fresh whole blood, or fresh frozen plasma

c. Albumin or plasma protein fractions, also hetastarch products (*pages 711–713*)
6. Febrile (*page 714*)

C. Patient Health Problems

1. Each parent, hypoxic (*page 715*)
2. Hemolysis or hemolytic anemia, thrombosis or ischemia or necrosis (*page 715*)
3. 100, 50 (*page 716*)
4. a. Shift of the oxygen hemoglobin dissociation curve to the right
   b. Redistribution of blood flow to those with higher oxygen demands
   c. Increased cardiac output
   d. Increased rate of erythrocyte synthesis (*page 717*)
5. Primary polycythemia (*page 721*)
6. a. Decrease
   b. Decrease
   c. Decrease
   d. Decrease (*page 723*)
7. 1500 μL, 500 μL (*page 724*)
8. Decreased, leukemic infiltrates (*pages 724–725*)
9. a. Acute lymphoblastic leukemia
   b. Acute nonlymphoblastic leukemia
   c. Chronic lymphocytic leukemia
   d. Chronic myeloid or granulocytic leukemia (*pages 724–729*)
10. Myeloma or M proteins or abnormal immunoglobulins, bone, nephrons, increased (*pages 729–730*)
11. Decreased, increased, Bence-Jones (*page 730*)
12. Reed-Sternberg cells, specific symptoms, lymph node and other organ involvement (*pages 731–732*)
13. a. No
    b. No
    c. Yes
    d. Yes
    e. Yes (*pages 732–733*)
14. Antigen-antibody, histamine (*page 734*)
15. Vasodilation, hypovolemia (*page 734*)
16. Helper T, 6 months, 5 years (*pages 735–736*)
17. a. 0 = Exposure (with negative HIV).
    b. 1 = Onset of infection (positive HIV from now on).
    c. 2 = Chronic lymphadenopathy developed.
    d. 3 = Subclinical immune dysfunction developed (decreased T_4 count).
    e. 4 = Asymptomatic defects in delayed hypersensitivity develops.
    f. 5 = Skin and mucous membrane defects develop with persistent fungal and viral infections. Anergy as well as failure of delayed hypersensitivity reactions may develop.
    g. 6 = Opportunistic infections develop. Now diagnosis is AIDS (*page 736*).
18. AIDS-related complex (ARC) (*page 737*)
19. Increased, decreased, decreased (*page 739*)
20. Prolonged, decreased, increased, strongly positive (*pages 740, 741*)
21. a. Both types of hemophilia (A and B)
    b. Von Willebrand's disease
    c. Hemophilia A
    d. Hemophilia B (*page 741*)
22. Partial thromboplastin (*page 742*)

D. Summary of Patient Health Problems

Refer to the following pages in the Core Curriculum

1. Sickle Cell Disease (*pages 715–717*)
2. Anemias (*pages 717–721*)
3. Polycythemia (*pages 721, 722*)
4. Neutropenia (*pages 722–724*)
5. Leukemia (*pages 724–725*)
6. Acute Lymphoblastic Leukemia (*pages 725–726*)
7. Acute Nonlymphoblastic Leukemia (*pages 726–727*)
8. Chronic Lymphocytic Leukemia (*pages 727–728*)
9. Chronic Myeloid Leukemia (*pages 728–729*)
10. Multiple Myeloma (*pages 729–731*)
11. Lymphomas (*pages 731–734*)
12. Anaphylaxis (*pages 734–735*)
13. Human Immunodeficiency Virus (*pages 735–739*)
14. Disseminated Intravascular Coagulation (*pages 739–741*)
15. Select Hereditary Bleeding States (*pages 741–742*)

HEMATOLOGY

Post Quiz

The following questions are designed to test understanding of some of the key points in the section. Select the one best answer for each. The correct answers are at the end of the test.

1. Reticulocytes are immature
   a. red blood cells
   b. platelets
   c. lymphocytes
   d. monocytes
2. Plasma cells are a specific type of
   a. red blood cells
   b. platelets
   c. lymphocytes
   d. monocytes
3. Erythrocytes, leukocytes, and thrombocytes are produced by the
   a. bone marrow
   b. spleen
   c. lymphatic system
   d. thymus
4. Humoral immunity
   a. is dependent on the thymus
   b. is a function of T cells
   c. is a delayed response
   d. involves immunoglobulins
5. Cellular immunity
   a. is thymic independent
   b. is a function of B cells
   c. is a more delayed response than reactions mediated by antibodies
   d. is accomplished through immunoglobulins
6. The complement system involves activation of proteins that
   a. are called reagins
   b. are anti-inflammatory
   c. enhance the immune response
   d. must precede antigen-antibody reaction
7. The normal inflammatory response may include
   a. an immediate decrease in local blood flow
   b. an attempt to isolate the injured area
   c. a fall in white blood cell count
   d. decreased capillary permeability
8. The extrinsic coagulation pathway
   a. is part of the vascular phase of hemostasis
   b. uses only factors found in the bloodstream
   c. is activated by tissue injury
   d. uses more clotting factors than the intrinsic pathway
9. Anticoagulation mechanisms include
   a. the process of thrombin formation
   b. the process of clot retraction
   c. the formation of plasmin
   d. the release of Coumadin from mast cells

10. The index used to evaluate the size of red blood cells is the
    a. MCV
    b. MCH
    c. MCHC
    d. reticulocyte count
11. Patients with blood type AO produce
    a. anti-A antibodies only
    b. anti-B antibodies only
    c. anti-A and anti-O antibodies
    d. neither anti-A nor anti-B antibodies
12. Platelets can be administered by which of the following?
    a. regular banked blood
    b. packed red blood cells
    c. fresh frozen plasma
    d. fresh whole blood
13. Eosinophilia is most likely to be related to
    a. allergic reactions
    b. chronic inflammation
    c. acute stress
    d. adrenocorticotropic hormone (ACTH) or steroid therapy
14. The primary stimulus for erythropoiesis seems to be
    a. tissue hypoxia or hypoxemia
    b. control centers in the medulla
    c. buildup of RBC breakdown products
    d. an elevation in 2,3-diphosphoglyceric acid (2,3-DPG)
15. The test that is most specific for the external coagulation pathway is the
    a. partial thromboplastin time
    b. prothrombin time
    c. bleeding time
    d. platelet count
16. Hemophilia A is a congenital condition in which the following element is lacking:
    a. hemoglobin A
    b. the Christmas factor
    c. factor IX
    d. factor VIII
17. Intravenous solutions containing albumin
    a. decrease the intravascular volume
    b. increase the interstitial fluid volume
    c. are hypo-osmolar
    d. spend a relatively long time in the vascular space
18. A major component of lymph fluid is
    a. platelets
    b. fibrinogen
    c. leukocytes
    d. erythrocytes
19. Mechanisms to compensate for anemia include
    a. increased production of erythropoietin
    b. decrease in cardiac output
    c. increased blood flow to the skin
    d. decreased production of 2,3 DPG
20. Human immunodeficiency virus
    a. infects B-cell lymphocytes primarily
    b. has a long asymptomatic and transmittable period
    c. increases the number of helper compared to suppressor T cells

d. is not a risk to health care practitioners unless they experience sticks from needles used on infected patients

21. The pathophysiology of anaphylaxis includes
    a. a late delayed reaction to an antigen-antibody reaction
    b. bronchodilation in response to histamine
    c. widespread vasoconstriction
    d. hypovolemia from increased capillary permeability
22. Disseminated intravascular coagulopathy
    a. is usually a primary disorder
    b. is widespread clotting that follows a bleeding tendency
    c. is a widespread clotting phenonemon that ultimately predisposes the patient to bleeding
    d. is diagnosed by decreased bleeding times and an increased level of clotting factors
23. When the patient has sickle cell disease
    a. the hemoglobin electrophoresis will reveal less than 50% HbS
    b. the peripheral smear will be normal
    c. thrombotic and necrotic events are possible
    d. there is usually no history of sickle cell disease in the family
24. A laboratory result that suggests the presence of multiple myeloma is
    a. urine positive for Bence-Jones protein
    b. hypocalcemia and hypophosphatemia
    c. decreased levels of plasma cells in bone marrow
    d. leukocytosis
25. Patients with Stage II Hodgkin's lymphoma
    a. have disease that has spread outside the lymph system
    b. are rarely cured and usually die within 10 years
    c. are usually treated with radiation therapy
    d. do not have Reed-Sternberg cells present
26. Patients with platelet counts of 10,000 to 30,000
    a. should have arterial lines inserted for proper monitoring
    b. are at a higher risk of bleeding when undergoing invasive procedures
    c. are placed on aspirin to stimulate platelet activity
    d. have an increased tendency to clot
27. Invasion and destruction of bony tissue is most likely to occur in
    a. sickle cell disease
    b. multiple myeloma
    c. non-Hodgkin's lymphoma
    d. Hodgkin's lymphoma
28. The presence of an abnormal Philadelphia chromosome is usually found in patients with
    a. chronic lymphocytic leukemia
    b. chronic myeloid leukemia
    c. acute lymphoblastic leukemia
    d. acute nonlymphoblastic leukemia
29. Unexplained weight loss, fever, and night sweats are common symptoms of
    a. lymphoma
    b. sickle cell anemia
    c. disseminated intravascular coagulapathy
    d. hemophilia
30. Hemathroses are more likely to occur as a complication of
    a. lymphoma
    b. multiple myeloma
    c. anaphylaxis
    d. hemophilia

Answers to Hematology Post Quiz

1. **a** (*page 678*)
2. **c** (*page 683*)
3. **a** (*page 675*)
4. **d** (*pages 684–685*)
5. **c** (*page 684*)
6. **c** (*page 687*)
7. **b** (*pages 688–689*)
8. **c** (*pages 691–692*)
9. **c** (*pages 692–693*)
10. **a** (*page 697*)
11. **b** (*pages 685–686*)
12. **d** (*pages 711–712*)
13. **a** (*page 681*)
14. **a** (*page 679*)
15. **b** (*page 698*)
16. **d** (*page 742*)
17. **d** (*pages 712–713*)
18. **c** (*page 677*)
19. **a** (*page 717*)
20. **b** (*pages 736–739*)
21. **d** (*page 734*)
22. **c** (*pages 739–741*)
23. **c** (*pages 715–716*)
24. **a** (*page 730*)
25. **c** (*pages 731–732*)
26. **b** (*pages 690–691*)
27. **b** (*page 729*)
28. **b** (*page 729*)
29. **a** (*page 732*)
30. **d** (*page 741*)

These are primarily the comprehend or recall, and apply or analyze levels of questions. Examples of synthesis or evaluate questions can be found in the comprehensive examination at the end of the book on pages 278 to 293.

7

The Gastrointestinal System

SECTION-RELATED TIPS FOR THOSE STUDYING TO TAKE THE CERTIFICATION EXAMINATION

The gastrointestinal anatomy and physiology are much easier to understand and visualize than most of the previous sections, especially at the level tested on the certification examination. There are only a few things that require memorizing. They include:

1. The names of cells that secrete substances such as hydrochloric acid from parietal cells and pepsinogen from chief cells in the stomach
2. The names of important enzymes involved in digestion such as amylase, trypsin, lipase, and pepsin
3. The simplest form of proteins (amino acids), carbohydrates (monosaccharides glucose, galactose, and fructose), and fats (triglycerides, glycerol)
4. The functions of the three main enzymes (gastrin, cholecystokinin, secretin).

It is unlikely that more than a few, if any, of these will appear on any given certification examination.

The other reasons this section may be easier to study are that the gastrointestinal complications of other diseases (stress ulcers, ileus, diarrhea, and constipation) have already been covered in preceding sections, as have the complications of gastrointestinal disorders (see the pulmonary section for acid-base imbalances and the renal section for fluid and electrolyte imbalances). Also, most of the disorders covered on the certification examination are commonly encountered in intensive care units.

Two other study-related tips are worth passing on. First, as you study the Patient Health Problems, remember that the examination does ask questions on the definitive symptoms, diagnosis, treatment, and complications. Second, make sure you save adequate time to study this section. Even though it may not be difficult, it is the last chapter and sufficient time must be allocated to these very important aspects of critical care.

The only other aspect of this section that may require amplification is nutritional support of the critically ill. Evaluating and meeting the patients' unique nutritional needs are briefly addressed below.

Evaluating Nutritional Requirements

Critically ill patients have altered metabolic rates that may change day to day. Formulas exist for predicting these needs based on patients' history, size, age, and problems, but they may be only estimates. Needs may be more accurately assessed by metabolic carts (direct calorimetry) that measure the amount of oxygen consumed and carbon dioxide produced per minute. The ratio yields information about the type of substrates being used. Nitrogen balance studies give information about whether the current demand for calories and proteins is being met. They may be inaccurate in patients with diarrhea since significant amounts of urea and nitrogen may then be lost in the stools.

Classic signs of chronic malnutrition (anergy, loss of lean body mass, and fat-fold studies) are relatively insensitive in cases of acute malnutrition. Measurement of serum proteins such as albumin, globulin, and transferrin are more sensitive but are almost universally low in seriously ill patients. Low lymphocyte counts are also used as a sign of acute malnutrition.

Meeting Nutritional Demands

Once a nutritional prescription is established, the next problem is to meet both protein and calorie needs. Immediate feeding of critically ill patients may be desirable but not often achieved. This is because of hormone and autonomic responses that tend to cause hyperglycemia and to channel the use of proteins for acute phase reactions rather than anabolic functions.

Although many physicians would prefer to use the gastrointestinal tract if at all possible to protect the patient from the potential for loss of mucosal integrity, stress ulcers, and septic syndrome, it may not be possible. Stress, hormone alterations, or the patient's problems may cause severe gastric hypomotility. Small bowel function is often intact or even hyperactive. In these patients, jejunostomy or small bore feeding tubes placed in the duodenum may be used to allow for early enteral nutrition.

Both enteral and parenteral nutrition have potential complications. The use of the enteral route may cause an added risk of aspiration or diarrhea, with resultant skin complications and fluid and electrolyte losses. The parenteral route carries a risk of infection, hyperglycemia, fluid shifts, osmotic diuresis, and electrolyte imbalances. Many enteral and parenteral products are available for use in various patient subsets. Research is ongoing into the effects of various types of amino acids and lipids in critically ill patients. The hospital nutrition team and the pharmacist are valuable resources in understanding their advantages, disadvantages, and differences.

Please see the instructions at the beginning of the book for important general suggestions that are relevant to the bulk of the *Core Curriculum* content. They apply to this section as well as all of the others.

FIGURES AND TABLES

Refer to these figures and tables while reading the gastrointestinal section of the Core Curriculum.

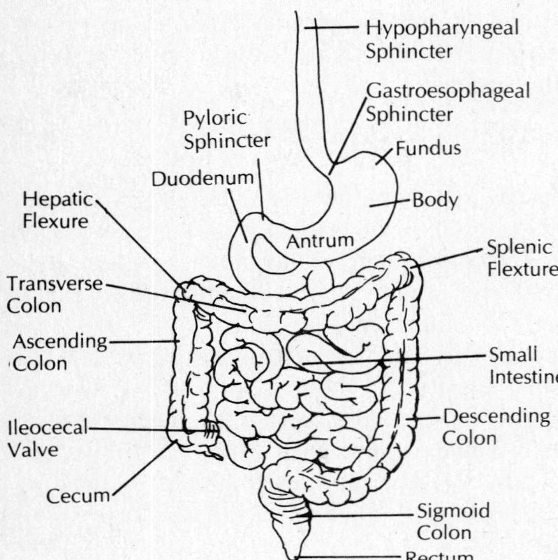

Figure 7–1. Structures of the gastrointestinal tract (*pages 748–757*).

Figure 7–2. Microscopic anatomy of the intestinal wall (*pages 754–757*).

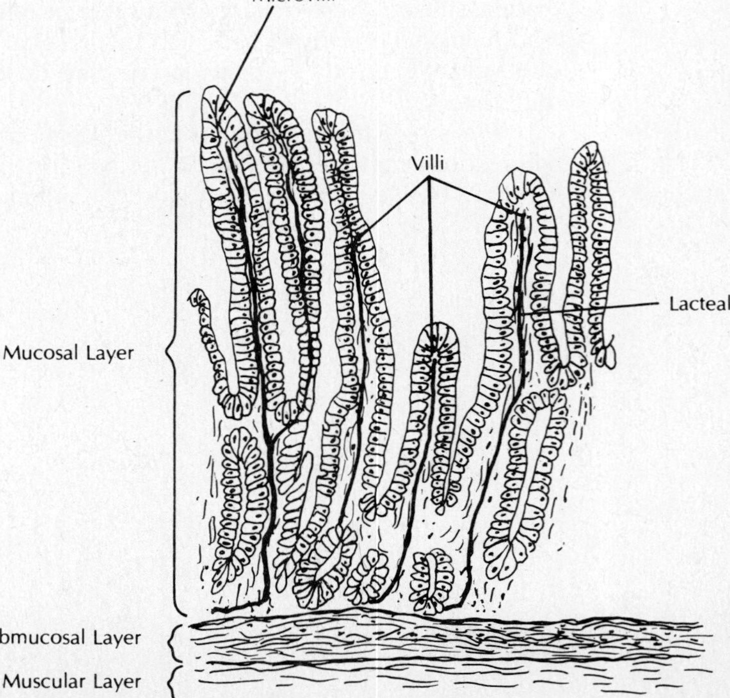

Table 7–1. MECHANICAL, SECRETORY, AND ABSORPTIVE FUNCTIONS OF THE GASTROINTESTINAL TRACT (*pages 748–759*)

Area (length)	Mechanical Functions	Secretory Functions			Absorption
		Substance	Site of Secretion	Action	
Oral Cavity	Ingestion } voluntary Mastication } Swallowing reflex	Saliva	Salivary glands stimulated by parasympathetic nerves	Amylase begins starch digestion	None
Pharynx	Swallowing reflex	None			None
Esophagus (10 in.)	Peristalsis reflex to swallowing and mechanical stimuli	Mucus	Mucous glands	Lubricate Protect	None
Stomach (10–12 in.)	Reservoir Mixing Regulated by autonomic nerves, reflexes, and hormones	Gastric acid (HC1) released in 3 phases: Cephalic Gastric Intestinal	Parietal cells stimulated by histamine, acetylcholine, and gastrin	Activates other enzymes (pepsin) Kills bacteria	Limited
	Emptying Increased with liquids, high gastric volume, anger and aggression, insulin	Pepsinogen (+HC1 = pepsin)	Chief cells	Protein breakdown	
		Intrinsic factor	Parietal cells	Vitamin B_{12} absorption in intestines	
	Decreased with lipids, high protein, starch, pain, sadness, depression, and duodenal hormones	Mucus	Cardiac cells Chief cells	Lubricate Protect	
	Vomiting Controlled by center in medulla and autonomic nerves Stimulated by gag, distention, increased intracranial pressure, dizziness, and pain				

Table continued on following page

Table 7–1. MECHANICAL, SECRETORY, AND ABSORPTIVE FUNCTIONS OF THE GASTROINTESTINAL TRACT (*pages 748–759*) *Continued*

Area (length)	Mechanical Functions	Secretory Functions			Absorption
		Substance	**Site of Secretion**	**Action**	
Small Intestine (Total = 12 ft.)	Segmental or mixing contractions Propulsive or peristaltic movements	Digestive enzymes	Intestinal cells and pancreas stimulated by the presence of chyme, nerves, and hormones	Digestion of nutrients	90% of nutrients 50% of water and electrolytes
		Mucus	Mucous cells	Lubricate Protect	
Large Intestine (5–6 ft.)	Increased by high fiber, irritation, high osmolality, and drugs Colonic motility Primary in fasting state is haustral shuttling (mixing) Primary in eating state is segmental or multihaustral propulsions and peristalsis (mass movement) Defecation	Mucus	Mucous cells	Lubricate Protect	Water Electrolytes

Note: Additional Functions of Large Intestine:
Bacterial cycles break down cellulose and synthesize vitamins
Urea is broken down into ammonia

Table 7–2. SUMMARY OF ABSORPTION IN THE INTESTINES (*pages 755, 756*)

Substrate	Type of Absorption	Sites
Electrolytes	Active transport	50% in small intestine Most of rest in large intestine
Water	Passive diffusion	50% in small intestine Most of rest in large intestine
Carbohydrate		90% in small intestine
Glucose	Active transport	
Galactose	Active transport	
Fructose	Facilitated diffusion	
Protein	Active transport	90% in small intestine (ileum and jejunum)
Fat	Small amount via passive diffusion Majority via facilitated diffusion	90% in small intestine (jejunum)
Vitamins		90% in small intestine
Water soluble	Passive diffusion (vitamin B_{12} requires intrinsic factor)	All parts
Fat soluble	Facilitated diffusion by bile salts	Jejunum
Minerals		90% in small intestine
Calcium	Facilitated diffusion	Duodenum
Iron	Active transport	All parts

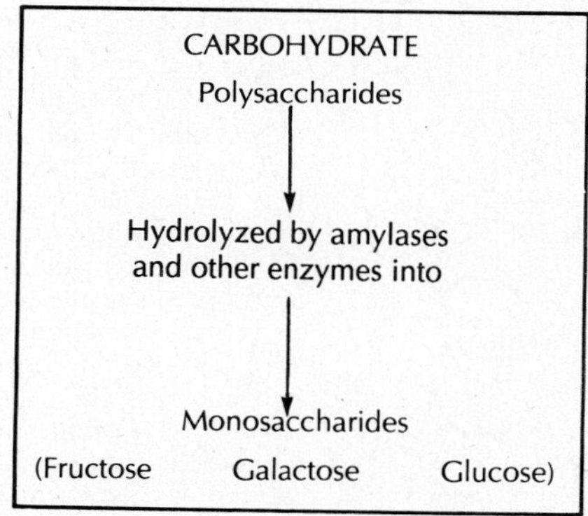

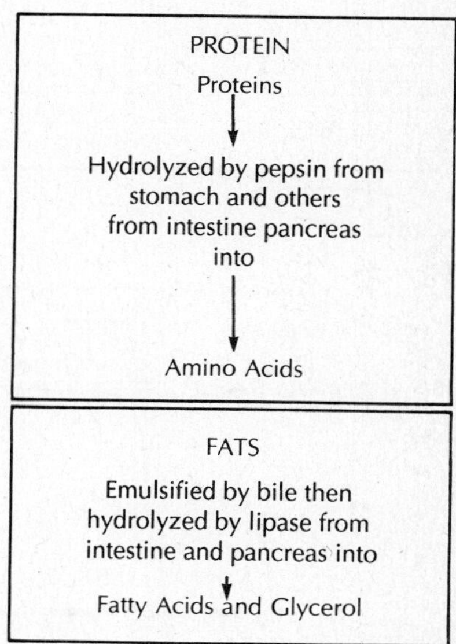

Figure 7–3. Progression of nutrient digestion (*pages 752–761*).

Table 7–3. SUMMARY OF THE PRIMARY COMPONENTS OF GASTROINTESTINAL CIRCULATION (*pages 759, 760*)

Vessel	Function
Celiac Artery	Supplies most of upper gastrointestinal tract, gall bladder, pancreas, and spleen
Superior Mesenteric Artery	Supplies gastrointestinal tract from jejunum through part of transverse colon
Inferior Mesenteric Artery	Supplies rest of transverse colon to rectum
Portal Vein	Drains venous return from entire gastrointestinal tract to liver

Table 7–4. FUNCTIONS OF THE PANCREAS (*pages 761–762*)

Type	Substance	Action
Exocrine Functions		
Acinar Cells	Trypsin	Protein breakdown
	Amylase	Starch breakdown
	Lipase	Triglyceride breakdown
	Ribonuclease, Deoxyribonuclease	Nucleic acid breakdown
Endocrine Functions		
Alpha Cells	Glucagon	Glucose production via glycogenolysis and gluconeogenesis
Beta Cells	Insulin	Glucose into cells to be oxidized or stored as glycogen or fat
Delta Cells	Somatostatin	Inhibits insulin, glucagon, and growth hormone

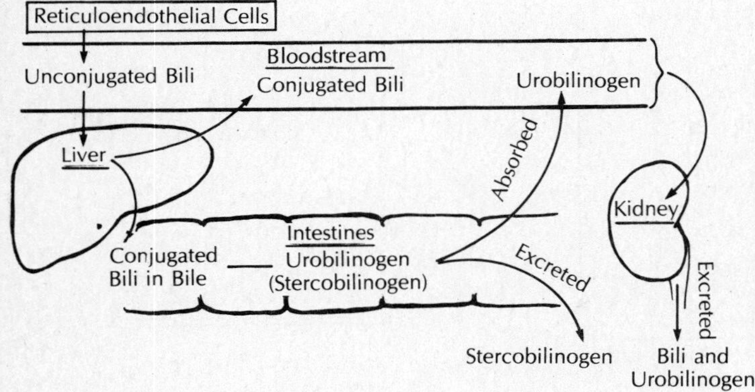

Figure 7–4. Bilirubin metabolism. Bilirubin is a breakdown product of red blood cells. The reticuloendothelial system creates the unconjugated form; the liver creates the conjugated form. The majority of the bilirubin produced by the liver is used to make bile, of which 80% is reabsorbed and returned to the liver for recycling. The bilirubin that remains in the intestine is converted to urobilinogen, most of which is excreted in stool. The urobilinogen that is absorbed, along with both conjugated and unconjugated circulating bilirubin, is excreted by the kidney (*pages 763–764*).

Table 7–5. SUMMARY OF THE FUNCTIONS OF THE LIVER (*pages 764–765*)

Cells	Functions
Kupffer cells (tissue phagocytes)	Hemolyze old erythrocytes Detoxify toxic substances, drugs, and hormones
Hepatocytes	Secrete bile Metabolize nutrients Synthesize amino acids, albumin, and globulin Synthesize glucose from glycogen and amino acids Catabolize fatty acids and neutral fats Synthesize lipoproteins, cholesterol, and phospholipids Synthesize clotting factors and antithrombin Form ammonia into urea Store fat soluble vitamins, B_{12}, copper, and iron

Table 7–6. FACTORS COVERED IN THE PHYSIOLOGIC ANATOMY SECTION THAT HAVE CLINICAL APPLICATIONS WORTH EMPHASIZING (*pages 748–765*)

Factor	Clinical Application	Page
Swallowing Reflex	The trigeminal (V), glossopharyngeal (IX), vagus (X), and hypoglossal (XII) cranial nerves are involved in the protective reflexes of gag and swallowing. Dysfunction of these nerves follows higher cranial nerve dysfunction in supratentorial lesions but may be an early finding in patients with lower brainstem disease (their origin) and in those with neck or mediastinal disorders (their peripheral path). Their function is recovered after spinal nerve function in patients recovering from general anesthesia.	749, 750
Fundus of the Stomach	The fundus is one of the most difficult aspects of the stomach to visualize on endoscopy and is often the sight of bleeding.	751
Hydrochloric Acid	The secretion of hydrochloric acid by the stomach makes it by far the most acidic part of the GI tract. The stomach normally has a pH of under 4.	752
The pH of GI Secretions	Since gastric secretions are acidic, nausea, vomiting and nasogastric suction can lead to metabolic alkalosis. Since small intestinal secretions are alkalotic, dumping syndrome and small-bowel obstruction or resections can led to metabolic acidosis. Both can lead to concomitant losses of fluid and electrolytes, such as potassium, sodium, and magnesium. One reason the gastric pH is so acidotic is its bacteroidal properties. The food we eat is full of flora. Drugs that raise the gastric pH is one method of preventing stress ulcers (antacids and histamine blockers like cimetidine, ranitidine, and pepsid) may result in colonizing the gut and increasing the risk of sepsis or secondary infections. Carafate may protect against stress ulcers without altering the gastric pH and the risk of secondary infection.	752–759
Autonomic Innervation of the GI Tract	In general, GI motility, secretion, and blood flow are stimulated by the parasympathetic nerves and inhibited by the sympathetic nerves. Prolonged critical illness may lead to prolonged periods of decreased motility, secretion, absorption, and blood flow. The resultant lack of protective mucus and ischemia may decrease mucosal wall integrity. The lack of secretion and motility have made it difficult to use the gut to feed patients.	753–760
Layers of the Small Intestinal Wall	The small intestinal mucosa is the only part of the body that does not get nourished by the bloodstream. Nutrients are absorbed from the intestinal lumen through it into the blood and lymph microcirculation, not vice versa. It is, therefore, primarily nourished by the nutrients passing through it. Prolonged NPO states may decrease mucosal integrity.	754
Mucosal Regeneration	The GI mucosal layer is regenerated approximately every 24 hours. The decrease in mucosal nutrition, protection, and oxygenation may lead to decreased integrity. This is under current investigation as a potential source of sepsis in critically ill patients.	754
Active Transport	Decreased blood flow to the GI tract may decrease the amount of ATP available for active transport. This is one of the many potential causes of diarrhea in patients on enteral feedings.	755
Colonic Motility	Morphine and other opiates or narcotics are more likely to cause inhibited rather than enhanced motility or, in other words, are more likely to cause constipation. Diarrhea that occurs in critically ill patients may be the result of an osmotic load, malabsorption, drugs, enterotoxins or infections, inflammations or irritations, hypoalbuminemia, and the type or temperature of enteral feedings.	757, 758
Colonic Synthesis of Vitamin K	The normal bacterial flora in the colon facilitate the synthesis of vitamin K. Antibiotics that decrease this flora may decrease the patient's vitamin K stores and contribute to bleeding tendencies.	758
Secretin	The first hormone released when chyme arrives in the duodenum is secretin. It stimulates the pancreas to release what is termed "the alkaline tide," to buffer gastric juices up to a pH approaching 8.0. This is important since the gastric mucosa is the only part of the GI tract capable of tolerating exposure to very acidic fluids.	759

Table continued on following page

Table 7–6. FACTORS COVERED IN THE PHYSIOLOGIC ANATOMY SECTION THAT HAVE CLINICAL APPLICATIONS WORTH EMPHASIZING (*pages 748–765*) *Continued*

Factor	Clinical Application	Page
Nervous System Innervation	The alpha sympathetic nerves in the GI tract cause vasoconstriction and dopaminergic sympathetic nerves cause vasodilation. Patients with bowel infarcts or ischemia may benefit from low-dose dopamine. Alpha dose dopamine and other drugs with alpha effects may be contraindicated.	760
Somatostatin	Somatostatin is now available as an injectable medication. It has been approved for use in controlling symptoms in patients with some metastatic tumors. Since it blocks many gastrointestinal and endocrine hormones, it is under investigation for many other conditions (pancreatitis, intestinal obstruction, some types of diarrhea, variceal bleeding, pancreatic fistulas, pseudocysts)	762
Control of Pancreatic Secretions	Stimulation of further pancreatic secretion may be contraindicated in patients with acute pancreatitis. Accordingly, stimulation of parasympathetic nerves or hormone secretion, especially by oral feedings, may be contraindicated.	762
Liver Functions	Learning the functions of the liver is one of the easiest ways to learn the signs of liver failure. The potential sequelae of liver failure that are not obvious from its functions are hypoglycemia, hyperdynamic cardiac output demands due to peripheral shunting, lack of testosterone production from cholesterol that can lead to feminizing changes in men, and increased intracranial pressure, which is not well understood. The increased intracranial pressure may be due to increased serum ammonia, intracranial bleeding, or a substance produced by the liver that is important to neurometabolism.	764, 765

Table 7–7. SUMMARY OF SELECT NORMAL FINDINGS IN PHYSICAL ASSESSMENT OF THE GASTROINTESTINAL TRACT (*pages 766–768*)

Technique	Normal Findings
Inspection	Symmetrical appearance Lack of scars, markings, or masses Only normal motion Peristalsis or aortic impulse in thin individuals Abdominal rise during inspiration (especially in men)
Auscultation	Gurgling and bubbling fairly continuous sounds
Percussion	
over liver	Dullness
over spleen	Dullness
over stomach	Tympany when empty
over gut	Hyperresonant or tympanic
Palpation	Normal-sized liver Nonpalpable spleen Lack of abdominal masses Lack of pain or tenderness

Table 7–8. SUMMARY OF THE MOST COMMON CAUSES OF SELECT ABNORMAL FINDINGS IN ASSESSMENT OF THE GASTROINTESTINAL TRACT (*pages 766–768*)

Finding	Common Causes
Visceral Pain (dull and diffuse pain)	Organic lesions or distention of organs
Somatic Pain (sharp and localized pain)	Inflammatory processes
Caput Medusae and/or Cutaneous Angiomata	Liver disease or portal hypertension
Borborygmi (loud, rushing, high-pitched bowel sounds)	Early intestinal obstruction or anxiety
Decreased or Absent Bowel Sounds	Peritonitis Ileus Ischemic bowel Late intestinal obstruction
Succussion Splash	Increased gastrointestinal air and fluid in stomach
Bruit (vascular murmur)	Partial arterial occlusion
Venous Hum	Portal hypertension
Abdominal Friction Rub (during respiratory cycle)	Peritonitis, inflammation or infarction
Decreased Dullness to Percussion over Liver	Free air below diaphragm
Increased Tympany to Percussion over Stomach	Upper abdominal distention
Change in Percussion from Tympany to Dullness over Left Subcostal Area	Splenic enlargement
Shifting Dullness (moves to dependent areas with changes in position)	Ascites
Fluid Wave (slight impact felt on opposite side when one side is clapped)	Severe ascites
Rebound Tenderness	Peritonitis
Abdominal Rigidity	Peritonitis
Enlarged, Smooth, Nontender Liver	Nonmalignant liver infiltrate
Enlarged, Smooth, Tender Liver	Hepatitis or liver congestion
Enlarged Irregular Liver	Liver malignancy or cirrhosis
Palpable Spleen	Spleen at least 3 times normal size

THE GASTROINTESTINAL SYSTEM

Exercises

After reading the gastrointestinal section of the Core Curriculum, *fill in the blanks in the following statements. It can be done one topic at a time or all at once. The answers are at the end of the exercises.*

A. Physiologic Anatomy (*pages 748–765*)

1. The amount of saliva secreted each day is about ______________ cc, and the only digestive enzyme it contains is ______________.
2. The three areas of the gastrointestinal tract involved in deglutition are the
   a. ______________
   b. ______________
   c. ______________
3. Swallowing is a motor activity controlled by the ______________, ______________, ______________, and ______________ cignial nerves.
4. The anterior esophagus shares a common membrane with the posterior ______________.
5. The stomach has two sphincters, the ______________ at the esophageal end and the ______________ at the duodenal end.

6. Secretions of the stomach include ______________ from the chief cells, and ______________ from the parietal cells.
7. The stomach secretes about ______________ cc of fluid per day.
8. Indicate what effect each of the following has on the rate of gastric emptying.
   a. Increased fat intake ______________
   b. Pain ______________
   c. High volume of liquids ______________
   d. Secretin ______________
   e. Feelings of aggression ______________
9. The three phases of gastric secretion are
   a. ______________
   b. ______________
   c. ______________
10. The small intestinal cells that participate in immunity are called ______________.
11. Indicate the type of absorption each one of the following undergoes in the small intestine.
    a. Most water-soluble vitamins ______________
    b. Glucose ______________
    c. Electrolytes ______________
    d. Water ______________
    e. Amino acids ______________
12. Carbohydrates are broken down into the three basic monosaccharides ______________, ______________, and ______________; proteins are broken down into ______________ and ______________; fats are broken down into ______________ and ______________.
13. The small intestine secretes ______________ cc of fluid per day.
14. Indicate whether the following increase or decrease colonic motility.
    a. Increased osmolality of contents ______________
    b. Increased bile salts ______________
    c. High-fiber diet ______________
    d. Atropine ______________
15. The two functions of the bacterial flora normally found in the large intestine are to break down ______________ and synthesize ______________.
16. The type of colonic motility most common in the fasting state is ______________.
17. The gastrointestinal hormone that stimulates the pancreas to release bicarbonate and water is ______________.
18. The gastrointestinal hormone that augments gastric secretion and emptying is ______________.
19. The gastrointestinal hormone that stimulates gall bladder contraction and release of enzymes from the pancreas is ______________.
20. Name the artery that supplies each of the following structures.
    a. Jejunum ______________
    b. Upper gastrointestinal tract ______________
    c. Ileum ______________
    d. Descending colon ______________

21. The ______________ vein carries blood from the gastrointestinal tract to the liver, while the ______________ vein carries blood from the liver to the vena cava.
22. The pancreas secretes approximately ______________ cc of fluid with a pH of ______________.
23. In the pancreas, digestive enzymes are secreted by ______________ cells, insulin by ______________ cells, and glucagon by ______________ cells.
24. Pancreatic secretion increases in response to stimulation of the ______________ nerve or release of the hormones ______________ and ______________.
25. ______________ percent of the bile salts are reabsorbed in the small intestine and the rest are ______________.
26. ______________ bilirubin is the type produced by the reticuloendothelial system, ______________ bilirubin is produced by the liver, and ______________ is a compound formed out of bilirubin present in the intestine.
27. The ______________ bilirubin increases in hepatocellular disease, and the ______________ bilirubin increases in biliary tract obstruction.
28. The two major types of liver cells are the ______________, which are phagocytic, and the ______________, which produce bile and metabolize nutrients.
29. The liver can form ______________ from ammonia, convert ______________ to glycogen, and store ______________-soluble vitamins.

B. Nursing Assessment Data Base (*pages 765–770*)

1. Auscultation of the abdomen should be done prior to assessment by ______________ or ______________.
2. To be sure of the absence of bowel sounds, it may be necessary to listen to the abdomen for ______________ minutes.
3. State the cause for each of the following physical findings.
   a. Venous hum over right upper quadrant ______________
   b. Borborygmi ______________
   c. Absent bowel sounds ______________
4. Indicate the normal percussion note elicited over each of the following.
   a. Liver ______________
   b. Spleen ______________
   c. Empty stomach ______________
5. ______________ pain from organic abdominal lesions is ______________ and ______________ localized.
6. ______________ pain from abdominal inflammation is ______________ and ______________ localized.
7. List the most likely causes of each of the following abnormal palpable findings.
   a. Rebound tenderness ______________
   b. Enlarged, smooth, tender liver ______________
   c. Enlarged, irregular liver ______________

C. Commonly Encountered Nursing Diagnoses (*pages 770–774*)

1. List two mechanisms that the nursing diagnosis of "potential for alteration in nutrition, less than body requirements" may be related to in the patient with gastrointestinal disorders.
   a. ____________________
   b. ____________________
2. List two mechanisms that the nursing diagnosis "potential for fluid volume deficit" may be related to in the patient with gastrointestinal disorders.
   a. ____________________
   b. ____________________
3. List two mechanisms that the nursing diagnosis "potential for alteration in bowel elimination, diarrhea" may be related to in the patient with gastrointestinal disorders.
   a. ____________________
   b. ____________________

D. Patient Health Problems (*pages 774–835*)

1. Name two enzymes thought to be involved in the pathophysiology of pancreatitis.
   a. ____________________
   b. ____________________
2. The two most common etiologic factors for pancreatitis are ____________________ and ____________________.
3. Urine that is dark amber or foamy may reflect the presence of ____________________.
4. Discoloration of the flanks, called ____________________, discoloration of the umbilicus, called ____________________, or pale, bulky, foul stools, called ____________________, may be present in hemorrhagic pancreatitis.
5. Indicate whether the following are more likely to be increased or decreased in patients with acute pancreatitis.
   a. Serum amylase ____________________
   b. Serum lipase ____________________
   c. Serum protein ____________________
   d. Serum potassium ____________________
   e. Serum calcium ____________________
   f. WBC ____________________
   g. Urine amylase ____________________
6. List five potential complications of acute pancreatitis.
   a. ____________________
   b. ____________________
   c. ____________________
   d. ____________________
   e. ____________________
7. Meperidine is ____________________ likely than morphine to cause contraction of the sphincter of Oddi.
8. Indicate whether each of the following is more true of hepatitis A or hepatitis B.
   a. Longer incubation period ____________________
   b. Spread via parenteral routes ____________________
   c. Affects primarily younger adults ____________________
9. The nursing diagnosis of "potential for impaired skin integrity" in the patient with hepatitis can be related to ____________________.

10. Cirrhosis of the liver occurs when damage and degeneration is followed by irregular and abnormal ______________________.
11. The major cause of cirrhosis is ______________________.
12. List two potential nursing diagnoses in a patient with cirrhosis of the liver.
    a. ______________________
    b. ______________________
13. Hepatic failure may cause secondary dysfunction of the ______________________ or ______________________.
14. In addition to cirrhosis, hepatic failure can be caused by ______________________, ______________________, and ______________________.
15. Indicate whether the following are more likely to be increased or decreased in patients with severe hepatic failure.
    a. Albumin ______________________
    b. Prothrombin time ______________________
    c. Respirations ______________________
    d. Reflexes ______________________
    e. Size of spleen ______________________
16. Hepatic failure may be associated with ______________________ levels of circulating ammonia, which can be treated by the administration of ______________________ and ______________________, and by the limitation of dietary ______________________.
17. Indicate whether each of the following is more likely to be related to ulcerative colitis or regional enteritis.
    a. Involvement of the terminal ileum ______________________
    b. Bloody diarrhea ______________________
    c. Intestinal fistulas and abscesses ______________________
    d. Increased risk of cancer of the colon ______________________
18. A complication of inflammatory bowel disease that is related to decreased intestinal contractility and severe dilation of the large colon is called ______________________.
19. The above complication can be precipitated by ______________________ or ______________________.
20. List the sequential pathophysiology of bowel infarction.
    a. ______________________
    b. ______________________
    c. ______________________
    d. ______________________
    e. ______________________
    f. ______________________
21. Nursing diagnoses commonly encountered in a patient with bowel infarct include
    a. ______________________
    b. ______________________
    c. ______________________
22. Abdominal trauma includes injuries from the ______________________ to the ______________________ of the patient.
23. Nursing diagnoses commonly encountered in a patient with abdominal trauma include
    a. ______________________
    b. ______________________
    c. ______________________
24. Cancer of the esophagus usually occurs in (male/female) patients over the age of ______________________ with a history of ______________________.

25. Nursing diagnoses commonly encountered in patients with cancer of the esophagus include
    a. ______________________
    b. ______________________
    c. ______________________
26. List two risk factors for cancer of the stomach.
    a. ______________________
    b. ______________________
27. Nursing diagnoses commonly encountered in patients with cancer of the stomach include
    a. ______________________
    b. ______________________
    c. ______________________
28. Potential pathologic consequences of cancer of the colon include ______________________ and ______________________.
29. Nursing diagnoses commonly encountered in patients with cancer of the colon include
    a. ______________________
    b. ______________________
    c. ______________________
30. The pathophysiology of bleeding peptic ulcers may involve an imbalance between the ______________________ and the ______________________.
31. Risk factors for the development of peptic ulcers include ______________________ and ______________________.
32. Nursing diagnoses commonly encountered in patients with peptic ulcers include
    a. ______________________
    b. ______________________
33. The etiology of esophageal varices involves the development of ______________________ hypertension and about ______________________ % of them eventually bleed.
34. The current therapy for bleeding esophageal varices includes ______________________ and ______________________.
35. Potential causes of acute abdomen include
    a. ______________________
    b. ______________________
    c. ______________________
    d. ______________________
36. Nursing diagnoses commonly encountered in patients with acute abdomen include
    a. ______________________
    b. ______________________
    c. ______________________
37. The classic surgical treatment for pancreatic cancer is a pancreatoduodenectomy, also called the ______________________ procedure.
38. Risk factors for cancer of the pancreas include ______________________ and ______________________.
39. Nursing diagnoses commonly encountered in patients with pancreatic cancer include
    a. ______________________
    b. ______________________
    c. ______________________

E. Summary of Patient Health Problems (*pages 774—835*)

After reading each disease, summarize the pathophysiology, nursing assessment data base, and nursing diagnoses. Since the certification examination holds you responsible for knowing the etiology and risk factors, the signs and symptoms, the collaborative diagnosis, the complications, the management and treatment goals, those preparing to take it should also summarize these areas. If they are not clearly covered in the Core, *a second resource may be necessary. The space allotted is purposefully limited to encourage concise descriptions of concepts and careful selection of key points. It is not as helpful to write the things you already know as it is to write those you need to study.*

1. Acute Pancreatitis

Pathophysiology	*Etiology/Risk Factors*	*Signs/Symptoms*

Collaborative Diagnosis	*Complications*	*Management/Goals*

2. Acute Hepatitis

Pathophysiology	*Etiology/Risk Factors*	*Signs/Symptoms*

Collaborative Diagnosis	*Complications*	*Management/Goals*

3. Cirrhosis of the Liver

Pathophysiology	*Etiology/Risk Factors*	*Signs/Symptoms*

Collaborative Diagnosis	*Complications*	*Management/Goals*

4. Hepatic Failure

Pathophysiology	*Etiology/Risk Factors*	*Signs/Symptoms*

Collaborative Diagnosis	*Complications*	*Management/Goals*

5. Ulcerative Colitis

Pathophysiology	*Etiology/Risk Factors*	*Signs/Symptoms*

Collaborative Diagnosis	*Complications*	*Management/Goals*

6. Regional Enteritis

Pathophysiology	*Etiology/Risk Factors*	*Signs/Symptoms*

Collaborative Diagnosis	*Complications*	*Management/Goals*

7. Toxic Megacolon

Pathophysiology	*Etiology/Risk Factors*	*Signs/Symptoms*

Collaborative Diagnosis	*Complications*	*Management/Goals*

8. Bowel Infarction

Pathophysiology	*Etiology/Risk Factors*	*Signs/Symptoms*

Collaborative Diagnosis	*Complications*	*Management/Goals*

9. Abdominal Trauma

Pathophysiology	*Etiology/Risk Factors*	*Signs/Symptoms*

Collaborative Diagnosis	*Complications*	*Management/Goals*

10. Esophageal Carcinoma

Pathophysiology	*Etiology/Risk Factors*	*Signs/Symptoms*

Collaborative Diagnosis	*Complications*	*Management/Goals*

11. Gastric Carcinoma

Pathophysiology	*Etiology/Risk Factors*	*Signs/Symptoms*

Collaborative Diagnosis	*Complications*	*Management/Goals*

12. Carcinoma of the Colon

Pathophysiology	*Etiology/Risk Factors*	*Signs/Symptoms*

Collaborative Diagnosis	*Complications*	*Management/Goals*

13. Peptic Ulcers

Pathophysiology	*Etiology/Risk Factors*	*Signs/Symptoms*

Collaborative Diagnosis	*Complications*	*Management/Goals*

14. Esophageal Varices

Pathophysiology	*Etiology/Risk Factors*	*Signs/Symptoms*

Collaborative Diagnosis	*Complications*	*Management/Goals*

15. Acute Abdomen

Pathophysiology	*Etiology/Risk Factors*	*Signs/Symptoms*

Collaborative Diagnosis	*Complications*	*Management/Goals*

16. Pancreatic Cancer

Pathophysiology	*Etiology/Risk Factors*	*Signs/Symptoms*

Collaborative Diagnosis	*Complications*	*Management/Goals*

F. Application to Clinical Practice

Care for patients with gastrointestinal disease. Relate the anatomy, physiology, assessment and pathophysiology found in this section to their individual clinical pictures. Make note of those instances where they correlate and those where they deviate from the expected presentation. Devise a care plan based on the data collected.

Answers to Gastrointestinal Exercises

A. Physiologic Anatomy

1. 1000–1500, amylase (*page 748*)
2. a. Oral cavity
   b. Pharynx
   c. Esophagus (*page 748*)
3. Trigeminal (V), glossopharyngeal (IX), vagus (X), hypoglossal (XII) (*page 750*)
4. Trachea (*page 750*)
5. Cardiac, pyloric (*page 751*)
6. Pepsinogen, hydrochloric acid and/or intrinsic factor (*page 752*)
7. 1500–3000 (*page 752*)
8. a. Inhibit
   b. Inhibit
   c. Accelerate
   d. Inhibit
   e. Accelerate (*page 752*)
9. a. Cephalic
   b. Gastric
   c. Intestinal (*page 752*)
10. Peyer's patches (*page 754*)
11. a. Passive
    b. Active
    c. Active
    d. Passive
    e. Active (*pages 755–756*)
12. Glucose, fructose, galactose; amino acids, small peptides; glycerol, fatty acids (*pages 755–756*)
13. As much as 3000 (*page 757*)
14. a. Increase
    b. Increase
    c. Increase
    d. Decrease (*pages 757–758*)
15. Cellulose, vitamins (*page 758*)
16. Haustral shuttling (*page 758*)
17. Secretin (*page 759*)
18. Gastrin (*page 759*)
19. Cholecystokinin (*page 759*)
20. a. Superior mesenteric
    b. Celiac
    c. Superior mesenteric
    d. Inferior mesenteric (*pages 759–760*)
21. Portal, hepatic (*page 760*)
22. 1500–2000, 8.3 (*page 761*)
23. Acinar, beta, alpha (*page 761*)
24. Vagus (parasympathetic), secretin, cholecystokinin (*page 762*)
25. 80, excreted in the feces (*page 763*)
26. Indirect or unconjugated, direct or conjugated, urobilinogen (*page 764*)
27. Unconjugated or indirect, conjugated or direct (*page 764*)
28. Kupffer cells, hepatocytes (*page 764*)
29. Urea, glucose, fat (*pages 764–765*)

B. Nursing Assessment Data Base

1. Percussion, palpation (*page 767*)
2. 2 to 5 (*page 767*)
3. a. Portal obstruction or liver disease
   b. Hyperperistalsis
   c. Ileus, ischemia of the bowel, peritonitis, or late intestinal obstruction (*page 767*)
4. a. Dull
   b. Dull
   c. Tympanic (*page 768*)
5. Visceral, dull, poorly (*page 768*)
6. Somatic, sharp, well (*page 768*)
7. a. Peritoneal inflammation
   b. Hepatitis or hepatic congestion
   c. Malignancy or cirrhosis (*page 768*)

C. Commonly Encountered Nursing Diagnoses

1. Any two of the following (*page 770*):
   a. Nausea, vomiting
   b. Anorexia
   c. Restricted intake
   d. Increased metabolic demand
2. Any two of the following (*pages 771–772*):
   a. Vomiting
   b. Gastric suctioning
   c. Third spacing
   d. Diarrhea
   e. Hemorrhage
   f. Decreased fluid intake
   g. Diuresis
3. Any two of the following (*pages 772, 773*):
   a. Type of dietary intake
   b. Intestinal dysfunction
   c. Intestinal stimulants
   d. Colonization with certain pathogens

D. Patient Health Problems

1. Any two of these (*page 774*):
   a. Trypsin
   b. Elastase
   c. Chymotrypsin
   d. Phospholipase A
2. Chronic alcohol ingestion, cholelithiasis (*page 774*)
3. Bile (*page 775*)
4. Grey-Turner's sign, Cullen's sign, steatorrhea (*page 776*)

5. a. Increased
   b. Increased
   c. Decreased
   d. Decreased
   e. Decreased
   f. Increased
   g. Increased (*page 776*)
6. Any five of these (*pages 776–780*):
   a. Sepsis
   b. Pseudocysts
   c. Abscess
   d. Fistulas
   e. Myocardial infarction
   f. Shock
   g. Renal failure
   h. Malnutrition
   i. Fluid volume deficit
   j. Electrolyte imbalance
   k. Respiratory failure (ARDS)
   l. Pleural fusion
   m. Chronic pancreatitis
7. Less (*page 780*)
8. a. B
   b. B
   c. A (*page 781*)
9. Deposition of bile salts (*page 783*)
10. Regeneration (*page 783*)
11. Chronic alcoholism (*page 784*)
12. Any two of these (*pages 787–790*):
    a. Alteration in nutrition, less than body requirements
    b. Fluid volume deficit
    c. Impaired skin integrity
    d. Ineffective breathing pattern
    e. Alteration in tissue perfusion (due to volume deficit or coagulation abnormalities)
13. Any two of these (*page 790*):
    a. Brain
    b. Lungs
    c. Kidneys
    d. Pancreas
14. Any two of these (*page 790*):
    a. Hepatitis
    b. Hepatotoxicity
    c. Hepatic ischemia
    d. Fatty liver of pregnancy
    e. Reyes syndrome
15. a. Decreased
    b. Increased
    c. Increased
    d. Increased
    e. Increased (*page 791*)
16. Increased, neomycin or kanamycin enemas, lactulose, protein (*page 792*)
17. a. Regional enteritis
    b. Ulcerative colitis
    c. Ulcerative colitis
    d. Regional enteritis (*pages 792–795*)
18. Toxic megacolon (*page 797*)
19. Any two of these (*page 797*):
    a. Barium enema during an exacerbation
    b. Opiates given patients with ulcerative colitis
    c. Anticholinergic agents
    d. Hypokalemia
20. a. Decreased blood flow
    b. Bowel spasm then flaccidity
    c. Accumulation of intraluminal fluid
    d. Full thickness necrosis
    e. Perforation
    f. Peritonitis or abscess formation (*page 799*)
21. Any three of these (*pages 800–803*):
    a. Potential for infection
    b. Alteration in nutrition, less than body requirements
    c. Alteration in comfort related to severe abdominal pain
    d. Alteration in tissue perfusion
22. Nipple line, mid-thigh (*page 803*)
23. Any three of these (*pages 805–809*):
    a. Potential for infection
    b. Potential for alteration in nutrition, less than body requirements
    c. Fluid volume deficit
    d. Potential for ineffective breathing pattern
    e. Alteration in comfort
    f. Anxiety/fear
24. Male, 50 years, alcohol abuse or cigarette smoking (*page 809*)
25. Any three of the following (*pages 811–812*):
    a. Alteration in nutrition, less than body requirements
    b. Ineffective breathing pattern
    c. Alteration in comfort
    d. Anxiety/fear
    e. Grieving
    f. Powerlessness
26. Any two of the following (*page 813*):
    a. Diet high in nitrates
    b. Genetic predisposition
    c. Blood type A
    d. Atrophic gastritis
    e. Polyps of the stomach
27. Any three of the following (*pages 814–815*):
    a. Alteration in nutrition, less than body requirements

b. Alteration in comfort
c. Potential grieving
d. Powerlessness
e. Anxiety/fear

28. Any two of the following (*pages 815, 816*):
a. Obstruction
b. Abscess formation
c. Peritonitis

29. Any three of the following (*pages 816, 817*):
a. Alteration in nutrition, less than body requirements
b. Ineffective breathing pattern
c. Alteration in comfort
d. Anxiety/fear
e. Grieving
f. Powerlessness

30. Irritating gastrointestinal secretions, normal protective mechanisms (*page 817*)

31. Any two of the following (*page 818*):
a. Gastritis
b. Stress
c. Aspirin ingestion
d. Alcoholism
e. Smoking
f. Chemotherapy, radiation
g. Endocrine factors
h. Familial tendency
i. Caffeine

32. Any two of the following (*pages 819–821*):
a. Alteration in nutrition, less than body requirements
b. Potential for fluid deficits related to upper GI bleeding
c. Anxiety/fear

33. Portal, 33 (*page 821*)

34. Any two of the following (*page 823*):
a. Lavage
b. Pitressin intravenously
c. Fluid and blood loss replacement
d. Tubes such as the Sengstaten-Blakemore

35. Any four of the following (*page 825*):
a. Perforated appendix
b. Perforated peptic ulcer
c. Perforated gall bladder
d. Perforated diverticulum
e. Diverticulitis
f. Foreign body perforation
g. Abdominal trauma
h. Ruptured ectopic pregnancy
i. Bowel obstruction
j. Ruptured abdominal aortic aneurysm
k. Bowel infarct

36. Any three of the following (*pages 827, 828*):
a. Potential for infection
b. Alteration in nutrition, less than body requirements
c. Fluid volume deficit
d. Alteration in comfort
e. Anxiety/fear

37. Whipple (*page 828*)

38. Any two of the following (*page 829*):
a. Smoking
b. Heavy alcohol consumption
c. Heavy fat consumption
d. Gall bladder disease
e. Bile duct disease

39. Any three of these (*pages 830–832*):
a. Potential for infection
b. Alteration in nutrition, less than body requirements
c. Impaired skin integrity
d. Potential for impaired gas exchange, altered breathing pattern
e. Anxiety/fear
f. Powerlessness
g. Grieving
h. Fluid volume deficit
i. Alteration in comfort

E. Summary of Patient Health Problems

Refer to the following pages in the Core Curriculum

---

1. Acute Pancreatitis (*pages 774–781*)
2. Acute Hepatitis (*pages 781–783*)
3. Cirrhosis of the Liver (*pages 783–790*)
4. Hepatic Failure (*pages 790–792*)
5. Ulcerative Colitis (*pages 792–794*)
6. Regional Enteritis (*pages 794–797*)
7. Toxic Megacolon (*pages 797–799*)
8. Bowel Infarction (*pages 799–803*)
9. Abdominal Trauma (*pages 803–809*)
10. Esophageal Carcinoma (*pages 809–812*)
11. Gastric Carcinoma (*pages 812–815*)
12. Carcinoma of the Colon (*pages 815–817*)
13. Peptic Ulcers (*pages 817–821*)
14. Esophageal Varices (*pages 821–825*)
15. Acute Abdomen (*pages 825–828*)
16. Pancreatic Cancer (*pages 828–832*)

THE GASTROINTESTINAL SYSTEM

Post Quiz

The following questions are designed to test understanding of some of the key points in the section. Select the one best answer for each. The correct answers are at the end of the test.

1. The most difficult portion of the stomach to visualize during endoscopy is the
   a. fundus
   b. body
   c. antrum
   d. cardiac sphincter
2. The substance secreted by chief cells in the stomach that participates in protein digestion is
   a. gastric acid
   b. pepsinogen
   c. peptidase
   d. amylase
3. Factors that accelerate gastric emptying include
   a. presence of large amounts of fat in gastric contents
   b. pain or depression
   c. hormones from the duodenum
   d. increased gastric volume
4. Which substance is secreted in the cephalic and gastric phases of gastrin secretion?
   a. gastric acid from the parietal cells
   b. pepsinogen from the chief cells
   c. mucus from the mucous glands
   d. intrinsic factor from the parietal cells
5. The most useful aspect of the evaluation of the location of the bleed in patients with bleeding peptic ulcers is
   a. the history
   b. the physical examination
   c. a barium enema
   d. endoscopy
6. Absorption of nutrients in the small intestine involves
   a. the passive diffusion of proteins and glucose
   b. the active transport of water
   c. the use of bile salts for absorption of fat-soluble vitamins
   d. the use of 1,25-dehydroxycholecalciferol for iron uptake
7. An example of a basic sugar is
   a. galactose
   b. sucrose
   c. lactose
   d. maltose
8. The gastrointestinal hormone that stimulates insulin release is
   a. secretin
   b. gastric-inhibiting polypeptide
   c. cholecystokinin
   d. gastrin
9. Factors that inhibit colonic motility include
   a. lactulose
   b. increased osmolality of the colon contents

c. the presence of bile salts in the colon
d. anticholinergic drugs

10. The functions of the large intestine include
a. absorption of most of the nutrients
b. secretion of sodium and chloride
c. cellulose breakdown and vitamin synthesis by bacteria
d. breakdown of ammonia into urea

11. The exocrine functions of the pancreas include
a. the release of insulin from the Islets of Langerhans
b. the secretion of a relatively acidic colorless fluid
c. an increase in secretion of digestive fluid in response to secretin
d. a decrease in secretion of digestive fluid in response to vagal stimuli

12. Bile is a substance that
a. is produced by the gall bladder
b. is responsible for the formation of fats into micelles
c. is lost in the feces because little is reabsorbed
d. is deconjugated into indirect bilirubin by the liver

13. The functions of the liver include
a. bile secretion by Kupffer cells
b. phagocytosis by hepatocytes
c. elimination of electrolytes
d. formation of urea from ammonia

14. Auscultation of the abdomen
a. should be performed after palpation
b. is best done with the bell of the stethoscope
c. should reveal a fairly continuous succession of clicking and bubbling sounds
d. is only done to evaluate bowel sounds

15. When percussing the abdomen, it should be remembered that tympanic notes are only normally heard
a. over an empty stomach
b. over the liver
c. over the spleen during expiration
d. over a full bladder

16. When palpating the liver in a patient with advanced cirrhosis, the findings include
a. rebound tenderness
b. an enlarged, soft, painful mass
c. an enlarged, painless mass
d. an enlarged, soft mass

17. Hepatitis B is more likely than hepatitis A to
a. be transmitted by fecal means
b. have an abrupt onset
c. affect all age groups
d. cause a positive in serum anti-HAV test

18. A diagnostic study that is relatively contraindicated in acute pancreatitis is
a. abdominal ultrasound
b. CT scan
c. endoscopy
d. chest x-ray

19. Severe hepatic failure is most likely to be associated with
a. decreased ammonia levels
b. increased serum colloid osmotic pressure
c. diffuse slowing of the EEG
d. low prothrombin time

20. Which of the following is least likely to be associated with the development of peptic ulcers?
    a. coffee
    b. alcohol
    c. aspirin
    d. acetaminophen
21. Positive Trousseau's sign in a patient with acute pancreatitis is suggestive of
    a. hyperglycemia
    b. hypoglycemia
    c. hypercalcemia
    d. hypocalcemia
22. Intensive care nurses are being advised to get the hepatitis A vaccine because of their association with
    a. patients admitted with acute hepatitis
    b. contact with potentially contaminated blood products
    c. contact with contaminated water
    d. contact with contaminated food
23. Consequences of cirrhosis of the liver may include
    a. thrombotic events
    b. decreased capillary permeability
    c. increased colloid osmotic pressure
    d. gynemastia
24. Methods used to decrease serum ammonia levels in patients with hepatic failure include
    a. high-protein diets
    b. use of narcotics and sedatives
    c. lactulose or neomycin
    d. maintaining dehydrated states
25. The most helpful laboratory test for the diagnosis of acute pancreatitis is the serum
    a. bilirubin
    b. amylase
    c. acid-phosphatase
    d. SGOT
26. Factors that can contribute to the development of toxic megacolon include
    a. a history of carcinoma of the colon
    b. anticholinergic agents or opiates
    c. hyperkalemia
    d. intestinal decompression
27. Bowel infarction or an acute abdomen may be difficult to diagnose in patients receiving paralyzing agents except for the presence of
    a. abdomen rigidity
    b. verbalization of abdominal pain
    c. hyperresonance to percussion
    d. hepatosplenomegaly
28. Laboratory findings in bowel infarction may include
    a. leukocytosis and hyperphosphatemia
    b. hyperphosphatemia and hypo-osmolality
    c. hypophosphatemia and hyperosmolality
    d. anemia and hyperphosphatemia
29. The normal amount of secretions released into the gastrointestinal tract every 24 hours is about
    a. 100–1000 cc
    b. 2000–4000 cc

c. 4000–8000 cc
d. 10,000–20,000 cc

30. Which of the following clinical manifestations is *least* likely to occur in hepatic cirrhosis?
    a. bleeding tendencies
    b. hypovolemia
    c. alterations in nutrition
    d. hyperkalemia

Answers to Gastrointestinal Post Quiz

1. **a** (*page 751*)
2. **b** (*page 752*)
3. **d** (*page 752*)
4. **a** (*page 752*)
5. **d** (*page 819*)
6. **c** (*page 755*)
7. **a** (*page 756*)
8. **b** (*page 759*)
9. **d** (*pages 757–758*)
10. **c** (*page 758*)
11. **c** (*pages 761–762*)
12. **b** (*page 763*)
13. **d** (*pages 764–765*)
14. **c** (*page 767*)
15. **a** (*page 768*)
16. **c** (*page 768*)
17. **c** (*pages 781–782*)
18. **c** (*pages 786–791*)
19. **c** (*pages 786, 791*)
20. **d** (*page 818*)
21. **d** (*page 779*)
22. **b** (*page 781*)
23. **d** (*pages 784–786*)
24. **c** (*pages 791, 792*)
25. **b** (*page 776*)
26. **b** (*pages 797–798*)
27. **c** (*pages 799–800, 825–826*)
28. **c** (*page 800*)
29. **c** (*pages 748–757*)
30. **d** (*pages 786–790*)

These are primarily the comprehend or recall, and apply or analyze levels of questions. Examples of synthesis or evaluate questions can be found in the comprehensive examination at the end of the book on pages 278 to 293.

8

Psychosocial Aspects

SECTION-RELATED TIPS FOR THOSE STUDYING TO TAKE THE CERTIFICATION EXAMINATION

Since 1985, the Certification Blueprint has not included a separate section on psychologic aspects. Instead, it has been based on a more holistic module. In other words, when a question is asked about the psychosocial aspects of care of a patient with a myocardial infarction, it counts as a cardiovascular question. This keeps the examination focused on the elements of psychosocial care more relevant to critical care nursing. They are well addressed in this chapter of the *Core Curriculum*.

The topic of psychosocial aspects of critical care is unique, and the content in this section is not subject to the same types of figures, diagrams, and exercises used to demonstrate concepts in the previous seven systems-oriented sections. The brevity of this part of the *Study Guide* is solely a reflection of this difference.

PSYCHOSOCIAL ASPECTS

Exercises

After reading the section on Psychosocial Implications in the Core Curriculum, *fill in the blanks or select the best alternative offered for the following statements. The answers are at the end of the exercises.*

A. Psychosocial Aspects (*pages 836–900*)

1. The perceptions of two people experiencing the same event are often ____________________.
2. Behavior is usually consistent with individuals' ____________________, an internalized perception of their unique characteristics.
3. The way individuals feel about their self-concept determines their level of self- ____________________.
4. List Maslow's five levels of human needs, beginning with the lowest and ending with the highest.
   a. ____________________
   b. ____________________
   c. ____________________
   d. ____________________
   e. ____________________
5. A better self-concept will result from focusing on ____________________ rather than ____________________.
6. The possible consequence of not developing the appropriate skills of one life stage is difficulty in ____________________.

7. Name and describe Selye's two types of stress.
   a. ______________________
   b. ______________________
8. It is (possible/impossible) for distress to lead to personal growth.
9. When distress is prolonged and inadequately met, the next psychologic step that may develop is ______________________.
10. The elements incorporated into most authorities' definitions of pain are
    a. ______________________
    b. ______________________
    c. ______________________
11. Pain is best identified by (the person experiencing it/a bystander).
12. Interpersonal communication (can/cannot) be avoided whenever two people meet.
13. Patients in critical care sometimes incorporate monitors and other devices into their ______________________.
14. Comparing sexuality in a 20-year-old and a 70-year-old patient, the concerns of the 70-year-old are ______________________ important and are more likely to be about ______________________.
15. When a patient is critically ill, family dynamics are altered in that the patient's family role is often ______________________.
16. The stressors inherent in the critical care environment can cause dysfunctional behavior in the ______________________, ______________________, and ______________________.
17. A crisis usually lasts a few ______________________.
18. The two general types of crisis are
    a. ______________________
    b. ______________________
19. List Fink's four phases of crisis.
    a. ______________________
    b. ______________________
    c. ______________________
    d. ______________________
20. The psychophysiologic symptoms of fear and anxiety are (essentially the same/distinctly different).
21. Confusion or even hallucinations in critically ill patients can result from feelings of ______________________ or ______________________, and from sensory ______________________ or ______________________.
22. Patients' feelings of ______________________ can be diminished by facilitating their sense of relatedness to body, psyche, significant other, familiar events, or the nurses.
23. Patients' feelings of ______________________ can be diminished by facilitating their beliefs that their behavior can make a difference in resulting outcomes.
24. ______________________ refers to the level of stimuli present in most critical care units that exposes all who are in the environment to the risk of feeling confused, restless, agitated, or angry.
25. The opposite of sensory overload is ______________________, which connotes a lack of a variety of meaningful and familiar input.
26. A person is ______________________ to something when it is inappropriately perceived as essential for self-maintenance and completeness.
27. (Most/Few) people at one time or another have entertained the possibility of suicide in response to perceived overwhelming threats.

28. The acute suicidal period usually lasts a few ________________ during which the individual (usually/never) gives hints to others about what is being considered.
29. The two types of burdens imposed on a dying patient are ________________ and ________________.
30. List Kübler-Ross' five stages of the dying process.
    a. ________________
    b. ________________
    c. ________________
    d. ________________
    e. ________________
31. Two primary mechanisms used to help cope with the process of dying are ________________ and ________________.
32. The differential diagnosis for psychologic causes of the nursing diagnosis of anxiety/fear in ICU patients includes:
    a. ________________
    b. ________________
    c. ________________
33. The differential diagnosis for psychologic causes of the confusion in an ICU patient includes:
    a. ________________
    b. ________________
    c. ________________

B. Summary of Psychosocial Aspects of Critical Care Nursing (*pages 836–899*)

1. Perception

Definition or Description:	*Key Aspects of Nursing History and Examination:*

Nursing Diagnosis of Sensory-Perceptual Alterations

Defining Characteristics	*Expected Outcome*	*Nursing Interventions*	*Evaluation of Nursing Care*

2. Self-Concept

Definition or Description:	*Key Aspects of Nursing History and Examination:*

Nursing Diagnosis of Self-Concept, Disturbance

Defining Characteristics	*Expected Outcome*	*Nursing Interventions*	*Evaluation of Nursing Care*

3. Self-Esteem

Definition or Description:	*Key Aspects of Nursing History and Examination:*

Nursing Diagnosis of Self-Concept, Disturbance in Self-Esteem

Defining Characteristics	*Expected Outcome*	*Nursing Interventions*	*Evaluation of Nursing Care*

4. Needs

Definition or Description:	*Key Aspects of Nursing History and Examination:*

Nursing Diagnosis of Need Disturbance

Defining Characteristics	*Expected Outcome*	*Nursing Interventions*	*Evaluation of Nursing Care*

5. Strengths, Potentials, Limitations

Definition or Description:	*Key Aspects of Nursing History and Examination:*

Nursing Diagnosis of Disturbance in Perception, Self-Concept, Self-Esteem, or Needs

Defining Characteristics	*Expected Outcome*	*Nursing Interventions*	*Evaluation of Nursing Care*

6. Growth and Development Patterns

Definition or Description:	*Key Aspects of Nursing History and Examination:*

Nursing Diagnosis of Growth and Development, Altered

Defining Characteristics	*Expected Outcome*	*Nursing Interventions*	*Evaluation of Nursing Care*

7. Stress

Definition or Description:	*Key Aspects of Nursing History and Examination:*

Nursing Diagnosis of Stress Level, Alteration

Defining Characteristics	*Expected Outcome*	*Nursing Interventions*	*Evaluation of Nursing Care*

8. Pain

Definition or Description:	*Key Aspects of Nursing History and Examination:*

Nursing Diagnosis of Comfort, Altered: Pain

Defining Characteristics	*Expected Outcome*	*Nursing Interventions*	*Evaluation of Nursing Care*

9. Interpersonal Communication

Definition or Description:	*Key Aspects of Nursing History and Examination:*

Nursing Diagnosis of Communication, Impaired

Defining Characteristics	*Expected Outcome*	*Nursing Interventions*	*Evaluation of Nursing Care*

10. Body Image

Definition or Description:	*Key Aspects of Nursing History and Examination:*

Nursing Diagnosis of Self-Concept, Disturbance in: Body Image

Defining Characteristics	*Expected Outcome*	*Nursing Interventions*	*Evaluation of Nursing Care*

11. Human Sexuality

Definition or Description:	*Key Aspects of Nursing History and Examination:*

Nursing Diagnosis of Human Sexuality: Altered Patterns

Defining Characteristics	*Expected Outcome*	*Nursing Interventions*	*Evaluation of Nursing Care*

12. Family

Definition or Description:	*Key Aspects of Nursing History and Examination:*

Nursing Diagnosis of Family Processes, Altered

Defining Characteristics	*Expected Outcome*	*Nursing Interventions*	*Evaluation of Nursing Care*

13. Critical Care Environment

Definition or Description:	*Key Aspects of Nursing History and Examination:*

Nursing Diagnosis of Impact of Critical Care Environment, Disturbance

Defining Characteristics	*Expected Outcome*	*Nursing Interventions*	*Evaluation of Nursing Care*

14. Crisis

Definition or Description:	*Key Aspects of Nursing History and Examination:*

Nursing Diagnosis of Crisis, Altered Response to Stress

Defining Characteristics	*Expected Outcome*	*Nursing Interventions*	*Evaluation of Nursing Care*

15. Fear and Anxiety

Definition or Description:	*Key Aspects of Nursing History and Examination:*

Nursing Diagnosis of Fear/Anxiety

Defining Characteristics	*Expected Outcome*	*Nursing Interventions*	*Evaluation of Nursing Care*

16. Loneliness

Definition or Description:	*Key Aspects of Nursing History and Examination:*

Nursing Diagnosis of Loneliness, Sense of Alienation

Defining Characteristics	*Expected Outcome*	*Nursing Interventions*	*Evaluation of Nursing Care*

17. Powerlessness

Definition or Description:	*Key Aspects of Nursing History and Examination:*

Nursing Diagnosis of Powerlessness

Defining Characteristics	*Expected Outcome*	*Nursing Interventions*	*Evaluation of Nursing Care*

18. Sensory Overload

Definition or Description:	*Key Aspects of Nursing History and Examination:*

Nursing Diagnosis of Sensory Overload

Defining Characteristics	*Expected Outcome*	*Nursing Interventions*	*Evaluation of Nursing Care*

19. Sensory Deprivation

Definition or Description:	*Key Aspects of Nursing History and Examination:*

Nursing Diagnosis of Sensory Deprivation

Defining Characteristics	*Expected Outcome*	*Nursing Interventions*	*Evaluation of Nursing Care*

20. Addictions

Definition or Description:	*Key Aspects of Nursing History and Examination:*

Nursing Diagnosis of Addiction

Defining Characteristics	*Expected Outcome*	*Nursing Interventions*	*Evaluation of Nursing Care*

21. Suicidal Phenomenon

Definition or Description:	*Key Aspects of Nursing History and Examination:*

Nursing Diagnosis of Suicidal Behavior

Defining Characteristics	*Expected Outcome*	*Nursing Interventions*	*Evaluation of Nursing Care*

22. Dying Process and Death

Definition or Description:	*Key Aspects of Nursing History and Examination:*

Nursing Diagnosis of Dying Process—Death

Defining Characteristics	*Expected Outcome*	*Nursing Interventions*	*Evaluation of Nursing Care*

C. Nurses Coping with Critical Care

1. In the space provided, identify these aspects of your current practice. Find a quiet place and spend about 10 minutes thinking about each one before you write anything.

   a. Identify your reasons for choosing the critical care setting for practice.

   b. Identify your strengths as a critical care nurse.

   c. Identify your professional potentials or goals.

   d. Identify your limitations as a critical care nurse.

   e. Identify the effect critical care nursing is having on you currently.

2. Reread each of the following sections of this chapter and then describe how you see them from a personal perspective. Find a quiet place and spend at least 10 minutes thinking about each one before you write anything.

   a. Your self-concept

   b. Your level of self-esteem

c. Your highest priority needs

d. Your strengths, potentials, limitations

e. Your interpersonal communications style and ability

f. Your body image

g. Your human sexuality

h. Your attitudes toward the dying process and death

3. Repeat Exercises 1 and 2 every year or so. Keep track of trends in these perceptions.

D. Application to Clinical Practice

Care for patients with specific psychosocial problems. Relate the manifestations found in this section to their individual clinical pictures. Make note of instances where they correlate and those where they deviate. Devise a care plan based on the data collected.

Answers to Psychosocial Aspects Exercises

A. Psychosocial Aspects

1. Different or unique (*page 836*)
2. Self-concept (*page 839*)
3. Esteem (*page 841*)
4. a. Physiologic
   b. Safety and security
   c. Love and belonging
   d. Self-esteem
   e. Self-actualization (*pages 843–844*)
5. Strengths or potentials, limitations or weaknesses (*page 847*)
6. Mastering skills of subsequent stages (*page 849*)
7. a. Distress—condition resulting from noxious stimuli
   b. Eustress—condition resulting from nonthreatening stimuli (*page 851*)
8. Possible (*page 851*)
9. Crisis (*page 852*)
10. a. There is a breakdown in the protective barrier.
    b. It is perceived as a danger signal.
    c. It is reflective of all previous painful experiences. (*page 854*)
11. The person experiencing it (*page 855*)
12. Cannot (*page 857*)
13. Body image (*page 860*)
14. As, being accepted as a sexual being (*page 863*)
15. Assumed by other members (*page 866*)
16. Patients, family, staff (*page 868*)
17. Weeks (*page 871*)
18. Situational, maturational (*page 871*)
19. a. Shock
    b. Defensive retreat
    c. Acknowledgment
    d. Adaptation and change (*page 871*)
20. Essentially the same (*pages 874, 881–886*)
21. Fear, anxiety, overload, deprivation (*page 874*)
22. Loneliness (*pages 876–877*)
23. Powerlessness (*pages 879–880*)
24. Sensory overload (*pages 881–882*)
25. Sensory deprivation (*page 885*)
26. Addicted (*page 887*)
27. Most (*page 890*)
28. Hours to days, usually (*page 891*)
29. Intrapsychic and interpersonal (*page 893*)
30. a. Denial or isolation
    b. Anger, rage, envy, or resentment
    c. Bargaining
    d. Depression
    e. Acceptance (*page 894*)
31. Denial, hope (*page 894*)
32. Any three of these:
    a. Self-concept, disturbance
    b. Need disturbance
    c. Stress level, alteration
    d. Comfort, altered: Pain
    e. Human sexuality, altered patterns
    f. Family processes, altered
    g. Psychosocial impact of the critical care environment, disturbance
    h. Powerlessness
    i. Sensory overload
    j. Sensory deprivation
    k. Addiction
    l. Dying process, grieving (*pages 838–899*)
33. Any three of these:
    a. Sensory-perceptual alterations
    b. Stress level, alteration
    c. Psychosocial impact of the critical care environment, disturbance
    d. Crisis, altered response to stress
    e. Sensory overload
    f. Sensory deprivation
    g. Addiction (*pages 836–890*)

B. Summary of Psychosocial Aspects

Refer to these pages in the Core Curriculum

1. Perception (*pages 836–838*)
2. Self-Concept (*pages 838–841*)
3. Self-Esteem (*pages 841–843*)
4. Needs (*pages 843–846*)
5. Strengths, Potentials, Limitations (*pages 846–849*)
6. Growth and Development Patterns (*pages 849–851*)
7. Stress (*pages 851–854*)
8. Pain (*pages 854–857*)
9. Interpersonal Communication (*pages 857–860*)
10. Body Image (*pages 860–862*)
11. Human Sexuality (*pages 862–865*)
12. Family (*pages 865–868*)
13. Critical Care Environment (*pages 868–871*)
14. Crisis (*pages 871–874*)

THE PSYCHOSOCIAL ASPECTS SECTION

Post Quiz

The following questions are designed to test understanding of some of the key points in this section. Select the one best answer for each. The correct answers are at the end of the test.

1. The manner in which all stimuli are experienced is called
   a. perception
   b. valuing
   c. communication
   d. sensory overload
2. The *feelings* a person has about his/her personal characteristics are called
   a. self-concept
   b. self-esteem
   c. body image
   d. validation
3. A prolonged period of overwhelming stress that results in difficulty coping is called
   a. fear
   b. anxiety
   c. disequilibrium
   d. crisis
4. Suicidal thoughts during periods of severe stress are
   a. very uncommon
   b. often ambivalent
   c. confined to specific demographic subsets
   d. a sign of mental illness
5. Patients who are addicted to chemical substances
   a. are not coping adaptively
   b. are rarely concerned with how others view them
   c. are not easily threatened
   d. are usually growing and developing
6. People's self-concepts
   a. are consistent with what others really think of them
   b. are usually not concerned with internal consistency
   c. do not have an important impact on behavior
   d. are not easily changed, especially during threatening events
7. The highest level in Maslow's hierarchy of human needs is
   a. safety and security
   b. physiologic
   c. self-actualization
   d. self-esteem
8. Threats to feelings of meaning most directly affect the patient's need for
   a. safety and security

b. love and belonging
c. self-actualization
d. self-esteem

9. The condition Selye refers to as "distress"
a. is a universal reaction to any given stimuli
b. is a motivating factor
c. usually becomes a crisis
d. cannot ultimately result in increased self-esteem

10. The perception of pain
a. is unaltered from birth
b. can only be properly assessed by a bystander
c. is a purely physiologic phenomenon
d. can be diminished by psychologic interventions

11. Human sexuality
a. is primarily a physiologic phenomenon
b. is only present a relatively small portion of a life span
c. is heavily impacted by a person's self-concept
d. is dormant during periods of physiologic stress

12. Depression is most likely to occur during the stage of crisis that Fink refers to as
a. shock
b. defensive retreat
c. acknowledgment
d. adaptation

13. Feelings of fear and anxiety
a. trigger only maladaptive physiologic responses
b. are not easily distinguished from each other
c. result in sleeplessness, which allows more time for better coping
d. are difficult for an individual to recognize

14. In her stages of the dying process, Kübler-Ross uses the statement "what's the use" to describe the feelings associated with the stage of
a. anger and resentment
b. denial or isolation
c. depression
d. acceptance

15. Dying patients often use denial and hope
a. when they reach the stage of acceptance
b. but should be actively discouraged from using either
c. only to help their family members cope
d. to help control the grieving process

Answers to Psychosocial Implications Post Quiz

1. **a** (*page 836*)
2. **b** (*page 838*)
3. **d** (*page 871*)
4. **b** (*page 890*)
5. **a** (*pages 887–888*)
6. **d** (*page 839*)
7. **c** (*page 844*)
8. **c** (*page 845*)
9. **b** (*page 851*)
10. **d** (*pages 854, 855*)
11. **c** (*pages 862, 863*)
12. **c** (*page 871*)
13. **b** (*page 874*)
14. **c** (*page 894*)
15. **d** (*pages 894, 895*)

9

Legal and Ethical Aspects of Critical Care Nursing

SECTION-RELATED TIPS FOR THOSE STUDYING TO TAKE THE CERTIFICATION EXAMINATION

Many aspects of a person's ethical code are universal, clear-cut, and not subject to controversy. Those aspects that vary from person to person, depending on cultural background, previous experience, religion, beliefs, and values, are subject to much debate without consensus on what is right or wrong. The latter type is difficult to incorporate into multiple-choice questions with one right answer. Similarly, the laws affecting nursing practice may vary from state to state, from year to year, and the interpretation of the law is subject to much debate. Accordingly, as of 1992 the legal/ethical questions are being deleted from the certification examination.

For both legal and ethical issues, it is useful to be comfortable with standards and definitions of terms. Many are included in this chapter. The American Hospital Association's "Patient's Bill of Rights" and the American Nursing Association's "Code of Ethics" are contained in this section of the *Core Curriculum* and are worth reviewing.

LEGAL AND ETHICAL ASPECTS

Exercises

After reading the chapter on "Legal and Ethical Aspects of Critical Care Nursing" of the Core Curriculum, *fill in the blanks in the following statements. It can be done one topic at a time or all at once. The answers are at the end of the exercises.*

A. Legal Aspects of Critical Care Nursing (*pages 905–912*)

1. The four sources of law are:
   a. ____________________
   b. ____________________
   c. ____________________
   d. ____________________
2. Sources of Standards of Care for the Critically Ill include:
   a. ____________________
   b. ____________________
   c. ____________________
   d. ____________________
   e. ____________________

3. The main objectives of the CCRN certification program are to:
   a. ____________________
   b. ____________________
   c. ____________________
4. Documentation requirements come from the following sources:
   a. ____________________
   b. ____________________
   c. ____________________
   d. ____________________
   e. ____________________
5. The three requisites to informed consent are:
   a. ____________________
   b. ____________________
   c. ____________________
6. The Uniform Determination of Death Act defines brain death as either ____________________ or ____________________.
7. The obligation to declare a brain-dead patient dead (does/does not) require the family's consent.
8. The two types of advanced directives are ____________________ and ____________________.
9. The federal law since 12/1/91 (requires/recommends) that all hospitals must ask patients on admission whether they have or know about advanced directives in order to qualify for medicare or medicaid reimbursement.
10. The acts enacted by states to provide immunity from liability to persons who provide emergency care at an accident scene are called ____________________.
11. The four elements of professional liability include:
    a. ____________________
    b. ____________________
    c. ____________________
    d. ____________________
12. ____________________ is the improper performance of professional duties that results in injury to another.

B. Ethical Aspects of Critical Care Nursing (*pages 912–926*)

1. ____________________ is the ethical principle that refers to patient self-determination and freedom of choice.
2. ____________________ is the ethical principle that refers to what is just, fair, or right.
3. ____________________ is the ethical principle that refers to honesty, integrity, or truth-telling.
4. ____________________ is the ethical principle that refers to keeping professional promises or obligations to patients.
5. ____________________ is an ethical theory that states that the right thing to do is the act that produces the greatest good for the most people.
6. ____________________ is an ethical approach that states that beneficence should supercede autonomy in some instances.
7. The three types of justice are:
   a. ____________________
   b. ____________________
   c. ____________________

8. List three nursing qualities described in the American Nursing Association's "Code of Ethics."
   a. ______________________
   b. ______________________
   c. ______________________
9. List three rights of patients described in the American Hospital Association's "Patient's Bill of Rights."
   a. ______________________
   b. ______________________
   c. ______________________
10. List three duties described in the American Association of Critical Care Nurses' (AACN's) "Position Statement on the Role of the Critical Care Nurse as Patient Advocate."
   a. ______________________
   b. ______________________
   c. ______________________
11. Withdrawal of medical care (does/does not) require withdrawal of nursing care.
12. A nurse (may/may not) morally refuse to participate in withdrawing or withholding therapy.
13. Nurses may reject a patient care assignment provided that they:
   a. ______________________
   b. ______________________
   c. ______________________
   d. ______________________
14. The three duties of the critical care nurse defined in the AACN's "Position Statement on the Clarification of Resuscitation Status in the Critical Care Setting" are:
   a. ______________________
   b. ______________________
   c. ______________________
15. The 1991 Joint Commission for Accreditation of Hospitals Organization (JCAHO) Standards (require/recommend) that institutions have a mechanism for all health care employees to have their ethical questions addressed.
16. The ______________________ grants sound individuals over the age of 18 the right to give all or part of their bodies upon death.
17. The sale of organs after a donor's death is forbidden by ______________________, not by ______________________.
18. According to an ANA position statement, nurses have the moral obligation to provide care to an AIDS patient whenever:
   a. ______________________
   b. ______________________
   c. ______________________
19. List three examples of different types of patient care where ethical dilemmas may arise.
   a. ______________________
   b. ______________________
   c. ______________________

C. Application to Clinical Practice

Care for patients with legal or ethical dilemmas. Relate the discussion and guidelines in this section to the patient's scenario. Devise a care plan based on these recommendations. Identify areas where issues were approached optimally and where they may have been improved.

Answers to Legal and Ethical Aspects Exercises

A. Legal Aspects of Critical Care Nursing

1. a. The Constitution
   b. Common law
   c. Statutory law
   d. Administrative law (*page 905*)
2. a. AACN Standards of Care for the Critically Ill
   b. ANA Standards
   c. Community or regional standards
   d. Hospital standards
   e. Unit standards/policies/procedures (*page 906*)
3. a. Establish the common body of knowledge necessary
   b. Test this body of knowledge needed to function effectively
   c. Recognize professional competence by granting CCRN status (*pages 906, 907*)
4. a. Federal requirements
   b. National voluntary requirements (JCACHO)
   c. State requirements
   d. Community standards
   e. Hospital requirements (*pages 907, 908*)
5. a. The patient must have decision-making capacity or substituted judgment doctrine is evoked.
   b. The decision must be made voluntarily without coercion.
   c. The patient must understand the risks and benefits involved. (*pages 908–909*)
6. Irreversible cessation of circulatory and respiratory function, or irreversible cessation of all functions of the entire brain, including the brainstem (*pages 909, 910*)
7. Does not (*page 910*)
8. Treatment directive, durable power of attorney (*page 911*)
9. Requires (Self Determination Act was passed after this chapter of the *Core* was written.)
10. Good Samaritan Acts (*page 911*)
11. a. Duty
    b. Breach
    c. Proximate cause
    d. Damages (*page 912*)
12. Malpractice (*page 912*)

B. Ethical Aspects of Critical Care Nursing

1. Patient autonomy (*page 912*)
2. Justice (*page 912*)
3. Veracity (*page 912*)
4. Fidelity (*page 912*)
5. Utilitarianism (*page 913*)
6. Paternalism (*page 913*)
7. a. Distributive
   b. Retributive
   c. Procedural (*page 913*)
8. Any three of these (*page 914*):
   a. Provides care with respect for patient dignity
   b. Provides care with respect for patient privacy
   c. Safeguards patients from incompetent, unethical, or illegal care practices
   d. Assumes responsibility and accountability for actions
   e. Maintains competence
   f. Competently seeks consultation, accepts responsibilities, and delegates activities
   g. Contributes to the development of the professional body of knowledge
   h. Participates in efforts to implement and improve standards
   i. Participates in efforts to maintain conditions of employment conducive to quality care
   j. Participates in efforts to maintain integrity of nursing
   k. Collaborates with colleagues and community to meet health care needs of the public
9. Any three of these (*pages 914–915*):
   a. To considerate and respectful care
   b. To information regarding diagnosis, treatment and prognosis
   c. To give informed consent for procedures
   d. To refuse treatment
   e. To privacy
   f. To confidentiality
   g. To a reasonable response to requests
   h. To information regarding the relationship between this hospital and others in terms of their care
   i. To refuse to participate in research
   j. To continuity of care
   k. To examine and question the bill

   l. To know relevant hospital rules and regulations
10. Any three of these (*page 916*):
   a. Support patient's right to autonomous, informed decision-making
   b. Intervene when the patient's best interests are in question
   c. Assist patients to obtain necessary care
   d. Respect patients' values, beliefs, and rights
   e. Assist patients as surrogates in decision-making through education and support
   f. Represent patients in accordance with their choice
   g. Support patients as surrogates in decision to transfer care to an equally qualified nurse
   h. Intercede for patients who cannot speak for themselves in situations requiring immediate action and act as liaison between patient, family, and health care providers
11. Does not (*page 917*)
12. May (*page 917*)
13. a. Understand the potential consequences
   b. Document concerns for patient safety
   c. Document how management was informed
   d. Use long-term strategies to prevent recurrence (*page 917*)
14. a. Ensure quality care regardless of resuscitation status
   b. Review resuscitation status clearly with the patient's physician
   c. Reflect the patient's resuscitation status in the plan of care (*page 918*)
15. Require (Published after this chapter of the *Core* was written.)
16. Uniform Anatomical Gift Act (*page 921*)
17. Ethical standards, law (*page 922*)
18. a. The patient is at significant risk if care is not given
   b. The nurse's intervention is directly related to preventing harm
   c. Patient gains outweigh any harm the nurse might incur (*page 923*)
19. Any three of these, but there are many more not necessarily mentioned here in the *Core Curriculum* (*pages 924–926*):
   a. Withholding treatment
   b. Code vs no-code
   c. Right to die at home vs remaining in the hospital
   d. Technology vs cost
   e. Nutritional dilemmas (withdrawal of food and fluid)

LEGAL AND ETHICAL ASPECTS OF CRITICAL CARE NURSING

Post Quiz

The following questions are designed to test understanding of some of the key points in this section. Select the one best answer for each. The correct answers are at the end of the test.

1. Most states' Nurse Practice Acts are:
   a. designed to protect the nurse more than the consumer
   b. a good example of constitutional law
   c. overseen by boards of nursing
   d. a primary source of standards of care
2. The AACN's CCRN certification examination is designed to:
   a. determine which of three levels a nurse's clinical skills have reached
   b. test the defined body of knowledge needed to function competently in critical care
   c. document possession of advanced clinical practice
   d. decrease the level of expectations placed on the practicing nurse

3. Which of the following is *not* a component of informed consent?
   a. patients must be of decision-making capacity
   b. surrogates making decisions must act in the patient's best interest
   c. decisions must be voluntary
   d. patients must consult significant others
4. Accepted definitions of brain death include:
   a. irreversible cessation of circulatory and respiratory functions
   b. irreversible cessation of all functions of the brain except those of the brainstem
   c. irreversible coma with vegetative processes intact
   d. unsuccessful resuscitation attempts when the family consents to discontinuing efforts
5. Which of the following has *not* been established by the courts?
   a. The right to refuse treatment
   b. The right to information
   c. The right to self-determination
   d. The right to active euthanasia
6. A document in which a competent person designates someone else to act on his/her behalf should he/she lose decision-making capacity is called a
   a. Good Samaritan Act
   b. treatment directive
   c. durable power of attorney
   d. Uniform Anatomical Gift Act
7. Professional misconduct that results in harm to a patient is legally referred to as:
   a. proximate cause
   b. breach of duty
   c. malpractice
   d. nonmalfeasance
8. The ethical philosophy that states that beneficence should take precedence over patient autonomy is:
   a. nonmalfeasance
   b. consequentialism
   c. utilitarianism
   d. paternalism
9. The ANA's Code of Ethics for Nursing:
   a. was originally written by Florence Nightingale
   b. only defines responsibilities to individual patients
   c. addresses responsibilities to the profession and community as well as to patients
   d. is used in lieu of the AHA's Patient's Bill of Rights
10. One recommended role of the critical care nurse in research involves:
    a. determining which patients should be exposed to risk
    b. allowing some patients to be treated against their will
    c. withholding information from patients that may make them decide not to participate
    d. participate on Institutional Review Boards
11. The role of the nurse caring for hopelessly critically ill patients with no chance of survival includes:
    a. insisting on immediate transfer from the ICU
    b. participating in withdrawal and withholding of therapy no matter what their personal moral code or ethics dictate
    c. providing futile care to brain-dead patients as long as one family member insists
    d. ensuring that the patient is not abandoned

12. The role of the critical care nurse in care of the potential organ donor involves:
    a. facilitating decision-making in families of potential donors, especially when state laws mandate "required request"
    b. altering care to meet the recipient's best interest over the donor's
    c. not resuscitating patients in whom consent for organ donation has been obtained
    d. notification of the media to put pressure on families reluctant to consent
13. Recommendations concerning institutional ethics committees is that they
    a. consist only of nurses and physicians
    b. serve both to educate and to develop guidelines
    c. deal in generalities rather than specific issues
    d. concentrate on protecting the hospital's liability

Answers to the Legal and Ethical Aspects Post Quiz

1. **c** (*page 905*)
2. **b** (*pages 906–907*)
3. **d** (*pages 908–909*)
4. **a** (*pages 909–910*)
5. **d** (*pages 910–911*)
6. **c** (*page 911*)
7. **c** (*page 912*)
8. **d** (*pages 912–913*)
9. **c** (*pages 913–914*)
10. **d** (*pages 916–917*)
11. **d** (*page 917*)
12. **a** (*page 919*)
13. **b** (*pages 919–921*)

Comprehensive Examination

The following questions are meant to integrate the knowledge gained from studying the Core Curriculum *into patient situations. Select the one best response for each. The answers are at the end of the section.*

Mr. A arrived in the emergency room complaining of severe shortness of breath. He had a history of chronic obstructive pulmonary disease. The initial findings were:

BP = 130/88	HR = 110/min	Temp = 38^{5}°C	RR = 34/min
pO_2 = 38 mm Hg	pH = 7.26	pCO_2 = 76 mm Hg	HCO_3 = 34 mEq

1. The interventions indicated by the results above were
   a. high-dose oxygen and intermittent positive pressure ventilation
   b. low-flow oxygen and measures to increase ventilation
   c. mechanical ventilation without supplemental oxygen
   d. nothing until the patient has gone to radiology for a chest x-ray
2. If mechanical ventilation is required, an important principle to consider in these patients is that
   a. pressure-cycled ventilation is preferred over volume-cycled ventilation in such patients
   b. the goal is to return the arterial pCO_2 to 35–45 mm Hg
   c. the goal is to return the pH toward normal
   d. PEEP must be part of the therapy

Three days into an uneventful recovery period from multiple trauma, Mr. B developed restlessness and increasing dyspnea. His breath sounds had not changed but his chest x-ray showed marked diffuse infiltrates. There was no fever but his heart rate and respiratory rate had increased.

3. The complication most likely to be developing in this patient was
   a. pneumothorax
   b. flail chest
   c. lobar pneumonia
   d. adult respiratory distress syndrome
4. The expected early blood gas findings in this pathologic condition are
   a. hypoxemia, hypocapnia, and alkalemia
   b. hypoxemia, hypercapnia, and acidemia
   c. stable hypoxemia and acidemia
   d. a decreased A-a gradient and percent shunt
5. Treatment goals for Mr. B included a
   a. PA wedge pressure of 16–20 mm Hg
   b. paO_2 of 60 mm Hg
   c. fall in the mixed venous oxygen
   d. rise in the A-a gradient

Mrs. C was admitted to the CCU anxious, diaphoretic, and pale. She was known to have chronic myocardopathy. A pulmonary artery catheter was inserted. The following parameters were obtained:

HR = 92/min	RAP = 10 mm Hg	BP = 100/70 mm Hg
RR = 30/min	PAw = 36 mm Hg	CO = 2.5 L/min

Intravenous nitroglycerin and dobutamine were begun.

6. Desired hemodynamic outcomes from this combination therapy include
   a. increased preload and afterload
   b. decreased preload and increased contractility
   c. decreased contractility and heart rate
   d. venodilation and arterioconstriction
7. Morphine sulfate was ordered. Before administration it was most important to reassess Mrs. C's
   a. heart rate
   b. respiratory rate
   c. skin color
   d. breath sounds

Mr. D was brought to the emergency room with chest pain. The ECG showed an acute injury pattern. Thrombolytic therapy was immediately considered.

8. Which of the following findings would make thrombolysis contraindicated?
   a. a history of surgery last week
   b. extensive anterolateral wall involvement
   c. a history of an infarction 2 years ago
   d. a history of hypertension
9. Streptokinase was administered. During therapy it was important to
   a. draw frequent arterial blood gas samples
   b. be prepared for allergic reactions, which are an expected routine outcome
   c. hold all antihypertensive medications
   d. observe for ventricular irritability and bleeding tendencies
10. If thrombolysis was successful, future interventions for this specific lesion
   a. would not include coronary artery bypass graft (CABG)
   b. would not include percutaneous transluminal coronary angioplasty (PTCA)
   c. would not include either CABG or PTCA
   d. might have included either CABG or PTCA

Mr. E, a construction worker, was hit in the back by a swinging beam. He was admitted to the intensive care unit with areflexia and loss of sensory and motor function from the neck down. He maintained a normal level of consciousness. He was hypotensive but a normal blood pressure was established after fluid therapy.

11. The most likely cause of his symptoms was
   a. spinal shock
   b. anterior cord syndrome
   c. autonomic dysflexia
   d. cerebral contusion
12. The hypotension was probably due to
   a. preexisting dehydration
   b. stress
   c. blood loss into the injured central nervous system tissues
   d. vasodilation

Mrs. F underwent repair of an intracerebral aneurysm yesterday. Her symptoms were at a Grade II level both pre- and postoperatively. Suddenly, she became restless and complained of severe headache. Within minutes she lost consciousness. A dilated pupil and respiratory depression were also noted.

13. The immediate therapy for Mrs. F was to
    a. administer a calcium-channel antagonist
    b. lower the head of the bed
    c. increase ventilation
    d. administer diuretics
14. The most likely cause of her change in status was
    a. intracerebral hemorrhage
    b. vasospasm
    c. cytotoxic cerebral edema
    d. global ischemia

Mrs. G arrested 7 days postmyocardial infarction and after 1 hour of resuscitation was transferred back to the coronary care unit. Two days later her vital signs were stable without pharmacologic support and her neurologic status was improving. The one problem that persisted was oliguria, despite normal blood pressure and preloads.

Relevant laboratory data included a BUN of 52 mg%, a serum creatinine of 4.6 mg, and a urinary sodium of 40 mEq/L with moderate cells and casts.

15. The etiologic classification of Mrs. G's oliguria was most likely to be
    a. prerenal failure
    b. intrarenal cortical failure
    c. intrarenal medullary failure
    d. postrenal failure

Mrs. G's BUN and creatinine continued to rise, and her serum potassium and pulmonary artery wedge became elevated. She no longer responded to diuretic therapy. Continuous arteriovenous hemofiltration was instituted.

16. The main goal of this therapy was to
    a. eliminate waste products alone
    b. decrease the serum potassium and phosphorus quickly
    c. treat the cause of this type of failure
    d. slowly remove water and small-size molecules
17. Mrs. G gradually developed a metabolic acidosis, which was partly due to
    a. potassium shifting from the cells to the serum
    b. decreased elimination of waste products
    c. increased renal reabsorption of bicarbonate
    d. increased renal secretion of hydrogen ions

Mrs. H had a colon resection and remained hospitalized 3 weeks later primarily because of pulmonary complications. At that point, her respiratory and gastrointestinal status seemed stabilized but her serum sodium was 157 mEq/L. On physical examination, her weight had increased, her neck veins were distended, and she had dependent peripheral edema.

18. The most likely cause of Mrs. H's change in serum sodium was
    a. dumping or short-bowel syndrome
    b. excess osmotic diuresis
    c. third spacing
    d. excess sodium administration and retention

19. Other findings confirming this diagnosis were
    a. low urine and serum osmolality
    b. an increased BUN and hematocrit
    c. oliguria and a high urine osmolality
    d. hyperkalemia and a high serum osmolality
20. Treatment for this disorder involved
    a. gradual diuresis and less sodium intravenously
    b. concentrated saline solutions
    c. rapid infusion of dextrose in water
    d. rapid aggressive intervention to prevent cerebral edema

Mr. I was hospitalized for the induction phase of chemotherapy for inoperable oatcell carcinoma of the lung. After a few days he became confused. His serum osmolality was 258 mosm/L and his urine osmolality was 1220 mosm/L. He was oliguric but his BUN was not elevated. He had gained 2 kg since admission.

21. The most likely cause of Mr. I's confusion was
    a. diabetes insipidus
    b. syndrome of inappropriate ADH
    c. nephrotoxicity from chemotherapy
    d. hyperosmolar syndrome
22. Because Mr. I developed seizures, his treatment involved
    a. a water-loading test
    b. a water-deprivation test
    c. lasix and hypertonic saline solutions intravenously
    d. lithium and dextrose in water intravenously

Mr. J was involved in an automobile accident and sustained multiple fractures and pulmonary contusions. His history was negative except for idiopathic pericarditis 6 months ago, which resolved with steroid therapy. His recovery from his injuries was going well when he developed the following: Increasing weakness and fatigue, weight loss, Glucose = 90 mg, Serum Na = 132, Serum K = 6.2, BUN = 42.

23. The diagnosis was
    a. adrenal insufficiency
    b. thyrotoxic crisis
    c. syndrome of inappropriate ADH
    d. diabetic ketoacidosis
24. The complications that can occur from this condition include
    a. arrhythmias and hypotension
    b. hyperosmolar coma
    c. congestive heart failure and pulmonary edema
    d. type II diabetes mellitus
25. Mr. J's therapy included
    a. daily steroid therapy for the rest of his life
    b. short-term hydrocortisone therapy and saline solutions
    c. insulin and saline solutions
    d. multipituitary hormone replacement therapy

Mrs. K delivered a healthy infant after a traumatic childbirth but continued to bleed profusely postpartum. A diagnosis of disseminated intravascular coagulation was made and she was transferred to intensive care.

26. The laboratory data supporting this diagnosis included
    a. a low prothrombin time and fibrinogen levels
    b. the presence of shistocytes and increased fibrin split products
    c. a low platelet count and decreased thrombin time
    d. increased clotting factors
27. The most important part of Mrs. K's treatment after arrival in the intensive care unit was
    a. treating the cause or trigger of her coagulopathy
    b. replacement of vascular volume losses and treatment of hypotension
    c. heparin
    d. streptokinase

Mr. L came to the emergency room with severe, persistent abdominal pain radiating to the back, accompanied by nausea and fever. Significant history included chronic use of moderate amounts of alcohol and no recent trauma, surgery, or change in dietary habits.

28. Laboratory tests used to help diagnose the disorder include
    a. serum and urinary amylase levels
    b. SGOT, SGPT, and LDH
    c. serum calcium, glucose and albumin
    d. serum lipase and BUN
29. Tests used to help monitor for complications of this disorder include
    a. serum and urinary amylase levels
    b. endoscopy
    c. serum calcium, glucose, and albumin
    d. serum lipase and BUN

Mr. L's symptoms continued for several days. During that time he was NPO with a nasogastric tube to intermittent suction and he received meperidine for pain. On the seventh day, parenteral nutrition and peritoneal lavage were initiated.

30. Important nursing implications during this time included
    a. suggesting interlipids to add to the parenteral regimen
    b. monitoring closely for hyperglycemia and increasing abdominal girth
    c. suggesting morphine be used instead of meperidine for pain relief
    d. piggybacking a CVP monitor to the central alimentation line to assess the volume status

Mrs. M had chronic congestive heart failure for several years and was admitted to the hospital with pulmonary edema after she decided to stop taking her digitalis and furosemide. The edema resolved with the usual aggressive therapy of cardiotonic, vasodilating, and diuretic agents. Assessment the day of planned discharge from the CCU revealed severely diminished bowel sounds and abdominal distention.

31. Mrs. M's paralytic ileus was most likely related to the
    a. cardiotonic agents
    b. diuretics
    c. vasodilators
    d. mucosal edema
32. The laboratory test that confirmed this suspicion was a serum
    a. potassium
    b. sodium
    c. albumin
    d. alpha-1 level

Mr. N, despondent over a prolonged period of unemployment, overdosed on a combination of salicylates and tranquilizers. He was brought to the emergency room unconscious, areflexic, hypotensive, and bradypneic. His arterial blood gases on admission were: pH = 7.55, pCO_2 = 22 mm Hg, and HCO_3 = 20 mEq.

33. The blood gas changes are primarily a reflection of
    a. the early effects of salicylates
    b. the late effects of salicylates
    c. the effects of the tranquilizer
    d. hepatorenal toxicity
34. The initial intervention appropriately undertaken included
    a. induction of vomiting
    b. naloxone
    c. acidification of the urinary pH
    d. airway protection
35. When Mr. N regained consciousness, one of the primary nursing concerns became convincing him that
    a. career counseling would have solved his problems
    b. suicide is the worst alternative to any seemingly insurmountable problem
    c. he really never wanted to die or he would have done a better job
    d. there are other ways to help reduce the terrible feelings he is having

Mrs. O had been in an extended care facility for 6 months after a massive cerebrovascular accident when she developed a urinary tract infection. Her physician transferred her to the acute care facility's intensive care unit when she began to develop fever, chills, vomiting, and decreased responsiveness. A pulmonary artery catheter was inserted and the following measurements were obtained:

CI = 4.5 L/min/m^2 $\quad$ $PA_{\overline{W}}$ = 8 mm Hg $\quad$ SVR = 600 dynes
BP = 90/60 mm Hg $\quad$ RR = 28/min

These findings, some laboratory data, and her history led to the diagnosis of early bacteremia and septic syndrome.

36. The primary causes of tissue hypoxia in this stage of septic syndrome are
    a. decreased oxygen content and increased oxygen demand
    b. increased oxygen demand and maldistribution of blood flow
    c. increased A-a gradient and intrapulmonary shunting
    d. decreased cardiac output and afterload
37. The key therapeutic interventions for Mrs. O included
    a. bicarbonate and volume replacement
    b. cardiovascular support and antibiotic therapy
    c. vasopressors and diuretics
    d. mechanical ventilation with positive end-expiratory pressure
38. The next day, the change in Mrs. O's status that caused the most concern was
    a. a decreased white blood cell count with a more pronounced shift to the left
    b. negative blood cultures despite continuing hyperthermia
    c. progressive hypoxemia and diffuse pulmonary infiltrates
    d. oliguria responsive to fluid therapy

Mr. P's admission diagnosis was upper gastrointestinal bleeding. He had a history of cirrhosis, angina, and congestive heart failure. His initial laboratory findings included:

BP = 108/86 mm Hg $\quad$ CVP = 7 mm Hg $\quad$ RR = 22/min $\quad$ UO = 40 cc/hr
Hgb = 10.8 gm $\quad$ Na = 131 mEq $\quad$ K = 3.2 mEq $\quad$ HCO_3^- = 24 mEq

His estimated blood loss, including that lost prior to hospitalization, was 1000 cc.

His course was complicated by the development of angina episodes that were difficult to control.

39. The initial treatment of Mr. P's gastrointestinal bleeding involved
    a. carafate
    b. gastric lavage
    c. high-dose antacids
    d. immediate surgery
40. Vasopressin administration was considered contraindicated owing to his
    a. hyponatremia
    b. history of angina
    c. hypervolemic status
    d. hyponatremia and anginal episodes
41. Mr. P's exacerbation of angina was expected to
    a. improve when his oxygen transport improved
    b. respond to thrombolytic therapy
    c. respond to higher doses of nitroglycerin and beta blockade
    d. improve when dopamine and norepinephrine were initiated
42. The source of Mr. P's bleeding was reliably diagnosed by
    a. endoscopy
    b. history and physical examination alone
    c. upper gastrointestinal x-rays
    d. his response to therapy

Mrs. Q visited her physician complaining of severe weakness and fatigue of gradual onset. Significant history included hypothyroidism since 1978 and prosthetic mitral valve replacement in 1981. She took Synthroid and Coumadin daily. Her hemoglobin was discovered to be only 6 gm. She was admitted to the hospital for further evaluation. The initial workup revealed no evidence of icterus, splenomegaly, or occult bleeds. Neither the bilirubin nor the reticulocyte count was elevated.

43. Based on these data, the most likely cause of Mrs. Q's anemia was thought to be
    a. bone marrow suppression related to her hypothyroidism
    b. bone marrow suppression related to prosthetic valve dysfunction
    c. hemolytic anemia related to her hypothyroidism
    d. hemolytic anemia related to prosthetic valve dysfunction
44. The decision was made to treat Mrs. Q's anemia with blood transfusions
    a. only if she became increasingly symptomatic
    b. immediately and aggressively
    c. before continuing the diagnostic workup
    d. until the hematocrit reached 12 gm
45. The nurses were aware that patients with hypothyroidism who are under severe physical stress are more likely to develop
    a. hyperthyroid crisis
    b. myxedema
    c. hypernatremia
    d. hyperosmolar crisis

Mr. R was being treated for a tooth abscess with antibiotics. Four days later he developed a persistent headache, return of fever, diplopia, and tinnitis.

46. To confirm the disorder suggested by this history, the emergency room physician

a. performed a spinal tap
b. checked for retinal changes
c. checked for Chvostek's and Trousseau's signs
d. ordered a CT scan for the morning

Mr. R's antibiotic therapy was altered based on the results of the culture of his abscess. Four days later his creatinine level was 3.2, double his initial creatinine.

47. Renal insufficiency in this setting would be most likely due to
  a. prerenal failure
  b. intrarenal cortical failure
  c. intrarenal medullary failure
  d. postrenal failure
48. Laboratory findings that often accompany this type of renal failure include
  a. excessive renal losses of protein and potassium
  b. excessive renal losses of sodium
  c. hypokalemia and hypernatremia
  d. renal tubular alkalosis

Mrs. S had been in the surgical intensive care for 12 hours after coronary artery bypass graft. She had been progressing as expected with the following findings:

HR = 96/min   RR = 16/min on mechanical ventilation
BP = 110/72 mm Hg   UO = 40 cc/hr
CVP = 10 mm Hg   PA$\overline{w}$ = 13 mm Hg   CO = 4.8 L/min

She then developed these changes:

HR = 110/min   BP = 100/84 mm Hg
CVP = 16 mm Hg   PA$\overline{w}$ = 16 mm Hg

49. The first thing the nurse checked was the chest tube drainage system, suspecting
  a. a sudden increase in drainage
  b. loss of chest tube patency
  c. an air leak
  d. a disconnection
50. This patient most likely required
  a. chest tube clamping
  b. massive transfusion therapy
  c. pericardiocentesis
  d. milking of the chest tubes
51. If the therapy was not successful, Mrs. S would have most likely developed
  a. increased cardiac output
  b. pulsus alternans
  c. hypotension with pulsus paradoxus
  d. hemorrhagic shock

Mrs. T called her obstetrician, complaining of sudden onset dyspnea. She was in the last trimester of pregnancy. She was instructed to come to the emergency room for evaluation, where she presented with increasing anxiety and moderately labored respirations at a rate of 30/min. Chest auscultation, palpation, and percussion findings were negative. Her vital signs were normal, and the fetal heart rate was somewhat increased. Results of arterial blood gas analysis were:

pH = 7.49 pO_2 = 65 mm Hg
pCO_2 = 30 mm Hg HCO_3^- = 22 mEq

52. Because of her history, clinical presentation, and blood gas results, the suspected diagnosis was
    a. pulmonary emboli
    b. hysteria
    c. fetal distress syndrome
    d. pneumonia
53. *Initial* diagnostic studies most likely to be ordered for Mrs. T include
    a. pulmonary angiography
    b. ventilation-perfusion scans
    c. ECG
    d. bronchoscopy
54. The initial plan for Mrs. T's management was
    a. admission for oxygen, entubation, and mechanical ventilation
    b. admission for oxygen, heparinization, and observation
    c. immediate thoracotomy to treat the primary problem and cesarean section to ensure a viable infant
    d. discharge on Coumadin therapy and bed rest

Mr. U was admitted to the ICU for acute polyneuritis, which had progressed to involve the respiratory muscles. His tidal volume and respiratory rate were decreasing and his most recent arterial blood gas results were:

pH	= 7.26	pO_2	= 72 mm Hg
pCO_2	= 57 mm Hg	HCO_3	= 24 mEq

55. The interpretation of his current respiratory status was
    a. hypoventilation due to a primary pulmonary obstructive disorder
    b. hypoventilation due to a primary neuromuscular disorder
    c. marked hypoxemia due to an increasing A-a gradient
    d. acute respiratory alkalosis due to hypoxic respiratory center drive

Mr. U was intubated and placed on a volume-cycled ventilator on assist/control mode at a tidal volume of 800 cc and a backup rate of 10 respirations/min.

56. Expected findings related to this therapy included
    a. correction of acute respiratory acidosis and acidemia
    b. high peak pressures to overcome decreased pulmonary compliance
    c. need for further increases in tidal volume as time goes on
    d. need for increasing FIO_2 as the pCO_2 decreases

Mr. U had been on continuous tube feedings and tolerated them well until an increase in heart rate, temperature, wheezing, and rales was noted. Aspiration was suspected.

57. The diagnosis was supported by the following results of blood gas, chest x-ray, and pulmonary function test findings:
    a. hypoventilation, increased pulmonary compliance and resistance
    b. increasing hypoxemia, pulmonary infiltrates
    c. respiratory acidosis, increasing intrapulmonary shunting
    d. decreasing peak pressure, increasing deadspace

Mrs. V had a history of chronic renal failure managed by hemodialysis in an outpatient dialysis center. She was admitted to the hospital after a pericardial friction rub was found during predialysis physical examination.

58. Other findings that may be present concurrently with pericardial friction rubs include:
    a. muffled heart sounds and pleuritic chest pain
    b. pulsus paradoxus and decreasing pulse pressure
    c. cardiomegaly and fever
    d. elevated ST segments in the precordial ECG leads
59. Modifications in dialysis therapy were most likely to include
    a. decreasing the length and amount of dialysis treatments
    b. increasing intradialysis heparin administration
    c. changing to slow continuous ultrafiltration temporarily
    d. increasing the length and amount of dialysis treatments using a nonheparin protocol

Miss W was a 16-year-old patient who had been found obtunded at home by her mother and was rushed to the hospital. The history was negative except for a family history of type I diabetes mellitus and a urinary tract infection, which she was treating herself by drinking large amounts of cranberry juice. She had been home alone all that day. Stat results of laboratory tests ordered in the emergency room included: pH = 7.16, pCO_2 = 28 mm Hg, pO_2 = 80 mm Hg, HCO_3^- = 10 mEq, Glucose = 870 mg/dL, and WBC = 20,000/μL.

60. Miss W's probable primary diagnosis was
    a. hyperglycemic hyperosmolar nonketotic coma
    b. septic shock
    c. diabetic ketoacidosis
    d. acute renal failure
61. Other expected laboratory findings at this point included
    a. increased serum and urine osmolality
    b. hypokalemia and hyponatremia
    c. negative serum and urine ketoacids
    d. increased serum amylase
62. The major components of therapeutic interventions were to
    a. quickly return the blood glucose toward normal
    b. administer enough bicarbonate stat to establish a normal pH
    c. aggressively replace fluid and electrolyte losses
    d. suppress hyperventilation with respiratory depressants

Mr. X was brought to the emergency room with sudden onset aphasia, left-sided facial weakness, and right-arm paralysis. The diagnosis of a stroke was made and he was admitted to the intermediate care unit for observation.

63. Mr. X's symptoms suggest that the site of this stroke is the
    a. right middle cerebral artery
    b. left middle cerebral artery
    c. left anterior cerebral artery
    d. left middle meningeal artery
64. Long-term symptoms or potential complications of lesions of this nature are most likely to include
    a. right-arm flaccidity
    b. right-arm spasticity
    c. autonomic dysreflexia
    d. left homonymous hemianopsia

Mr. Y is a 16-year-old who was admitted to the ICU after a motor vehicle accident that caused a left frontal skull fracture, contusion, and hematoma. The hematoma was treated surgically and his ICP was monitored via an intraventricular catheter. His ICP suddenly increased from 22 to 30 mm Hg.

65. Interventions that are most likely to decrease the ICP the quickest are
    a. hyperventilation and furosemide
    b. CSF drainage and mannitol
    c. hyperventilation and CSF drainage
    d. furosemide and lowering the head of the bed
66. Nursing action in this situation included making sure that the transducer connector to the intraventricular catheter was level with
    a. the phlebostatic axis
    b. the foramen of Monro
    c. the midaxillary line
    d. the aqueduct of Sylvius

The nurse noticed that the dressing over Mr. Y's cranial incision had increasing amounts of yellow-orange drainage fluid.

67. To differentiate serous from bloody CSF, the most definitive test would be
    a. the ring or halo sign
    b. the Battle's sign
    c. to send fluid to the lab for a glucose test
    d. the Waterhouse-Friderichsen's test

The ICP remained at about 30 mm Hg until Mr. Y began to have generalized seizures. It rose to over 50 mm Hg during each episode.

68. Seizures can cause elevations in ICP by
    a. hypoventilation and increased intrathoracic pressure
    b. hyperventilation and hypoxemia
    c. decreased neuro metabolic rate and decreased cerebral blood flow
    d. hypotension and vasoconstriction

Mr. Y's physicians are considering barbiturate coma to control his intracranial pressure and his seizures.

69. Barbiturates may decrease intracranial pressure by
    a. decreasing neuro metabolic rate
    b. increasing cerebral blood flow
    c. increasing the rate of CSF synthesis
    d. increasing blood-brain barrier permeability
70. Potential complications include
    a. hypertension and arrhythmias
    b. hypertension and hypoventilation
    c. hypotension and hyperventilation
    d. hypotension and hypoventilation

Mrs. Z was brought to the cardiovascular ICU immediately after triple coronary artery bypass grafts. She is receiving dopamine at 10 μg/kg/min and her hemodynamic data include

CO = 4.0 L/min	BP = 140/80 mm Hg	$PA\overline{w}$ = 15 mm Hg
CI = 2.0 L/min/m^2	MAP = 100 mm Hg	SVR = 1760 dynes

71. The intervention most likely to be ordered to improve her hemodynamic status is
    a. intra-aortic counterpulsation balloon pump
    b. increase the dopamine from 10 to 15 μg
    c. increase the D_5 in ¼ normal saline solution from 50 to 150 cc this hour
    d. begin a nitroprusside drip at 2 μg/min

After the above intervention, Mrs. Z's hemodynamic data were

CO	= 5.0 L/min	BP	= 130/70 mm Hg	PA$\overline{w}$	= 12 mm Hg
CI	= 2.5 L/min/m^2	MAP	= 90 mm Hg	SVR	= 1280 dynes

She was then given a fluid challenge of 200 cc over 10 min.

72. The expected outcomes from the above intervention are
    a. increased preload and afterload
    b. decreased preload and afterload
    c. increased preload and stroke volume
    d. decreased preload and stroke volume

Mr. A awakened with severe pressure in his chest, called 911, and was brought to the emergency room. His admission ECG showed ST segment elevation in leads II, III, and AVF and a sinus bradycardia. His creatinine kinase MB fraction was elevated. He had no history of heart disease.

73. The site of Mr. A's myocardial infarction is the
    a. anterior wall
    b. lateral wall
    c. inferior wall
    d. subendocardial surface
74. This wall of the myocardium is supplied by the
    a. left anterior descending artery
    b. left circumflex artery
    c. right coronary artery
    d. coronary sinus
75. This presence of sinus bradycardia
    a. is a potential complication of this type of myocardial infarction
    b. is probably a vasovagal response to pain
    c. is treated whether or not it is symptomatic
    d. is treated with verapamil if it is symptomatic
76. Patients with this type of myocardial infarction have an increased risk of developing
    a. right-axis deviation
    b. right ventricular failure
    c. infranodal blocks
    d. bundle-branch blocks

Mrs. B developed ARDS 4 days after a colon resection. She is 73 years old and has a history of congestive heart failure and occasional episodes of exertional angina. She is on a mechanical ventilator with an FIO_2 of .50, a minute ventilation of 15 L, and PEEP of 10 mm Hg. She is receiving continuous intravenous nitroglycerin and parenteral nutrition. Her data include:

CO	= 5.0 L/min	paO_2	= 48	Hgb	= 9 gm
PA$\overline{w}$	= 8 mm Hg	$paCO_2$	= 32		
BP	= 108/78 mm Hg	pH	= 7.48	Temp	= 37°C
SVR	= 1280	HCO_3^-	= 20		

77. Mrs. B's arterial saturation is most likely to be
    a. 50%
    b. 84%
    c. 90%
    d. 99%
78. Mrs. B's arterial oxygen content is about
    a. 5 cc/100 cc blood
    b. 10 cc/100 cc blood
    c. 20 cc/100 cc blood
    d. 24 cc/100 cc blood
79. Mrs. B's oxygen transport is about
    a. 50 cc/min
    b. 600 cc/min
    c. 1200 cc/min
    d. 5000 cc/min
80. Increasing the PEEP to treat this patient's hypoxemia has the potential risk of
    a. decreasing the oxygen content
    b. decreasing the oxygen transport
    c. increasing the intrapulmonary shunt
    d. shifting the oxygen-hemoglobin curve to the left
81. Increasing the FIO_2 to treat this patient's hypoxemia has a potential risk of
    a. oxygen toxicity
    b. decreasing the percent of intrapulmonary shunting
    c. decreasing the A-a gradient
    d. retrolental fibroplasia

Mr. C had a cholecystotomy that was complicated by postoperative pneumonia and a history of COPD. He has been on mechanical ventilation for 2 weeks and his current parameters include:

paO_2 = 80 mm Hg	HCO_3^- = 34 mEq	RR = 10 breaths/min
$paCO_2$ = 58 mm Hg	SaO_2 = 95%	FIO_2 = .30
pH = 7.37	TV = 1000 cc	PEEP = 0

82. The appropriate response to the data above is to
    a. increase Mr. C's tidal volume or respiratory rate
    b. increase Mr. C's FIO_2
    c. start Mr. C on PEEP therapy
    d. continue the therapy as outlined

The next day bedside pulmonary function studies are done to assess whether or not Mr. C is ready to be weaned from the mechanical ventilator.

83. Trends that indicate Mr. C may be ready to be weaned include:
    a. decreasing pulmonary compliance
    b. decreasing FEV_1
    c. increasing vital capacity
    d. decreased maximum inspiratory force

Attempts to wean Mr. C were not successful.

84. Factors that may contribute to failure to wean patients like Mr. C include:
    a. more acidotic CSF
    b. high-calorie/high-glucose feedings
    c. inadequate sedation
    d. hyperphosphatemia

Mrs. D has a history of chronic renal failure secondary to diabetes mellitus. She is admitted to the telemetry unit for evaluation and management of fever, weakness, and fluid overload.

Her laboratory data include:

BUN	= 66 mg	K	= 6.0 mEq
Cr	= 6.0 gm	Na	= 158 mEq
Glucose	= 180 mg/dL	HCO_3^-	= 18 mEq
		Cl	= 120 mEq

85. Mrs. D's serum osmolality is most likely to be
    a. 270 mosm
    b. 290 mosm
    c. 310 mosm
    d. 350 mosm
86. The elevation in BUN is most likely to be due to
    a. catabolic metabolism
    b. prerenal failure
    c. postrenal failure
    d. intrarenal failure
87. Since her pH was 7.30, Mrs. D also has
    a. respiratory acidosis
    b. respiratory alkalosis
    c. metabolic acidosis
    d. metabolic alkalosis

Mr. E was brought to the emergency room after he succumbed to a witnessed cardiac arrest shortly after a bee sting. Bystander CPR efforts were hampered by edema of the face and neck.

88. The first drug Mr. E was given on arrival was
    a. corticosteroids
    b. dopamine
    c. epinephrine
    d. Benadryl (diphenhydramine)
89. Immediate therapeutic goals for this patient will include:
    a. increasing intravascular volume
    b. decreasing intravascular volume
    c. vasodilation and bronchodilation
    d. vasoconstriction and bronchoconstriction
90. The pathophysiology of this reaction involves the release of
    a. histamine from B cells
    b. IgE from lymphocytes
    c. IgA from T cells
    d. eosinophils from the liver

Mrs. F developed a hypermetabolic septic response 4 days after resection of a bowel infarction. She is 84 years old and has no history of other serious preexisting disease.

91. The expected cardiovascular features of this early phase of the septic syndrome include:
    a. increased stroke volume and decreased vascular resistance
    b. decreased stroke volume and increased vascular resistance
    c. increased stroke volume and increased vascular resistance
    d. decreased stroke volume and decreased vascular resistance

92. The changes in fluid status caused by the disorder include the shifting of fluid from the
    a. vascular to the interstitial space
    b. interstitial to the vascular space
    c. cells to the plasma
    d. third space into the bloodstream
93. Goals in supportive care in Mrs. F would include:
    a. a PA wedge of 20–25 mm Hg
    b. an SVR of 2000 dynes
    c. a cardiac output above normal
    d. a GFR of 10 cc/min
94. Drugs that are relatively contraindicated when used alone because of the type of surgery Mrs. F had include
    a. dobutamine and nitroglycerin
    b. nitroglycerin and nitroprusside
    c. furosemide and mannitol
    d. dopamine at higher doses or norepinephrine

Three days later Mrs. F develops bleeding via her nasogastric tube and rectum. A coagulation panel reveals
PT = 10 sec Platelets = 80,000
PTT = 40 sec Hgb = 6.8 gm
Clotting time = 8 min

95. Based on these data, the most likely cause of Mrs. F's bleeding is:
    a. loss of integrity at the surgical site
    b. thrombocytopenia
    c. anticoagulation
    d. liver failure
96. Immediate supportive care is most likely to include
    a. packed red blood cells
    b. platelet units
    c. fresh frozen plasma
    d. cryoprecipitate

Mr. G has a history of severe coronary artery disease, which has limited his activity for 5 years. He was brought to the emergency room with abdominal pain that had been intermittent all day but became progressively more continuous and more severe. He has been vomiting large amounts of yellow-green fluid. Intestinal obstruction was the admission diagnosis.

97. Physical assessment of the abdomen in Mr. G is most likely to reveal:
    a. hyperresonance and distention
    b. hyporesonance and a fluid wave
    c. shifting dullness and visible veins
    d. Cullen's and Grey-Turner's signs
98. Physical assessment of fluid status is most likely to reveal hypovolemia related to
    a. third-spacing and vomiting
    b. decreased capillary hydrostatic pressure
    c. increased serum colloid osmotic pressure
    d. shifting dullness and ascites fluid

Mr. G went to the operating room for surgical intervention and was then brought directly to the intensive care unit on a mechanical ventilator and an intra-aortic counterpulsation balloon pump.

99. Potential complications of the intra-aortic counterpulsation balloon include
    a. increased coronary perfusion
    b. decreased afterload
    c. thrombocytosis
    d. decreased femoral artery perfusion

Mr. G had a prolonged course involving multiple complications and never regained consciousness. After a series of discussions with his family, it was decided that no further heroic efforts would be initiated. Mr. G had left prior instructions regarding his desire to donate organs. The hospital transplant coordinator determined that he met donor criteria for some organs.

100. When Mr. G goes into cardiac arrest, it is important to
    a. honor the no-code order and not resuscitate
    b. initiate CPR and call the transplant team
    c. call the transplant team to resuscitate the patient
    d. do a chemical code only

A few days later, cortical and brainstem death is firmly documented in Mr. G.

101. At this point, we are obligated to
    a. continue life-support equipment until the patient arrests
    b. withdraw life-support equipment immediately
    c. continue life-support until the transplant team arrives
    d. ask the family for permission to withdraw support

Answers to Comprehensive Examination

1. **b**
2. **c**
3. **d**
4. **a**
5. **b**
6. **b**
7. **b**
8. **a**
9. **d**
10. **d**
11. **a**
12. **d**
13. **c**
14. **a**
15. **c**
16. **d**
17. **b**
18. **d**
19. **c**
20. **a**
21. **b**
22. **c**
23. **a**
24. **a**
25. **b**
26. **b**
27. **b**
28. **a**
29. **c**
30. **b**
31. **b**
32. **a**
33. **a**
34. **d**
35. **d**
36. **b**
37. **b**
38. **c**
39. **b**
40. **d**
41. **a**
42. **a**
43. **a**
44. **a**
45. **b**
46. **a**
47. **c**
48. **b**
49. **b**
50. **d**
51. **c**
52. **a**
53. **c**
54. **b**
55. **b**
56. **a**
57. **b**
58. **d**
59. **d**
60. **c**
61. **a**
62. **c**
63. **b**
64. **b**
65. **c**
66. **b**
67. **a**
68. **a**
69. **a**
70. **d**
71. **d**
72. **c**
73. **c**
74. **c**
75. **a**
76. **b**
77. **b**
78. **b**
79. **b**
80. **b**
81. **a**
82. **d**
83. **c**
84. **b**
85. **d**
86. **d**
87. **c**
88. **c**
89. **a**
90. **b**
91. **a**
92. **a**
93. **c**
94. **d**
95. **a**
96. **a**
97. **a**
98. **a**
99. **d**
100. **b**
101. **c**

APPENDIX A

NAMES TO REMEMBER

There are several items with proper names that might appear on the certification examination. Many are often difficult to remember. Here is a list of the more important ones and where in the *Core* you can find them.

PULMONARY SYSTEM	PAGE
1. Herring-Breuer	11
2. Ohm's law	17
3. Henderson-Hasselbach equation	22
4. Angle of Louis	31
5. Cheyne-Stokes	33
6. Venturi	78
7. Virchow's Triad	98

CARDIOVASCULAR SYSTEM	PAGE
1. Bachmann's bundle	138
2. Laplace's law	136
3. Purkinje's system	138
4. Bainbridge reflex	144
5. Frank-Starling's law	150
6. Bowditch's law	151
7. Korotkoff's sounds	155
8. Erb's point	157
9. Lewis lead	174
10. Wenckebach	184
11. Mobitz II type A-W block	184
12. Wolff-Parkinson-White syndrome	186
13. Fick method	191
14. Prinzmetal's angina	208
15. Dressler's syndrome	247
16. Janeway lesions	252
17. Osler's nodes	252
18. Quincke's sign	269
19. Hill's sign	269
20. Marfan's syndrome	268, 291

NEUROLOGIC SYSTEM

RENAL SYSTEM

ENDOCRINE SYSTEM

HEMATOLOGIC SYSTEM

GASTROINTESTINAL SYSTEM

APPENDIX B

DRUGS TO REMEMBER

Knowledge of the action of drugs is an important aspect of critical care nursing and the certification examination. Here is a list of commonly used agents and where in the *Core Curriculum* they appear. Not all drugs listed are covered specifically in the *Core*.

	PAGE
BRONCHODILATORS	71

Methylxanthines (theophylline, Aminophylline)
β-Agents (epinephrine, isoproterenol)
β_2 Agents (salbutolol, isoetharine, Terbutaline, albuterol, bitolterol)
Anticholinergic agents (Ipratropium)
Antibronchoconstriction (cromolyn)

PARALYZING AGENTS 70

Nondepolarizing agents (Tubocurarine, pancuronium, vecuronium, atracurium)
Depolarizing agents (succinylcholine)

NARCOTICS 70

Morphine
Meperidine
Fentanyl

SEDATIVES, CNS DEPRESSANTS 70, 384, 435

Diazepam
Lorazepam
Midazolam
Haloperidol

ANTICONVULSANTS 435

Phenobarbital
Phenytoin

DIRECT VASODILATORS 215–216, 288

Nitroglycerine
Nitroprusside
Apresoline

INOTROPIC AGENTS

β_1 (middose dopamine, dobutamine)	215
α-β (epinephrine, norepinephrine)	307, 480, 621
Digitalis glycosides	222
Amrinone	245

β-BLOCKERS 220

Propranolol
Metoprolol
Nadolol
Timolol
Atenolol
Esmolol

α-AGENTS (VASOCONSTRICTORS)

Neosynephrine
Dopamine (high-dose)

α-BLOCKERS (VASODILATORS)

Prazosin	508
Phentolamine	288

α-β BLOCKERS

Labetalol

CALCIUM-CHANNEL BLOCKERS 221

Verapamil
Diltiazem
Nifedipine
Nicardipine
Nimodipine

ACE INHIBITORS 510

Captopril
Enalopril
Lisinopril

DRUGS TO SUPPRESS TACHYCARDIA

Class I–A (quinidine, procainamide, disopyramide, cifenline)	219
Class I–B (lidocaine, phenytoin, tocainide, mexiletine)	220
Class I–C (flecainide, encainide, propafenone)	220
Class II (β-blockers)	220
Class III (amiodarone, bretylium)	221
Class IV (calcium-channel blockers)	221
Digitalis Glycosides	222
Adenosine	

DRUGS TO INCREASE SA RATE AND AV CONDUCTION

Atropine
Isoproterenol

DIURETICS 507–508

Osmotic Agents (mannitol)
Loop Inhibitors (furosemide, ethacrynic acid, bumetanide)
Thiazides (hydrochlorothiazides, metolazone)
Carbonic Anhydrase Inhibitors (acetazolamide)
Dopaminergic Agents (low-dose dopamine)

THROMBOLYTIC AGENTS 228

Steptokinase
Urokinase
Tissue-Plasminogen Activator

ANTICOAGULANTS

ASA
Heparin
Warfarin

OTHERS WITH SPECIFIC APPLICATIONS IN CRITICAL CARE

Corticosteroids (anti-inflammatory)	384, 619
Vasopressin and desmopressin or DDAVP (water retention, vasoconstriction, procoagulant)	629
Propylthiouracil and methimasol (thyroid synthesis inhibition)	640
Tensilon, neostigmine, pyridostigmine, and ambenonium (anticholinesterase agents)	445
Mithramycin and calcitonin (serum calcium-reducing agents)	588
Cimetidine, ranitidine (H_2 blockers that raise gastric pH)	
Kayexalate (potassium-reducing agent)	575
Erythropoietin (increased red cell synthesis)	489